Femoral Revision Arthroplasty

Springer Nature More Media App

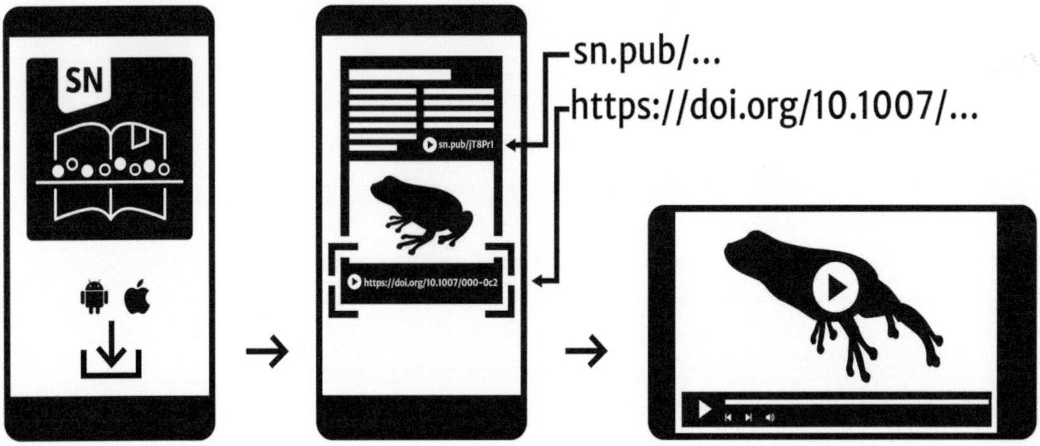

1. Download → **2. Scan Link** → **3. Enjoy Video**

Support: customerservice@springernature.com

Bernd Fink

Femoral Revision Arthroplasty

Springer

Bernd Fink
Orthopaedic Clinic Markgröningen
Markgröningen, Baden-Württemberg, Germany

This work contains media enhancements, which are displayed with a "play" icon. Material in the print book can be viewed on a mobile device by downloading the Springer Nature "More Media" app available in the major app stores. The media enhancements in the online version of the work can be accessed directly by authorized users.

ISBN 978-3-030-84820-0 ISBN 978-3-030-84821-7 (eBook)
https://doi.org/10.1007/978-3-030-84821-7

English translation of the original German edition published by Springer-Verlag GmbH Deutschland 2021 With German-language titles: Femorale Revisionsendoprothetik by Bernd Fink

Translation from the German language edition: Femorale Revisionsendoprothetik by Bernd Fink, © The Editor(s) (if applicable) and The Author(s), under exclusive license to Springer Nature Switzerland AG 2021. Published by Springer Berlin Heidelberg. All Rights Reserved

This Springer imprint is published by the registered company Springer Nature Switzerland AG
The registered company address is: Gewerbestrasse 11, 6330 Cham, Switzerland

Preface

Revision arthroplasty of the hip joint represents a great challenge for the surgeon, and numerous problems such as firmly seated implants, axial deviations, and bone defects of the femur have to be addressed. In this context, it is necessary to weigh up the different surgical techniques with regard to the approach, the chosen fixation method of the new prosthetic stem, and the implant to be selected. Often, small details are decisive in determining the success or failure of the chosen procedure, and it is frequently the case that the "devil is in the detail." Therefore, it is essential to know the specific features of the different surgical procedures together with their potential complications and, above all, the different revision stems. This book will focus on these details in particular and is therefore intended to be an aid to the surgeon in achieving reproducibly good outcomes and avoiding complications.

Baden-Württemberg, Germany Bernd Fink

Contents

1 **Introduction** . . . 1
References . . . 2

2 **Reasons for Femoral Revision** . . . 3
2.1 Aseptic Loosening . . . 3
2.2 Instability . . . 6
2.3 Periprosthetic Infection . . . 6
2.4 Periprosthetic Fractures . . . 7
References . . . 8

3 **Classification of Femoral Bone Defects** . . . 11
3.1 Paprosky Classification . . . 11
3.1.1 Paprosky Type I Defect . . . 13
3.1.2 Paprosky Type II Defect . . . 13
3.1.3 Paprosky Type IIA Defect . . . 13
3.1.4 Paprosky Type IIB Defect . . . 14
3.1.5 Paprosky Type IIC Defect . . . 14
3.1.6 Paprosky Type III Defect . . . 14
3.1.7 Paprosky Type IV Defect . . . 15
3.2 AAOS Classification by D'Antonio . . . 15
3.3 Endo-Clinic Classification . . . 16
References . . . 18

4 **Principles of Femoral Revision** . . . 19

5 **Cemented Revision Stems** . . . 21
5.1 Cemented Fixation of Stems Analogous to Primary Implantation . . . 21
5.1.1 Surgical Technique . . . 21
5.1.2 Outcomes . . . 22
5.2 Cement-in-Cement Revision . . . 24
5.2.1 Surgical Technique . . . 24
5.2.2 Outcomes . . . 25
5.3 Impaction Bone Grafting . . . 26
5.3.1 Surgical Technique . . . 27
5.3.2 Outcomes . . . 30
References . . . 31

6 Cementless Revision Stems 35
6.1 Nonmodular Cementless Revision Stems for Proximal Fixation 35
6.1.1 Surgical Technique 36
6.1.2 Outcomes 37
6.2 Cementless Proximal-Fixing Modular Revision Stems 37
6.2.1 Surgical Technique 40
6.2.2 Outcomes 41
6.3 Cementless Nonmodular Revision Stems for Distal Fixation 44
6.3.1 Extensively Porous-Coated Stems 44
6.3.2 Corundum-Blasted, Tapered Titanium Stems 47
6.3.3 Cementless Distal Fixation Modular Revision Stems 51
References 69

7 Principles of Cementless Distal Fixation 75
7.1 Scratch Fit (Cylinder-in-Cylinder Fixation) 75
7.2 Cone-in-Cylinder Fixation 76
7.3 Cone-in-Cone Fixation 76
7.3.1 Length of Fixation Zone 82
7.3.2 Distal Interlocking 84
References 87

8 Differences in Distal Fixated Revision Stems 89

9 Allograft Prosthesis Composite (APC) and Megaprostheses 99
9.1 Allograft Prosthesis Composite (APC) 99
9.1.1 Surgical Technique 99
9.1.2 Outcomes 101
9.2 Proximal Femoral Replacement (Megaprostheses) 101
9.2.1 Surgical Technique 103
9.2.2 Outcomes 105
9.3 Total Femoral Replacement 105
9.3.1 Surgical Technique 105
9.3.2 Outcomes 110
References 110

10 Choice of the Implant Depending on the Type of Defect 113
10.1 Paprosky Type I Defects 113
10.2 Paprosky Type IIA Defects 114
10.3 Paprosky Type IIB Defects 115
10.4 Paprosky Type IIC Defects 115
10.5 Paprosky Type IIIA Defects 116
10.6 Paprosky Type IIIB Defects 117
10.7 Paprosky Type IV Defects 120
References 122

11 Preoperative Planning 125

11.1 Exclusion of a Periprosthetic Infection 126
11.2 Prosthesis Planning 127
11.3 Re 1: Analysis of the Shape of the Femur 129
11.4 Re 2: Analysis of the Mechanical Stability of the Femur 130
11.5 Re 3: Necessity for Osteotomies 130
11.6 Re 4: Selection of Prosthesis Shape (Curved or Straight) 130
11.7 Re 5: Selection of the Method of Fixation (Proximal or Distal) 133
11.8 Re 6: Selection of Component Sizes 137
11.9 Preparation of the Preoperative Planning Sketch 141
11.9.1 Step 1: Mapping the Axes and, Where Necessary, the Osteotomies 141
11.9.2 Step 2A: Mapping the Distal Components for Distally Fixed Stems 141
11.9.3 Step 2B: Mapping the Distal Components for Proximally Fixed Stems 145
11.9.4 Step 3A: Mapping the Proximal Component for Distally Fixed Stems 146
11.9.5 Step 3B: Mapping the Proximal Component for Proximally Fixed Stems 147
11.9.6 Step 4: Mapping Reference Points and Distances . . . 148
11.9.7 Step 5: Further Steps in Digital Planning 148
References 149

12 Choice of the Surgical Approach 151
12.1 Factors Influencing the Choice of Access 152
12.2 Anterior Approaches 153
12.3 The Transgluteal Approach 153
12.4 Trans-Trochanteric Access 155
12.5 The Posterior Approach 155
12.6 Extended Approaches 157
References 161

13 Removal of the Old Stem 163
13.1 Instrumentation 166
13.2 Techniques of Stem Removal 166
13.3 Advanced Special Techniques 166
13.3.1 Longitudinal Femoral Osteotomy 166
13.3.2 Extended Trochanteric Osteotomy (ETO) and/or Transfemoral Access 169
13.3.3 Ventral Bone Window 170
13.4 Removal of Broken Stems 170
References 172

14 Removal of the Cement 173
14.1 Endofemoral, Proximal Techniques 174
14.2 Extended Techniques for Removal of Cement 175
References 179

15 Technical Implementation of the Transfemoral Approach 181

15.1 Indications for Transfemoral Access 181
15.1.1 Broken Prosthetic Stem 182
15.1.2 Thin Bone Prone to Fracture 182
15.1.3 Long Cement Mantle 183
15.1.4 Firmly Fixed or Only Partially Loosened Cementless Stem 184
15.1.5 Axial Deviation of the Femur 185
15.1.6 Periprosthetic Fracture of the Femur (Vancouver B2 or B3 Type) 186
15.1.7 Periprosthetic Infection with Firmly Seated Implant or Cement or Hard-to-Reach Osteolyses 187
15.1.8 Cup Protruding into the Lesser Pelvis 189
15.2 Transfemoral Access Technique 190
15.3 Variations 198
15.3.1 Double Osteotomy 198
15.3.2 Osteotomy Through the Femur After Prior Removal of the Implanted Stem 199
15.3.3 Extended Trochanteric Osteotomy 199
15.4 Complications 200
15.5 Outcomes 200
References 206

16 Technical Implementation of the Stem Implantation of Modular Revision Stems with Distal Fixation 209
16.1 Scratch-Fit Distal Fixation of a Modular Revision Stem. . . . 210
16.2 Cone-in-Cylinder Distal Fixation of a Modular Revision Stem 212
16.3 Cone-in-Cone Distal fixation of a Modular Revision Stem 212
16.3.1 Basic Sequence of Surgical Steps for a Modular Straight Stem (Arcos) 213
16.3.2 Surgical Procedures with a Tapered Modular Revision Stem (Revitan Curved) 215
16.4 Comments on Surgical Descriptions or Assembly of Modular Stems 233
References 235

17 Necessary Length of the Revision Stems 237
References 244

18 Stem Revision in Periprosthetic Fractures 245
18.1 Principles of Stem Revision in Periprosthetic Fractures 246
18.2 Treatment of Vancouver Type B2 Fractures (UCS Type IV.3-B2) 250
18.3 Treatment of Vancouver Type B3 Fractures (USC Type IV.3-B3) 251
18.4 Surgical Techniques of Revision Prostheses in Periprosthetic Fractures 251

1 Introduction

Content

References 2

Total hip replacement (THR) is one of the most successful and frequent operations in medicine and has been called "the operation of the century" [1]. The number of implantations has increased steadily in recent years due to a progressively aging society. Currently, about 240,000 primary THRs are carried out in Germany every year and this number is expected to increase further.

Due to mainly technical advances, the 10-year survival rate in the Swedish Prosthesis Registry increased from 86% between 1979 and 1981 to 96% between 2000 and 2002 [2]. In addition, a patient satisfaction rate of 96% after 16 years has been reported [3]. Nevertheless, the increased number of hip endoprostheses implanted annually and the demographic trends mean that the number of hip revision arthroplasties is also increasing. It is estimated that more than 50,000 hip endoprosthesis revision procedures are performed annually in the USA and about 60,000 in Europe, of which about 16,000 are performed in Germany alone [4, 5]. Indeed, an increase of 137% in hip joint revision procedures was projected for the USA for the period 2005 through 2030 [6].

In this context, revision procedures on the hip joint in general and on the femur in particular pose a great challenge for the surgeon. Firmly seated implants and cement may have to be removed, and the new implant must be firmly fixed without complications in the often weakened bone of the femur.

The primary goals of revision procedures on the hip joint are to re-establish a stable implant, to restore the biomechanics of the hip joint as effectively as possible, to avoid bone loss or to reconstruct bone loss that has already occurred, and to recover the functionality of the hip joint during walking. The aim should be to achieve good results in a reproducible manner. Clear strategies and concepts are necessary for this, and these involve correct treatment of the bone, its blood circulation, and the surrounding musculature.

Therefore, several key questions must already be addressed during the planning of such revision surgery: Which surgical approach should be taken? How can the implant be removed without complications? Which fixation principle and which implant type should be used for reimplantation? How can the new implant be firmly fixed? How should existing bone defects be dealt with?

B. Fink, *Femoral Revision Arthroplasty*, https://doi.org/10.1007/978-3-030-84821-7_1

This book aims to answer all these questions by presenting the different concepts for femoral revision arthroplasty, with an emphasis on cementless revision procedures. First, the scientific basis of the concepts will be discussed and then the technical implementation will be described in detail. In particular, the differences between the various stem systems available on the market will be explained and advice given for avoiding the most common complications.

In an analysis of the results of the Swedish Prosthesis Register, Weiss et al. [7] found that the survival rate in the first three postoperative years was significantly worse for the commonly used modular, distally fixed, cementless revision stem MP (Waldemar Link, Hamburg, Germany) than for three widely used cemented revision stems. This situation was reversed after a longer follow-up. The early failure of the cementless revision stems resulted from complications and suboptimal surgical outcomes. This book contains an in-depth study of the specifics of the individual cementless revision stems, which, together with the details of the actual operation, is intended to help reduce the rate of early failure of cementless revision stems.

In order to keep each chapter self-contained and understandable to the reader, the occasional reiteration of the advantages and disadvantages of individual techniques is intended. The discussion of these advantages and disadvantages will be primarily supported by relevant literature citations. Secondly, they will be based on personal experience and preferences for certain concepts. Thus, this book contains a number of personal opinions, which are identified as such and do not claim to be exclusive. However, I will endeavor to justify my views as they arise.

References

1. Learmonth ID, Young C, Rorabeck C. The operation of the century: total hip replacement. Lancet. 2007;370:1508–19.
2. Forster-Horvath C, Egloff C, Valderrabano V, Nowakowski AM. The painful primary hip replacement—review of the literature. Swiss Med Wkly. 2014;144:w13974.
3. Mariconda M, Galasso O, Costa GG, Recano P, Cerbasi S. Quality of life and functionality after total hip arthroplasty: a long-term follow-up study. BMC Musculoskelet Disord. 2011;12:222.
4. Puhl W, Kessler S. Which factors influence the long term outcome of total hip replacement? In: Rieker C, Oberholzer S, Urs W, editors. World tribology forum in arthroplasty. Bern: Hans Huber; 2001. p. 35–47.
5. HCUPnet, Healthcare cost and utilization project. Agency for Healthcare Research and Quality, Rockville. United States Department of Health & Human Services v 2009. http://hcupnet.ahrq.gov/
6. Kurts S, Ong K, Lau E, Mowat F, Halpern M. Projections of primary and revision hip and knee arthroplasty in the United States from 2005 to 2030. J Bone Joint Surg Am. 2007;89-A:780–5.
7. Weiss RJ, Stark A, Kärrholm J. A modular cementless stem vs. cemented long-stem prostheses in revision surgery of the hip. A population-based study from the Swedish hip arthroplasty register. Acta Orthop. 2011;82:136–42.

2 Reasons for Femoral Revision

Contents

2.1 Aseptic Loosening 3
2.2 Instability 6
2.3 Periprosthetic Infection 6
2.4 Periprosthetic Fractures 7
References 8

Several studies have shown that the most frequent causes of hip endoprosthesis failure are aseptic loosening, followed by dislocations, periprosthetic infections, and periprosthetic fractures (Table 2.1). In a literature review of 9952 hip prosthesis revision surgeries, Kenney et al. [1] identified aseptic loosening in 23.2%, instability in 22.4%, and periprosthetic infection in 22.1% as reasons for revision surgery. Instability and periprosthetic infection were the most common causes of early revision within 5 years of primary implantation, and aseptic loosening was the most common cause of late revision after more than 5 years [1]. In an analysis of the data from the Swedish Prosthesis Registry with 77,036 hip prosthesis replacement procedures, the main causes were aseptic loosening in 55.2%, instability in 11.8%, periprosthetic infections in 7.5%, and periprosthetic fractures in 6%. Prokopetz et al. [2] identified lower age (<60 years), secondary diseases (higher Charlson Comorbidity Index), and aseptic femoral head necrosis as primary diagnosis (as opposed to osteoarthritis), and smaller prosthesis heads and a low number of operations performed by the surgeon as risk factors for revision surgery of the hip endoprosthesis. Regarding specific causes of prosthesis failure, the male gender was found to be a risk factor for aseptic loosening and infection, longer surgery times for infection, and smaller prosthesis heads for joint instability [2].

2.1 Aseptic Loosening

Several factors and processes can lead to aseptic loosening of the hip prosthesis. A lack of osteointegration of a cementless hip implant leads to the formation of a connective tissue layer at the bone–implant interface and thus to early failure of the prosthesis [13]. Causes of this lack of osteointegration include low biocompatibility of implants (not the case with today's titanium implants), unfavorable surface characteristics of

B. Fink, *Femoral Revision Arthroplasty*, https://doi.org/10.1007/978-3-030-84821-7_2

Table 2.1 Indications for hip prosthesis revision surgery

Author	Prostheses	Aseptic loosening	Instability	Periprosthetic infection	Periprosthetic fracture	Osteolysis
Fink [3]	116	62.4%		26.7%	15.5%	
Sadoghi [4]	77,036	55.2%	11.8%	7.5%	6.0%	4.2%
Ulrich [5]	237	51.9%	16.9%	15.6%	5.5%	
Lachiewicz [6]	100	38%	2%	10%	2%	1%
Clohisy [7]	439	55%	14%	7%	5%	13%
Weeden [8]	188	82%	14%	8%	5%	
Lind [9]	87	95.4%		4.6%		
Ullmark [10]	62	95.2%		4.8%		
Böhm [11]	129	75.2%		12.4%	10.1%	
Kenney [1]	9952	23.2%	22.4%	22.1%		
Sandiford [12]	104	48%	7%	24%	15%	2%

the prosthesis and implant design, incorrect surgical technique, adverse weight-bearing situations, and poor bone quality with insufficient bone turnover (e.g., renal or hepatic osteopathy) [14].

The greater rigidity of cementless prosthetic stems results in a significant difference in the stiffness of the metal and bone. This leads to an unfavorable distribution of load between the metal and bone and causes stress shielding [15, 16]. Stress shielding results in increased bone resorption around the implant, a reduction in bone remodeling processes, and increased aseptic loosening [17]. Among cementless revision stems, stress shielding is more frequently observed in the rigid cobalt–chromium stems with a higher modulus of elasticity than in the more elastic titanium stems.

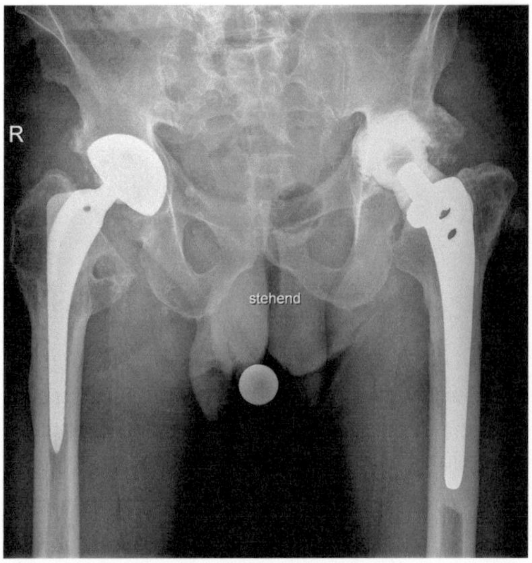

Fig. 2.1 Osteolysis in the region of the right stem due to polyethylene wear debris with loosening of the stem

The production of wear particles (polyethylene of the cup or inlay, ceramic, and metal) in and around the articulating hip prosthesis leads to local tissue reactions, which ultimately result in osteolysis and aseptic prosthesis loosening (Fig. 2.1). Every articulating artificial joint produces wear particles, regardless of their design or material properties [18]. Usually, the particles produced by an implant are eliminated by the cells of the immune system, and there is an equilibrium between their production and elimination. When the amount of particles exceeds the elimination capacity of the immune system, the decompensation process begins. This decompensation process is highly individual and depends on many factors (number and type of particles, but also on genetic, predisposing characteristics of the prosthesis bearer) [19, 20]. Oparaugo et al. [21] reported that polyethylene acetabular cups with annual wear rates of less than 80 mm^3 were associated with very low osteolysis, that cups with annual wear rates between 80 and 140 mm^3 showed low-to-moderate osteolysis, and that cups with annual wear rates above 140 mm^3 exhibited significantly increased levels of osteolysis.

The particles are caused by wear and corrosion. Wear is the loss of material from two surfaces sliding against each other while under load and can be caused by abrasion, adhesion, and fatigue. This results in the release of particles from articulating surfaces or from the surface of interfaces used for prosthesis fixation in bone [22]. The wear particles may be polyethylene (PE), bone, cement, metal, metallic corrosion products, ceramics, or hydroxyapatite particles [23]. Different combinations of type, size, and density of the wear particles affect the nature of the immune response of the host [22]. For example, particles resulting from metal-on-metal (MoM) combinations trigger B and T lymphocytes and cell-mediated delayed type hypersensitivity reactions or type 4 hypersensitivity reactions associated with plasma cells [22].

Corrosion is the chemical interaction between metals and their environment and their subsequent electrochemical breakdown and is caused by the release of metal ions from the metal of the implant into the surrounding tissue. Corrosion can also occur in modular assemblies due to fretting between the stem and head taper surfaces or between stem components, creating another tapered interface as a source of relative movement (besides the actual articulation between the prosthesis head and cup/inlay). The use of modular prostheses (head/stem), which represent the standard today, thus results in a constant deposition of metal oxide debris at the interface [24–26]. This is the case for both modular metal and ceramic heads and for modular stem configurations. The clinical and histological findings in periprosthetic tissues are very similar in periprosthetic reactions of metal-on-metal (MoM) and non-MoM combinations [25]. However, there is evidence to support the hypothesis that taper-derived particles may be biologically more active and destructive to soft tissue [27]. A variety of local factors, including metal solubility, pH, and organic component properties, lead to the occurrence of a variety of corrosion products, which may be soluble or insoluble salts, metal–protein complexes, or free radicals [28] .

The wear debris particles lead to a local inflammatory reaction in the tissue around the prosthesis. This inflammatory reaction is independent of the type of particle, and its purpose is to eliminate the foreign material [17, 29]. Studies have shown that this is a cumulative and chronic inflammatory response that includes in particular macrophages, fibroblasts, lymphocytes, and osteoclasts. These processes lead to a chronic disruption of the balance between bone tissue formation and degradation, to the detriment of the former. There are three main mechanisms responsible for this imbalance. The first mechanism involves excessive inflammation induced by activated macrophages and osteoclasts. The second is the disruption of periprosthetic bone formation, and the third mechanism is the discontinuation of bone regeneration as a result of the increased cytotoxic response of mesenchymal osteoprogenitor cells [30]. These processes, with shifts in balance from osteogenesis to bone resorption, then result in macroscopically visible osteolysis around the implant [31]. The extent of bone resorption is at least partially a function of the number, size, and origin of the prosthesis-derived particles [32].

The properties of the particles, particularly particles in the most biologically active submicron size range, including their composition, size, shape, and number, significantly affect overall cell and tissue responses [33]. These particles initially cause inflammation, which increases the number of inflammatory cells and especially the number of macrophages and fibroblasts in the synovial fluid. Intra-articular pressure increases and the wear particles can migrate from the surfaces of the prosthesis, even if it is firmly attached, out of this area and eventually spread into the joint cavity [28, 34–36]. Thus, particles resulting from wear or corrosion can spread both locally and systemically [28].

Each point in contact with the prosthesis encompasses the effective joint space, and this space encloses the cup, the stem, and, if present, the screws. The joint space fluid, and with it the particles, migrates to areas of lower pressure [33]. As a result, particle responses can spread to new sites, contributing to the overall extension of osteolytic sites and weakening of the bone–implant interface [33]. Screw holes in the socket, surfaces around the screws, and areas of bone cement detachment or cement mantle covering defects are the most likely sites for particle accumulation. The pressure of synovial fluid can also directly induce bone resorption [37]. When the synovial fluid and wear debris particles penetrate between the bone and the prosthesis, a synovial-like membrane develops in this area, which expands aggressively. This interfacial membrane is a type of granulation tissue that is rich in fibroblasts, macrophages, endothelial cells, and inflammatory mediators and provides an environment for cellular activity and enzymatic processes that may destroy adjacent bone [38–40].

Corrosion leads to increased formation of connective tissue [41]. This impairs the formation of solid bone bridges by osteoblasts during osteointegration of the implant. In addition, cytotoxic metal ions can directly damage the osteoblasts [41].

2.2 Instability

Recurrent dislocations may necessitate prosthesis revision. The position of the cup must usually be corrected in such cases. More rarely, a malrotated stem is the cause of the dislocation and therefore requires correction. However, a too small offset of the hip prosthesis stem can lead to dislocation via impingement by reducing the distance of the greater trochanter to the os ileum and that of the lesser trochanter to the os ischium [42].

2.3 Periprosthetic Infection

Periprosthetic infections with an incidence between 1 and 2% after primary implantation represent a rare but serious complication [43, 44]. Infections are significantly more common after revision surgery with an incidence of 2–6% [45–47]. Due to the relevance for further therapy, a periprosthetic infection should always be considered in cases of painful hip total endoprostheses until the contrary is proven.

Four different types of infections can be distinguished based on the classification developed by Coventry in 1975 [48] and its further development by Estrada and Tsukayma in the early 90s: positive intraoperative cultures, early infections, late infections, and acute hematogenic infections [49, 50].

The borderline between early and late infections is defined by Estrada et al. [49] and Tsukayma et al. [50] at 4 weeks, but has been extended up to 3 months by other authors [51–55]. Classic signs of an infection appear in early infection. This is not the case with late infections. Since an undetected periprosthetic infection as the reason for a revision endangers the success of the latter, the diagnosis of a periprosthetic infection should always be made before any prosthesis revision is carried out. The different diagnostic procedures available for detecting or excluding late periprosthetic infections can be divided into direct or specific procedures, in which the pathogen is detected and the sensitivity to antibiotics for therapy is tested, and indirect or nonspecific procedures, in which neither of these is determined. Indirect, nonspecific methods only provide an indication or proof of an infection, but they leave the questions of the identity of the pathogen and its sensitivity to antibiotics unanswered [56]. Thus, specific examination methods should be an integral part of the diagnosis of a periprosthetic infection (see Table 2.2). Since none of the tests is 100% accurate, several tests should always be combined to achieve the highest possible accuracy of diagnosis. Ideally, direct

Table 2.2 Classification of diagnostic procedures for verification or exclusion of periprosthetic infections (Fink and Lass 2016)

Direct or specific tests	Indirect or nonspecific tests
Laboratory: PCR (but no resistance determination)	**Laboratory:** CRP, BSR. IL-6
Joint aspiration: With incubation	**Joint aspiration:** With cell count in joint fluid and/or alpha-defensin and/or leukocyte esterase test
Biopsy: With incubation	**Biopsy:** Histological examination using normal technique or frozen sections
	Imaging: X-ray, sonography, scintigraphy, leukocyte scintigraphy, FDG-PET

and indirect diagnostic procedures should also be combined [57].

While the implant can be left in place for early infections (infections within 4 weeks of prosthesis implantation), late infections (infections more than 4 weeks after primary implantation) require an implant revision [56, 58–60]. A distinction is made between so-called one-stage and two-stage implant revisions. In one-stage revision, after removal of all foreign material and radical debridement of the tissue, a new implant is inserted during the same operation, usually with antibiotic-containing cement. In the two-stage revision, all foreign material is removed in a first operation and a Girdlestone situation is left for an interim phase of usually 6–12 weeks, or a cement spacer is implanted, before the final revision prosthesis is implanted in the second operation (see Chap. 14). The success rate of both concepts averages around 90% and appears to be discretely, but not significantly, higher for two-stage changes [61–63].

A challenge in the treatment of late periprosthetic hip joint infections is the precise removal of infected implants without unnecessarily traumatizing and devascularizing muscle and bone structures. Appropriate techniques are discussed in this book in the corresponding chapters (Chaps. 8, 9, and 10).

2.4 Periprosthetic Fractures

Postoperative periprosthetic fractures of the femur are reported to occur at rates below 1% after primary implantation and between 1.5 and 4.2% after revision surgery [64–69]. Lewallen et al. [66] report incidences after primary implantation of 0.6% for cemented stems and 0.4% for cementless stems. For revision surgery, the incidence after classification according to the stem endoprosthesis used is 2.8–4% for cemented and 1.5% for cementless stems [64–66, 68, 69].

The main cause of postoperative periprosthetic fractures is minor trauma in loosened stem endoprostheses, where the loosening process has led to weakening of the bone. Therefore, a periprosthetic fracture caused by minor trauma must always be associated with a loosening of the prosthesis, even if this is not clearly visible radiologically.

In the case of postoperative fractures, the risk factors can be divided into patient-related, general, and local ones.

The general risk factors for postoperative fractures are metabolic bone diseases with weakening of the mechanical properties of the bone, such as osteoporosis, osteomalacia, and renal and hepatic osteopathy [70–73].

Local risk factors include loosened implants, heterotopic ossification, and stress risers [12, 74]. Heterotopic ossification leads to an acute arrest of movement and usually causes long spiral fractures through a kind of hypomochlion. Stress risers include old screw holes, osteolyses, perforations, bone apertures (for cement removal), leaked cement, the ends of osteosynthesis plates, varus positioning of the stem with stress peaks at the lateral prosthesis tip, and impingement of loose stem implants against the lateral femoral cortex [75, 76].

Stem revision in periprosthetic fractures is necessary in the case of a loosened endoprosthesis (Vancouver type B2 and B3 fractures) and in the case of concomitant fractured implants (Fig. 2.2) [74, 76–78]. Bethea et al. [70] found

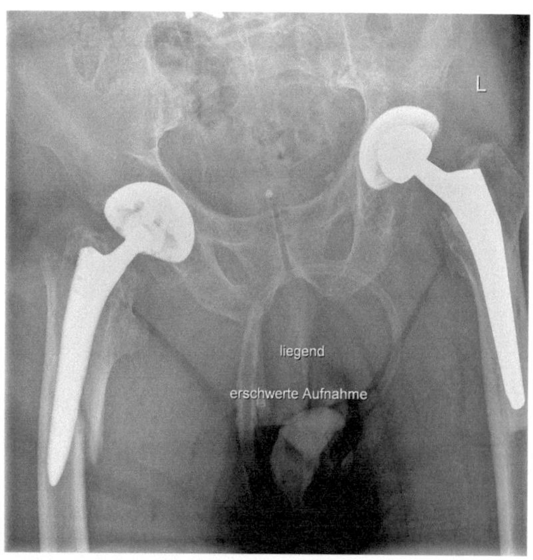

Fig. 2.2 Periprosthetic fracture with loosened, subsided stem on the right (Vancouver B2 type)

loosened implants in 75% of postoperative periprosthetic fractures, while Duncan et al. [76] reported loosened implants in 82% of type B fractures.

References

1. Kenney C, Dick S, Lea J, Liu J, Ebraheim NA. A systematic review of the causes of failure of revision hip arthroplasty. J Orthop. 2019;16:393–5.
2. Prokopetz JJZ, Losina E, Bliss RL, Wright J, Baron JA, Katz JN. Risk factors for revision of primary total hip arthroplasty: a systematic review. BMC Musculoskelet Disord. 2012;13:251.
3. Fink B, Urbansky K, Schuster P. Mid term results with the curved modular tapered, fluted titanium Revitan stem in revision hip replacement. Bone Joint J. 2014;96-B(7):889–95.
4. Sadolghi P, Liebensteiner M, Agreiter M, Leithner A, Böhler N, Labek G. Revision surgery after total joint arthroplasty: a complicated-based analysis using worldwide arthroplasty registers. J Arthroplasty. 2013;28:1329–32.
5. Ulrich SD, Seyler TM, Bennett D, Delanois RE, Saleh KJ, Thongtrangan I, Kuskowski M, Chen EY, Sharkey PF, Parvizi J, Stiehl JB, Mont MA. Total hip arthroplasties: what are the reasons for revision? Int Orthop. 2008;32:597–604.
6. Lachiewsicz PF, Soileau ES. Changing indications for revision total hip arthroplasty. J Surg Orthop Adv. 2005;14:82–4.
7. Clohisy JC, Calvert G, Tull F et al., Reasons for revision hip surgery: a retrospective review. Clin Orthop Relat Res. 2004;(429):188–192.
8. Weeden SH, Paprosky WG. Minimal 11-year follow-up of extensively porous-coated stems in femoral revision total hip arthroplasty. J Arthroplasty. 2002;17(Suppl 1):134–7.
9. Lind M, Krarup N, Mikkelson S, et al. Exchange impaction allografting for femoral revision hip arthroplasty: results in 87 cases after 3.6 years' follow-up. J Arthroplasty. 2002;17:158–64.
10. Ullmark G, Hallin G, Nilsson O. Impacted corticocancellous allografts and cement for revision of the femur component in total hip arthroplasty. J Arthroplasty. 2002;17:140–9.
11. Böhm P, Bischel O. Femoral revision with the Wagner SL revision stem: evaluation of one hundred and twenty-nine revisions followed for a mean of 4.8 years. J Bone Joint Surg Am. 2001;83-A:1012–31.
12. Sandiford NA, Garbuz DS, Masri BA, Duncan CP. Nonmodular tapered fluted titanium stems osseointegrate reliably at short term in revision THAs. Clin Orthop Relat Res. 2017;(475):186–192.
13. Mavrogenis AF, Dimitriou R, Parvizi J, et al. Biology of implant osseointegration. J Musculoskelet Neuronal Interact. 2009;9:61–71.
14. Parithimarkalaignan S, Padmanabdhan TV. Osseointegration: an update. J Indian Prosthodont Soc. 2013;13:2–6.
15. Oldani C, Domingeuz A Titanium as a biomaterial for implants, recent advances in arthroplasty. In: Kokter S (Ed.), Intech; 2012. isbn:978-953-307-990-5. http://www.intechopen.com/books/recent-advances-in-arthroplasty/titanium-a-abiomaterial-for-implants
16. Niinomi M, Nakai M. Titanium-based biomaterials for preventing stress shielding between implant devices and bone. Int J Biomater. 2011;2011:1–10.
17. Bitar D, Parvizi J. Biological response to prosthetic debris. World J Orthop. 2015;6(2):172–89.
18. Holt G, Munraghan C, Reilly J, Meek RMD. Biology of aseptic osteolysis. Clin Orthop Relat Res. 2007;460:240–52.
19. Wilkinson JM, Hamer AJ, Stockley I, Eastell R. Polyethylene wear rate and osteolysis: critical threshold versus continuous dose-response relationship. J Orthop Res. 2005;23:520–5.
20. Wilkinson JM, Wilson AD, Stockley I, Scott IR, MacDonald DA, Hamer AJ, Gordon WD. Variation in the TNF gene promoter and risk of osteolysis after total hip arthroplasty. J Bone Miner Res. 2003;18:1995–2001.
21. Oparaugo PC, Clarke IC, Malchau H, Herberts P. Correlation of wear debris-induced osteolysis and revision with volumetric wear-rates of polyethylene: a survey of 8 reports in the literature. Acta Orthop Scand. 2001;72(1):22–8.
22. Davies AP, Willert HG, Campbell PA, Learmonth ID, Case CP. An unusual lymphocytic perivascular infiltration in tissues around contemporary metal-on-metal joint replacements. J Bone Joint Surg Am. 2005;87(1):18–27.
23. Sinha RK, Shanbhag AS, Maloney WJ, Hasselman CT, Rubash HE. Osteolysis: cause and effect. Instr Course Lect. 1998;47:307–20.
24. Duisabeau L, Combrade P, Forest B. Environmental effect on fretting of metallic materials for orthopaedic implants. Wear. 2004;256:805–16.
25. Jauch SY, Huber G, Sellenschloh K, et al. Micromotions at the taper interface between stem and neck adapter of a bimodular hip prosthesis during activities of daily living. J Orthop Res. 2013;31(8):1165–71.
26. Schramm M, Wirtz DC, Holzwarth U, Pitto RP. The Morse taper junction in modular revision hip replacement—a biomechanical and retrieval analysis. Biomed Tech (Berl) 2000; 45(4): 105–109.
27. Pastides PS, Dodd M, Sarraf KM, Willis-Owen CA. Trunnionosis: a pain in the neck. World J Orthop. 2013;4:161–6.
28. Morawietz L, Classen RA, Schröder JH, et al. Proposal for a histological consensus classification of the periprosthetic interface membrane. J Clin Pathol. 2006;59(6):591–7.
29. Rujitanaroj PO, Jao B, Yang J, et al. Controlling fibrous capsule formation through long-term

down-regulation of collagen type I (COL1A1) expression by nanofiber-mediated siRNA gene silencing. Acta Biomater. 2013;9(1):4513–24.
30. Wataha JC. Materials for endosseous dental implants. J Oral Rehabil. 1996;23(2):79–90.
31. Messier SP, Gutekunst DJ, Davis C, DeVita P. Weight loss reduces knee-joint loads in overweight and obese older adults with knee osteoarthritis. Arthritis Rheum. 2005;52(7):2026–32.
32. Gallo J, Goodman SB, Konttinen YT, Raska M. Particle disease: biologic mechanisms of periprosthetic osteolysis in total hip arthroplasty. Innate Immun. 2013;19(2):213–24.
33. Aspenberg P, van der Vis H. Fluid pressure may cause periprosthetic osteolysis. Particles are not the only thing. Acta Orthop Scand. 1998;69(1):1–4.
34. Mert M, Oztürkmen Y, Ünkar EA, Erdoğan S, Uzümcügil O. Sciatic nerve compression by an extrapelvic cyst secondary to wear debris after a cementless total hip arthroplasty: a case report and literature review. Int J Surg Case Rep. 2013;4(10):805–8.
35. Berend ME, Ritter MA, Hyldahl HC, Meding JB, Redelman R. Implant migration and failure in total knee arthroplasty is related to body mass index and tibial component size. J Arthroplasty. 2008;23(6 Suppl 1):104–9.
36. Wong J, Steklov N, Patil S, et al. Predicting the effect of tray malalignment on risk for bone damage and implant subsidence after total knee arthroplasty. J Orthop Res. 2011;29(3):347–53.
37. Pap G, Machner A, Rinnert T, et al. Development and characteristics of a synovial-like interface membrane around cemented tibial hemiarthroplasties in a novel rat model of aseptic prosthesis loosening. Arthritis Rheum. 2001;44(4):956–63.
38. Gallo J, Raska M, Mrázek F, Petrek M. Bone remodeling, particle disease and individual susceptibility to periprosthetic osteolysis. Physiol Res. 2008;57(3):339–49.
39. Goldring SR, Jasty M, Roelke MS, Rourke CM, Bringhurst FR, Harris WH. Formation of a synovial-like membrane at the bone-cement interface. Its role in bone resorption and implant loosening after total hip replacement. Arthritis Rheum. 1986;29(7): 836–42.
40. Windisch C, Windisch B, Kolb W, Kolb K, Grützner P, Roth A. Osteodensitometry measurements of periprosthetic bone using dual energy X-ray absorptiometry following total knee arthroplasty. Arch Orthop Trauma Surg. 2012;132(11):1595–601.
41. Sansone V, Pagani D, Melaot M. The effects on bone cells of metal ions released for orthopaedic implants. A review. Clin Cases Miner Bone Metab. 2013;10:34–40.
42. Fackler CD, Poss R. Dislocation in total hip arthroplasties. Clin Orthop. 1980;151:169–78.
43. Li C, Renz N, Trampuz A. Management of periprosthetic joint infection. Hip Pelvis. 2018;30:138–46.
44. Pulido L, Ghanem E, Joshi A, Purtill JJ, Parvizi J. Periprosthetic joint infection: the incidence, timing, and predisposing factors. Clin Orthop Relat Res. 2008;466:1710–5.
45. Parvizi J, Ghanem E, Menashe S, Barrack RL, Bauer TW. Periprosthetic infection: what are the diagnostic challenges? J Bone Joint Surg. 2006;88-A:138–47.
46. Portillo ME, Salvado M, Alier A, Sorli L, Martinez S, Horcajada JP, Puig L. Prosthesis failure within 2 years of implantation is highly predictive of infection. Clin Orthop Relat Res. 2013;471:3672–8.
47. Gallo J, Kolar M, Novotny R, Rihakova P, Ticha V. Pathogenesis of prosthesis-related infection. Biomed Pap Med Fac Univ Palacky Olomouc Czech Repub. 2003;147:27–35.
48. Coventry MB. Treatment of infections occurring in total hip surgery. Orthop Clin North Am. 1975;6:991–1003.
49. Estrada R, Tsukayama D, Gustilo R. Management of THA infections. A prospective study of 108 cases. Orthop Trans. 1993;17:1114–5.
50. Tsukayma DT, Estrada R, Gustilo RB. Infection after total hip arthroplasty. A study of the treatment of one hundred and six infections. J Bone Joint Surg Am. 1996;78-A:512–23.
51. Zimmerli W, Widmer AF, Blatter M, Frei R, Ochsner PE. Role of rifampin for treatment of orthopedic implant-related staphylococcal infections: a randomized controlled trial. Foreign-Body Infection (FBI) Study Group. JAMA. 1998;279:1537–41.
52. Martínez-Pastor JC, Muñoz-Mahamud E, Vilchez F, García-Ramiro S, Bori G, Sierra J, Martínez JA, Font L, Mensa J, Soriano A. Outcome of acute prosthetic joint infections due to gram-negative bacilli treated with open debridement and retention of the prosthesis. Antimicrob Agents Chemother. 2009;53: 4772–7.
53. Berdal JE, Skramm I, Mowinckel P, Gulbrandsen P, Bjornholt JV. Use of rifampicin and ciprofloxacin combination therapy after surgical debridement in the treatment of early manifestation prosthetic joint infections. Clin Microbiol Infect. 2005;11:843–5.
54. Aboltins CA, Dowsey MM, Buising KL, Peel TN, Daffy JR, Choong PFM, Stanley PA. Gram-negative prosthetic joint infection treated with debridement, prosthesis retention and antibiotic regimes including a fluoroquinolone. Clin Microbiol Infect. 2011;17:862–7.
55. Soriano A, Garcia S, Bori G, Almela M, Gallart X, Macule F, Sierra J, Martinez JA, Suso S, Mensa J. Treatment of acute post-surgical infection of joint arthroplasty. Clin Microbiol Infect. 2006;12:930–3.
56. Fink B, Lass R. Diagnostischer Algorithmus für die Fehleranalyse bei schmerzhaften Hüfttotalendoprothesen. Z Orthop Unfall. 2016;154:527–44.
57. Garvin KL, Hanssen AD. Current concepts review: infection after total hip arthroplasty. J Bone Joint Surg Am. 1995;77-A:1576–88.
58. Cui Q, Mihalko WM, Shields JS, Ries M, Saleh HJ. Antibiotic-impregnated cement spacers for the treatment of infection associated with total

hip or knee arthroplasty. J Bone Joint Surg Am. 2007;89-A:871–82.
59. Hanssen AD, Osmon DR. Evaluation of a staging system for infected hip arthroplasty. Clin Orthop Relat Res. 2002;(403):16–22.
60. Mont MA, Waldman BJ, Hungerford DS. Evaluation of preoperative cultures before second-stage reimplantation of a total knee prosthesis complicated by infection: a comparison-group study. J Bone Joint Surg Am. 2000;82:1552–7.
61. Fink B. Revision of late periprosthetic infections of total hip endoprostheses: pros and cons of different concepts. Int J Med Sci. 2009;6:287–95.
62. Fink B. Treatment of infected total hip arthroplasty. Min Orthop Traumatol. 2010;61:123–33.
63. George DA, Logoluso N, Castellini G, Gianola S, Scarponi S, Haddad FS, Drago L, Romano CL. Does cemented or cementless single-stage exchange arthroplasty of chronic periprosthetic hip infections provide similar infection rates to a two-stage? A systematic review. BMC Infect Dis. 2016;16:553.
64. Morrey BF, Kavanagh BF. Complications with revision of the femoral component of total hip arthroplasty: comparison between cemented and uncemented techniques. J Arthroplasty. 1992;7:71–9.
65. Kavanagh BF. Femoral fractures associated with total hip arthroplasty. Orthop Clin North Am. 1992;23:249–57.
66. Lewallen DG, Berry DJ. Periprosthetic fracture of the femur after total hip arthroplasty: treatment and results to date. Instr Course Lect. 1998;47:243–9.
67. Pivec R, Issa K, Kapadia BH, Cheriari JJ, Maheshwari AV, Bonutti M, Mont MA. Incidence and future projections of periprosthetic femoral fracture following primary total hip arthroplasty: an analysis of international registry data. J Long Term Eff Med Implants. 2015;25:269–75.
68. Abdel MP, Watts CD, Houdek MT, Lewallen DG, Berry DJ. Epidemiology of periprosthetic fracture of the femur in 32644 primary total hip arthroplasties: a 40-year experience. Bone Joint J 2016;98-B: 461–467.
69. Abdel MP, Houdek MT, Watss CD, Lewallen DG, Berry DJ. Epidemiology of periprosthetic femoral fracture in 5417 revision total hip arthroplasties: a 40-year experience. Bone Joint J. 2016;98-B: 468–74.
70. Bethea JS, DeAndrade JR, Fleming LL, Lindenbaum SD, Welch RB. Proximal femoral fractures following total hip arthroplasty. Clin Orthop. 1982;170: 95–106.
71. Partridge AJ. Nylon straps for internal fixation of bone. Lancet. 1976;2:1252.
72. Tower SS, Beals RK. Fractures of the femur after hip replacement. The Oregon experience. Orthop Clin North Am. 1999;30:235–47.
73. Larsen E, Menck H, Rosenklint A. Fractures after hemialloplastic hip replacement. J Trauma. 1987;27:72–4.
74. Namba RS, Rose NE, Amstutz HC. Unstable femoral fractures in hip arthroplasty. Orthop Trans. 1991;15:753.
75. Haddad FS, Duncan CP, Berry DJ, Lewallen DG, Gross AE, Chandler HP. Periprosthetic femoral fractures around well-fixed implants: use of cortical onlay allografts with or without a plate. J Bone Joint Surg. 2002;84-A:945–50.
76. Duncan DP, Masri BA. Fractures of the femur after hip replacement. Instr Course Lect. 1995;44:293–304.
77. Cooke PH, Newman JH. Fractures of the femur in relation to cemented hip prostheses. J Bone Joint Surg. 1988;70-B:386–9.
78. Adolphson P, Jonsson U, Kalen R. Fractures of the ipsilateral femur after total hip arthroplasty. Arch Orthop Trauma Surg. 1987;106:353–7.

3 Classification of Femoral Bone Defects

Contents

3.1 **Paprosky Classification** ... 11
3.1.1 Paprosky Type I Defect ... 13
3.1.2 Paprosky Type II Defect ... 13
3.1.3 Paprosky Type IIA Defect ... 13
3.1.4 Paprosky Type IIB Defect ... 14
3.1.5 Paprosky Type IIC Defect ... 14
3.1.6 Paprosky Type III Defect ... 14
3.1.7 Paprosky Type IV Defect ... 15

3.2 **AAOS Classification by D'Antonio** ... 15

3.3 **Endo-Clinic Classification** ... 16

References ... 18

Many classifications of bony defects of the femur have been described for use in planning stem revision surgery. In general, these classifications are based on the description of the extent of the bone defect in the various anatomical regions of the femur and/or on the description of axial deviations of the femur. This involves an analysis of preoperative radiographs, which means that the actual biomechanical characteristics of the surrounding bone are not taken into account. But the extent of the bone defect as determined radiologically is not always the only decisive factor in the selection of the fixation procedure for the new prosthesis, but also the mechanical stability of the remaining bone. For example, the mechanical stability of the metaphyseal bone is of primary importance for proximal cementless fixation of the new revision stem or for impaction grafting. Ultimately, this can only be determined intraoperatively. Nevertheless, the preoperative analysis of defects during the planning stage is the key criterion for the selection of the type of fixation and preparation of the new prosthetic implant. Of the numerous classifications described, the most frequently used in practice and in the scientific literature will be described here.

3.1 Paprosky Classification

Wayne Paprosky described a classification in 1990 that was designed to determine whether the revision stem Solution™ (DePuy Synthes, Warsaw, IN) used by Paprosky for distal scratch-fit fixation in the isthmus of the femur was still

B. Fink, *Femoral Revision Arthroplasty*, https://doi.org/10.1007/978-3-030-84821-7_3

functional for the more severe defect types [1, 2]. It recognizes 4 defect types that were originally classified into subtypes for defect types II and III. Later, Paprosky amalgamated the different subtypes of type II into a single type II [3, 4] (Fig. 3.1).

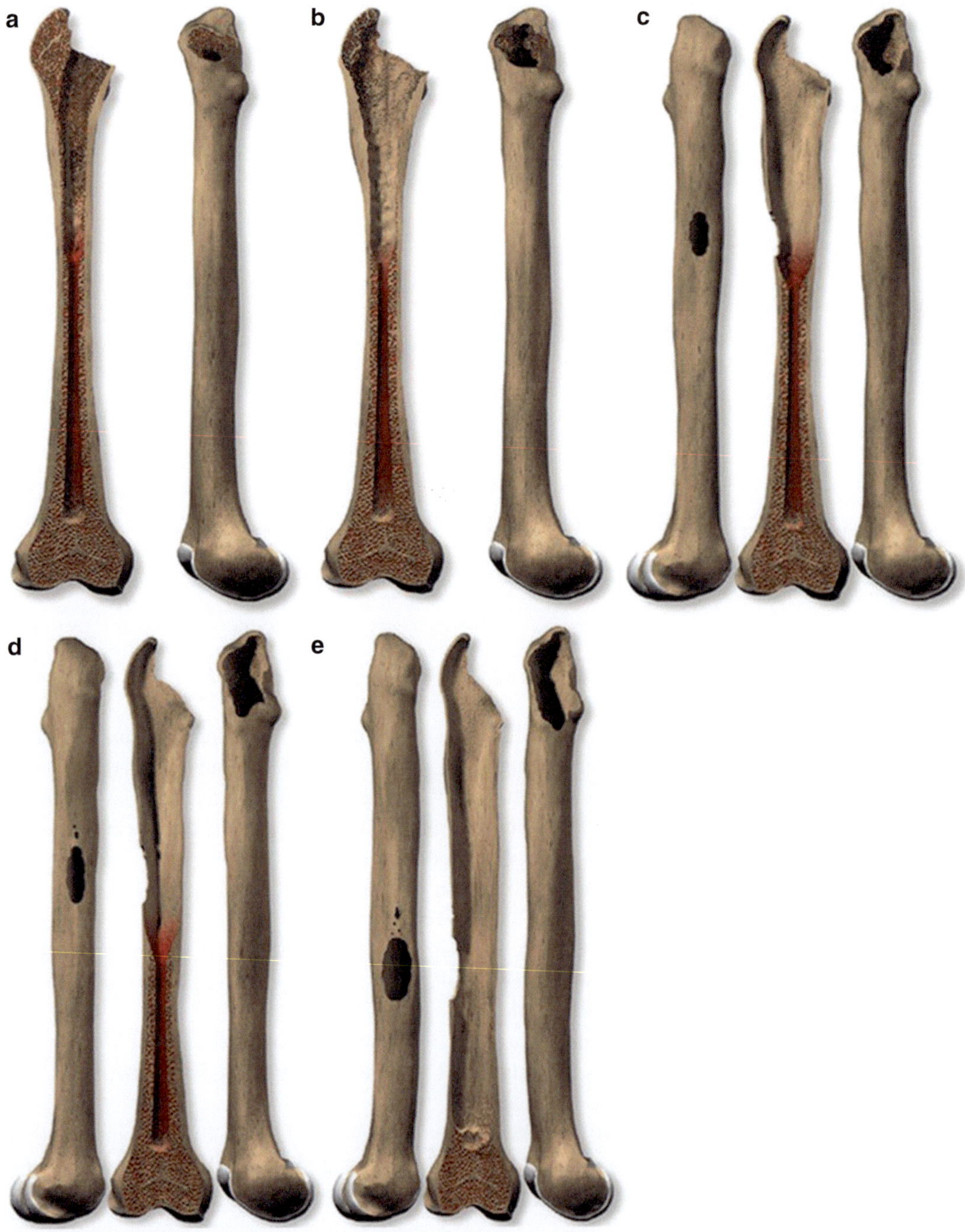

Fig. 3.1 Defect classification according to Paprosky I-IV (a = type I, b = type II, c = type IIIA, d = type IIIB, e = type IV) (with permission of DePuy Synthes, Warsaw, IN, USA)

3.1.1 Paprosky Type I Defect

Type I defects comprise only minimal defects in the calcar and metaphyseal anteroposterior bone. The metaphysis and diaphysis are sufficiently intact for bony support (Fig. 3.2).

3.1.2 Paprosky Type II Defect

Type II defects are characterized by more extensive defects in the metaphysis. The calcar of the femur is deficient, and there are defects of varying extent anteroposteriorly in the metaphysis (Fig. 3.3). The diaphysis is intact.

In the original classification, three subtypes were differentiated here, type IIA to type IIC [1, 2] (Fig. 3.4). Although this subclassification has long since fallen out of use, it will be discussed here, as it can be a useful aid in deciding whether to use proximally fitting stems (see Chap. 5).

3.1.3 Paprosky Type IIA Defect

The type IIA defect is a metaphyseal defect in the calcar region of the medial femur, but it does not extend beyond the subtrochanteric region of the femur (lesser trochanter) (Fig. 3.4). Although the subtrochanteric bone is still biomechanically

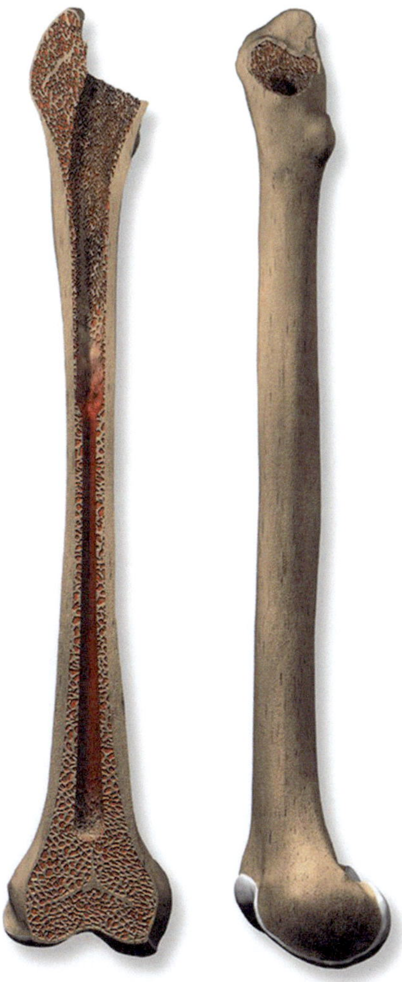

Fig. 3.2 Paprosky type I defect

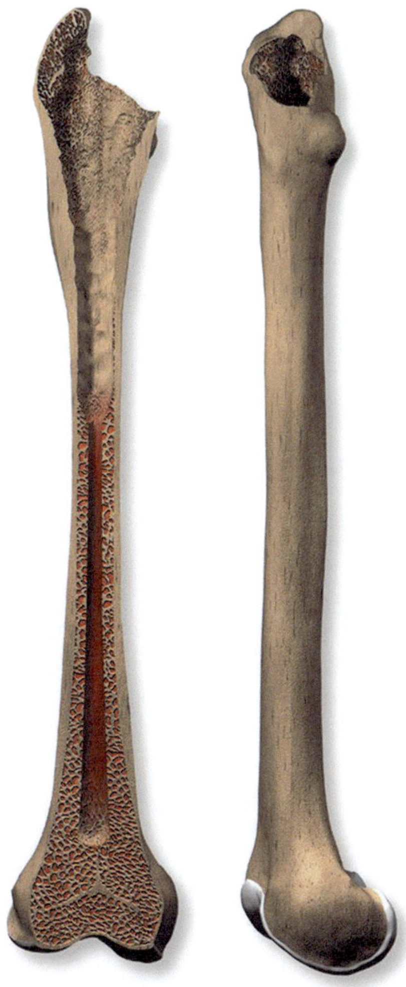

Fig. 3.3 Paprosky type II defect

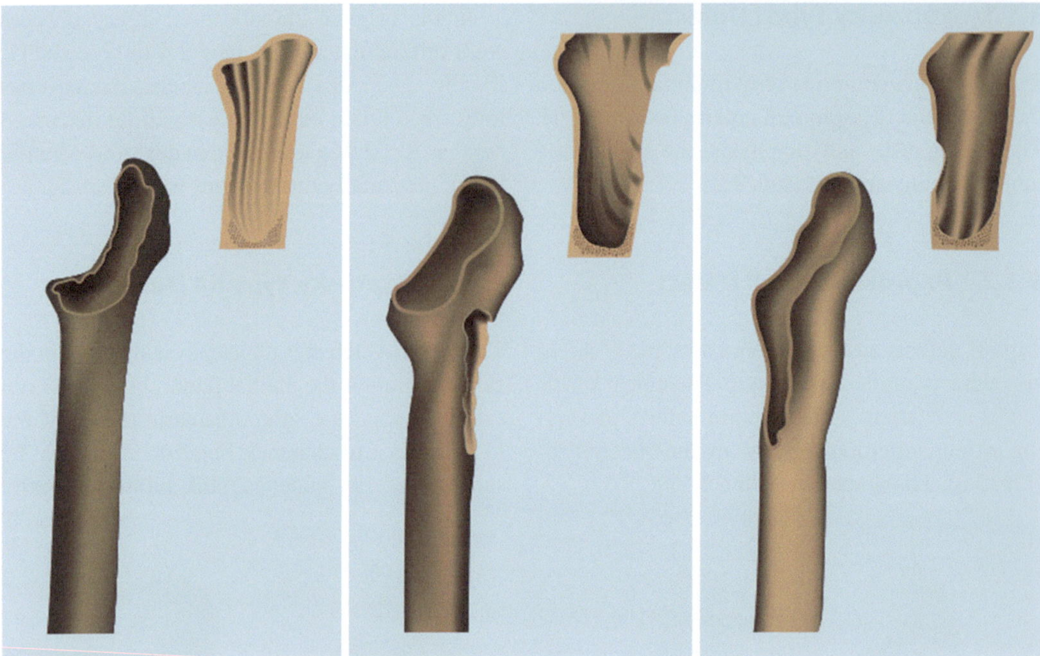
Typ IIA Typ IIB Typ IIC

Fig. 3.4 Subclassification of the Paprosky type II defect into types IIA to IIC

supportive, the area of metaphyseal bone that is still present only provides a low level of proximal rotational stability, partly due to the lack of anteroposterior bone.

3.1.4 Paprosky Type IIB Defect

Here, the lateral metaphyseal region of the femur below the greater trochanter is deficient. The anteroposterior bone loss is significant. The remaining metaphyseal bone no longer provides sufficient rotational stability for a proximal fixation stem with a standard length primary stem (Fig. 3.4). Longer prosthetic stems are required, or the bone can be reconstructed by impaction grafting.

3.1.5 Paprosky Type IIC Defect

The medial metaphyseal wall is defective and no longer stable enough for mechanical support or fixation (Fig. 3.4). Longer stem prostheses must be used, and, if necessary, the medial bone defect may need to be reconstructed with a medial strut graft in the case of metaphyseal fixation of the prosthesis.

3.1.6 Paprosky Type III Defect

Paprosky type III has extensive defects of the metaphysis that no longer allow proximal fixation. The diaphysis is also deficient. Depending on the length of diaphyseal bone in the isthmus of the femur that is still available for distal fixation, these defects are divided into Paprosky type IIIA defects (with at least 4 cm of intact isthmus) (Fig. 3.5) and Paprosky type IIIB defects (with less than 4 cm of intact isthmus) (Fig. 3.6) [4, 5]. The threshold between the IIIA and IIIB defects is 4 cm, based on Paprosky's experience with his Solution™ Stem (DePuy Synthes, Warsaw, IN, USA), which is fixed in the distal femur with a so-called scratch fit (personal communication) (see Chap. 4B). We were able to show that a minimum fixation length of 3 cm is sufficient for a

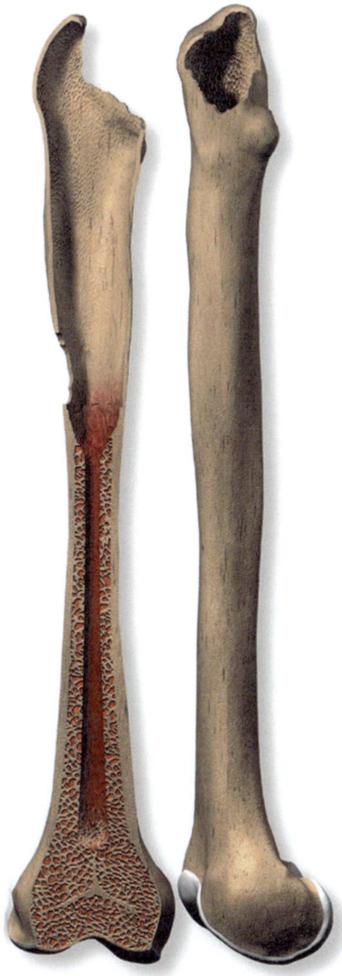

Fig. 3.5 Paprosky type IIIA defect

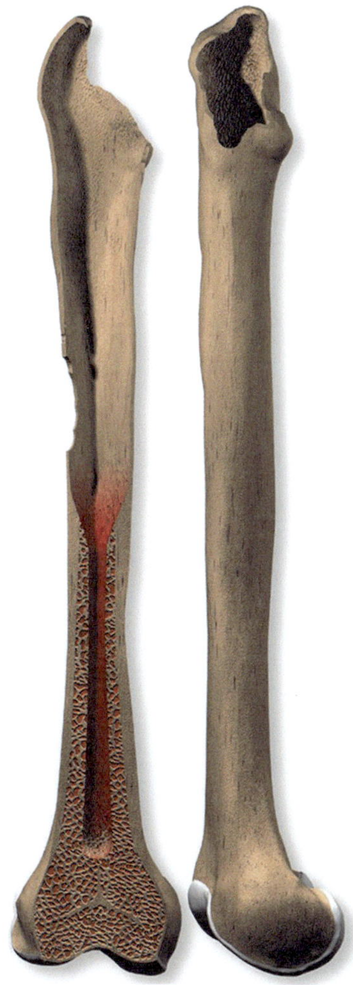

Fig. 3.6 Paprosky type IIIB defect

taper-to-taper locked, distally fixed titanium revision stem with a 2-degree taper [6]. Therefore, it might be useful to consider a modification of the defect classification for distally fixed conical revision stems.

3.1.7 Paprosky Type IV Defect

This is an extensive metaphyseal and diaphyseal defect of the femur. The entire femoral canal is expanded, and the remaining cortical bone is thin. The isthmus of the femur is no longer present and is unsuitable for normal distal fixation of a revision stem (Fig. 3.7).

3.2 AAOS Classification by D'Antonio

This classification of femoral defects published by the American Society of Orthopedic Surgeons first differentiates between segmental (type I) and cavitary defects (type II) (Fig. 3.8) [7]. Segmental defects are then defined as those with any loss of the cortical bone layer. Proximal segmental defects can be further divided into partial or complete defects. Type I segmental defects can be divided into three levels in terms of their extent. Level I is above the lesser trochanter, level II is within 10 cm of the distal border of the lesser trochanter, and level III is distal to 10 cm below the

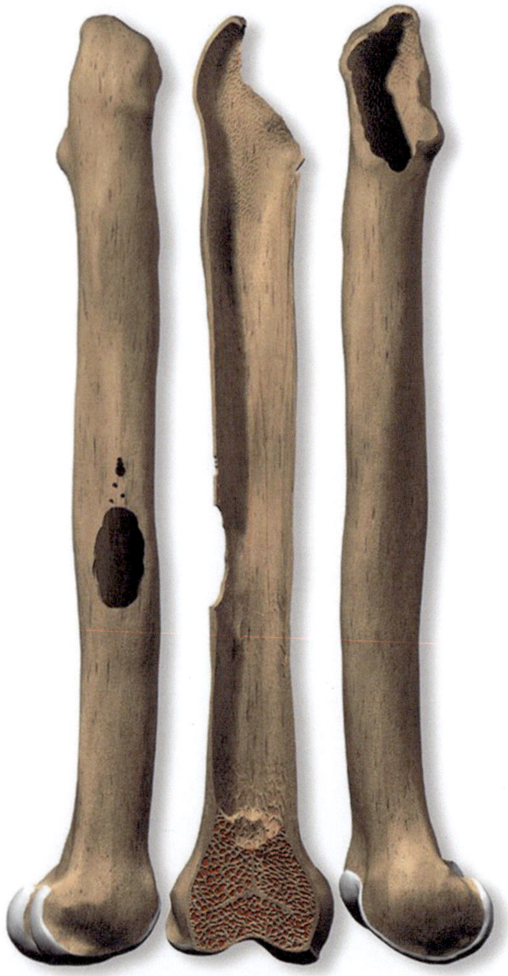

Fig. 3.7 Paprosky type IV defect

lower edge of the lesser trochanter [7] (Fig. 3.8). The greater trochanter is managed as a separate segmental defect due to its specific and difficult to address problems in femoral revision arthroplasty. The type II cavitary defect presents as a thinning of the cancellous and internal cortical bone wall, but without discontinuity or injury to the cortical margins (Fig. 3.8). Depending on the extent of the cavitary defect, a distinction can be made between purely cancellous defects and those with accompanying thinning of the inner cortical bone wall (type IIA). If the cortex of the femur is also expanded or bulging at the same time (an ectasia), this is called cavitary type IIB. If cavitary and segmental defects occur together, the combination of type I and type II is classified as type III (Fig. 3.8). In a type IV defect, there is an axial deviation of the femur caused by the loosening process, which usually shows additional cavitary and segmental defects (Fig. 3.8). If there is a femoral stenosis below the implanted prosthesis, this is referred to as type V, whereas type VI describes a discontinuity of the femur, i.e., a periprosthetic fracture resulting in a defect of the femur (Fig. 3.8). In these cases, levels I to III are again used for defining the location of the defects (level I above the lesser trochanter, level II within 10 cm below the distal edge of the lesser trochanter, and level III distally 10 cm below the distal edge of the lesser trochanter). In addition, a severity rating is also described in this classification to assist the surgeon in selecting the cementless revision implant in question. Grade I corresponds to a situation in which complete proximal contact of the revision implant with host bone is possible, and no additional bone grafting is required. Grade II describes an incomplete contact of the revision implant with the host bone, but in which a sufficiently stable anchorage in the proximal zone can be achieved with the host bone, and any bone grafting that may be performed only serves to fill the free spaces between the implant and the bone. Grade III has only incomplete contact with the host bone and is no longer sufficient for the proximal stability of the revision implant. Here, D'Antonio et al. [7] recommend the use of proximal femoral strut allografts to reconstruct the defect.

3.3 Endo-Clinic Classification

The endo-clinic classification was developed by Engelbrecht and Heinert [8] to assess bone defects in cemented, loosened stems (Fig. 3.9).

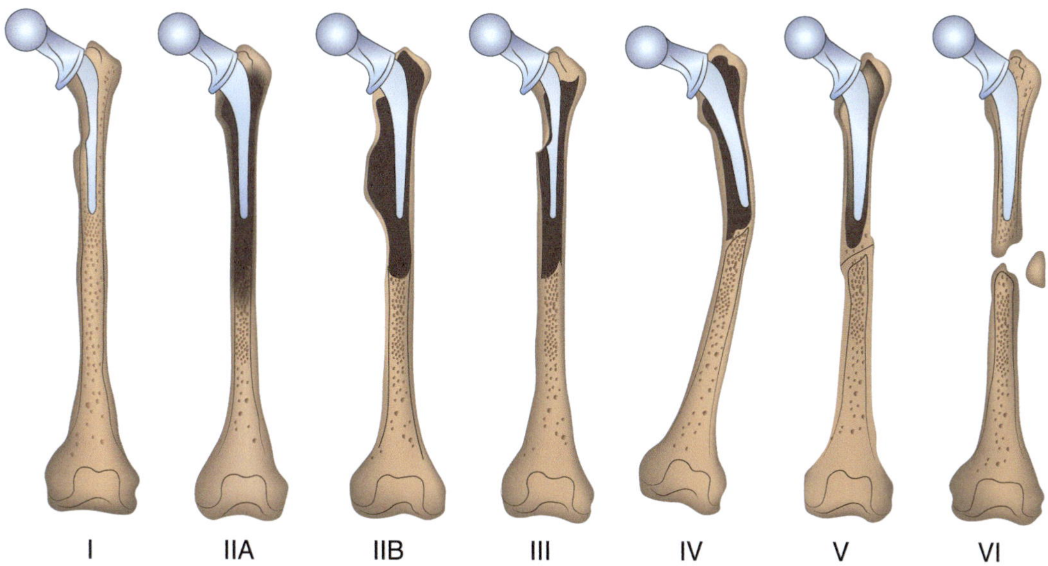

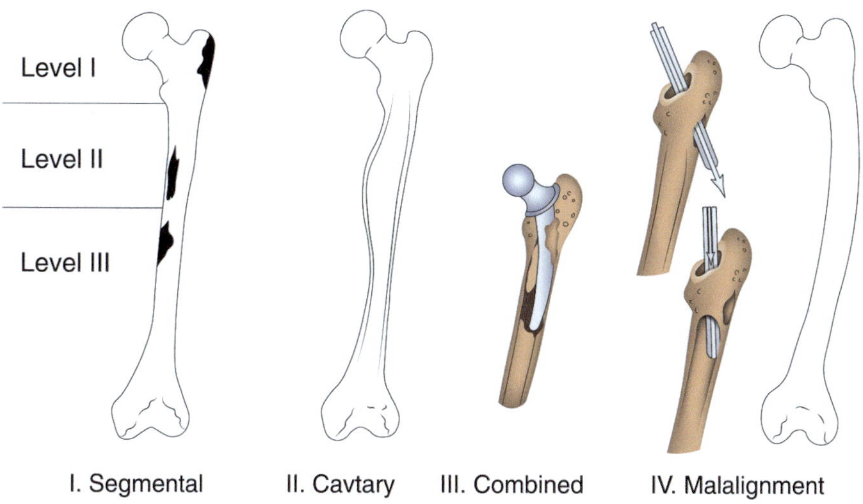

Fig. 3.8 AAOS classification of femoral defects

It is often used in studies to analyze the results of defect reconstruction by impaction grafting.

Grade 1 describes radiolucent margins as a sign of loosening in the upper half of the cement mantle (Fig. 3.9).

Grade 2 shows a generalized loosening zone around the entire prosthetic stem with an endosteal reaction and expansion of the medullary canal (Fig. 3.9).

Grade 3 describes an expansion of the proximal femur over the entire area of the inserted prosthetic stem (Fig. 3.9).

Grade 4 corresponds to extensive destruction of at least the proximal two-thirds of the femur (Fig. 3.9).

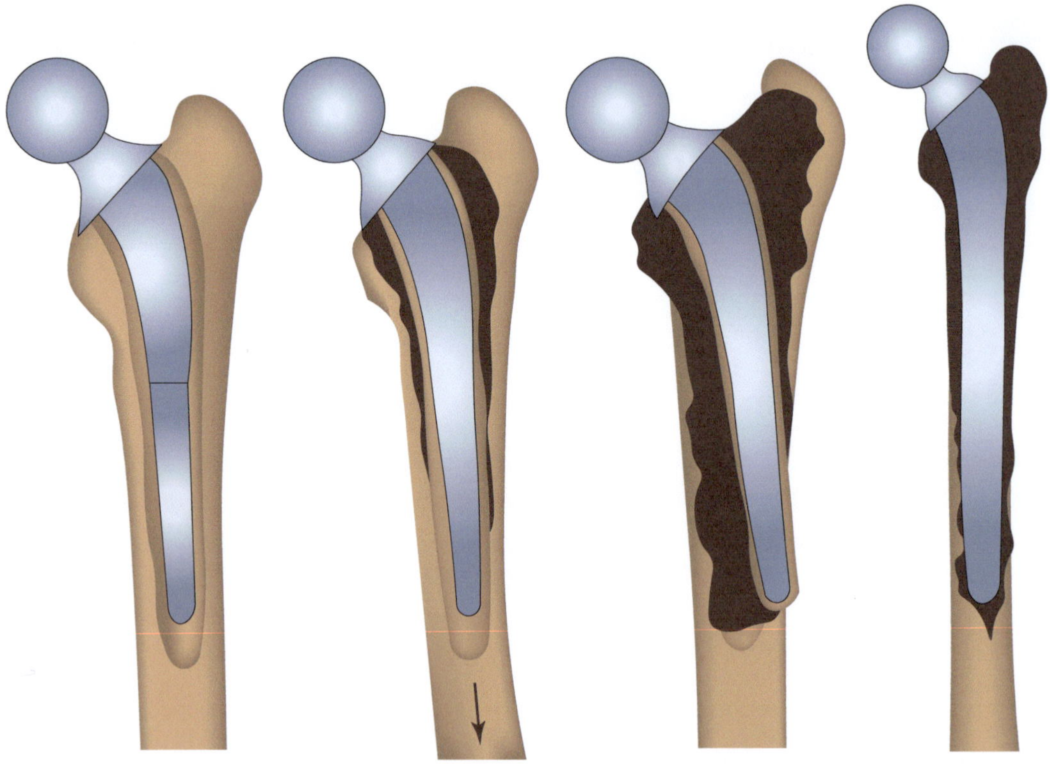

Fig. 3.9 Endo-clinic classification of femoral defects according to Engelbrecht and Heinert [8]

References

1. Pak JH, Paprosky WG, Jalonsky WS, Lawrence JM. Femoral strut allografts in cementless revision total hip arthroplasty. Clin Orthop Relat Res. 1993;(295):172–178.
2. Paprosky WG, Lawrence J, Cameron H. Femoral defect classification: clinical application. Orthop Rev. 1990;19(Suppl 9):9–15.
3. Paprosky WG, Greidanus NV, Antoniou J. Minimum 10-year-results of extensively porous-coated stems in revision hip arthroplasty. Clin Orthop. 1999;369:230–42.
4. Paprosky WG, Aribindi R. Hip replacement: treatment of femoral bone loss using distal bypass fixation. Instr Course Lect. 2000;49:119–30.
5. Della Valle CJ, Paprosky WG. Classification and an algorithmic approach to the reconstruction of femoral deficiency in revision total hip arthroplasty. J Bone Joint Surg Am. 2003;85-A(Suppl4):1–6.
6. Fink B, Grossmann A, Schubring S, Schulz MS, Fuerst M. Short-term results of hip revisions with a curved cementless modular stem in association with the surgical approach. Arch Orthop Trauma Surg. 2009;129:65–73.
7. D'Antonio J, McCarthy JC, Bargar WL, Borden LS, Cappelo WN, Collis DK, Steinberg ME, Wedge JH. Classification of femoral abnormalities in total hip arthroplasty. Clin Orthop Relat Res. 1993;(296):133–139.
8. Engelbrecht E, Heinert K. Klassifikation und Behandlungsrichtlinien von Knochensubstanzverlusten bei Revisionsoperationen am Hüftgelenk—mittelfristige Ergebnisse. In: Endo-Kliinik (ed.) Primär- und Revisionsalloarthroplastik Hüft und Knieglenk. Berlin: Springer; 1987:189–201.

4 Principles of Femoral Revision

There are several concepts and stem systems available for the revision of the femoral component of the hip joint (Fig. 4.1). When revising a loosened femoral component, it is possible to achieve implant stability of the new femoral component by cementing it in or by using cementless fixation. The cemented fixation can be performed with normal stems, with longer revision stems, with cement-in-cement techniques, with impaction grafting, or with megaprostheses. Cementless fixation can be performed proximal or distal in the femur with monoblock or modular stems in straight or curved versions. There are different concepts of distal cementless fixation. In the following, the different principles will be discussed in the next chapters with reference to stems that have been mentioned in numerous references, without attempting to provide a complete list of the implants available on the market.

Moreover, in cases of pronounced defects of the proximal femur, it can be replaced by an allograft, as a so-called allograft prosthesis composite (APC), or by a prosthetic component acting as a proximal femoral replacement. The former technique (APC) is more likely to be considered in younger patients and the proximal femoral replacement in older patients. If it is no longer possible to anchor a prosthetic stem in the femur, an intramedullary (push-through prosthesis) or extramedullary total endoprosthetic femoral replacement is required. The stems in these concepts of APC and megaprostheses mostly rely on a cemented fixation.

B. Fink, *Femoral Revision Arthroplasty*, https://doi.org/10.1007/978-3-030-84821-7_4

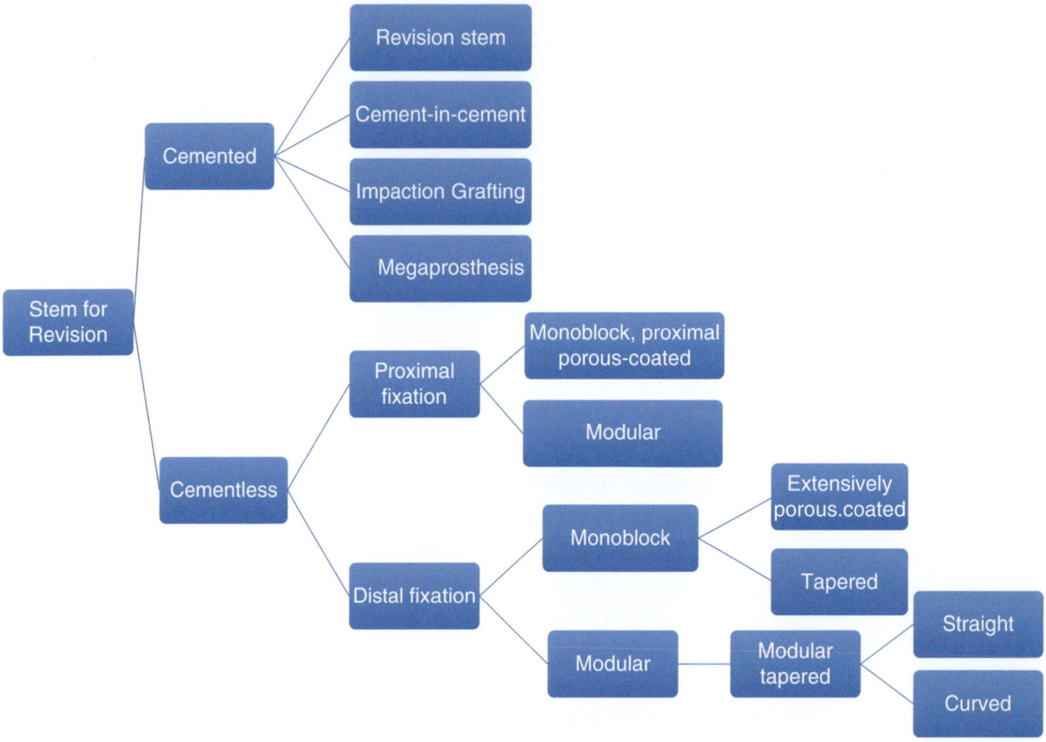

Fig. 4.1 Summary of the different revision stem systems

5 Cemented Revision Stems

Contents

5.1 **Cemented Fixation of Stems Analogous to Primary Implantation** 21
5.1.1 Surgical Technique 21
5.1.2 Outcomes 22

5.2 **Cement-in-Cement Revision** 24
5.2.1 Surgical Technique 24
5.2.2 Outcomes 25

5.3 **Impaction Bone Grafting** 26
5.3.1 Surgical Technique 27
5.3.2 Outcomes 30

References 31

There are three principles for the cemented fixation of stems in revision arthroplasty:

1. Cemented fixation of stems analogous to primary implantation.
2. Cement-in-cement revision.
3. Impaction bone grafting.

5.1 Cemented Fixation of Stems Analogous to Primary Implantation

In this procedure, after removal of the old, loosened stem and any cement from the primary implantation, a new fixation is achieved by cementing a standard or revision stem with interdigitation of the cement into the cancellous bone structure. The cemented revision stems are usually elongated standard stems with a straight form (e.g., Weber stem, Zimmer Biomet GmbH, Winterthur, Switzerland; Spectron stem, Smith & Nephew, London, UK; CSL stem, Smith & Nephew) (Fig. 5.1) or curved form (e.g., SP II stem, Waldemar Link, Hamburg, Germany) (Fig. 5.2). With the exception of the stem described by Crawford et al. [1], these stems are not modular. They achieve their stability through the use of cement to bond the stem to the bone over a longer distance.

5.1.1 Surgical Technique

These cemented revision prostheses are implanted using either the shorter rasps of the

B. Fink, *Femoral Revision Arthroplasty*, https://doi.org/10.1007/978-3-030-84821-7_5

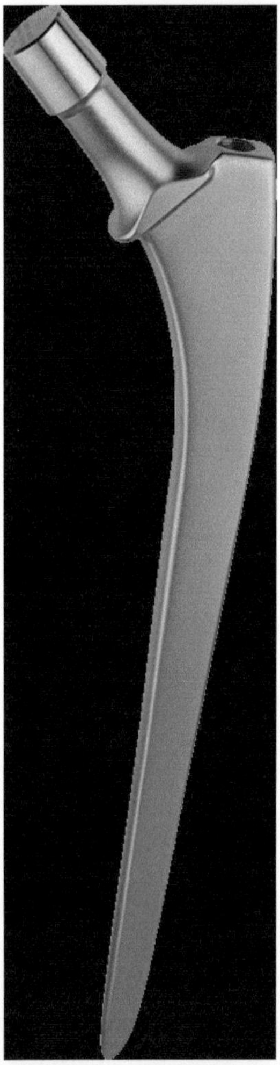

Fig. 5.1 Cemented straight revision stem (CSL, Smith & Nephew, Memphis, TN, USA)

corresponding standard stem or special, longer rasps used to prepare the new prosthetic bed. This must be done with appropriate care to avoid periprosthetic fractures and perforations. At the same time, the rasps can be used as trial prostheses as they are in primary arthroplasty. After satisfactory testing, the corresponding prosthesis is cemented in place using a modern, third-generation cementing technique (pulse lavage of the bone, distal cement plug, retrograde filling of the femoral canal with cement, solid cement compaction (pressure)).

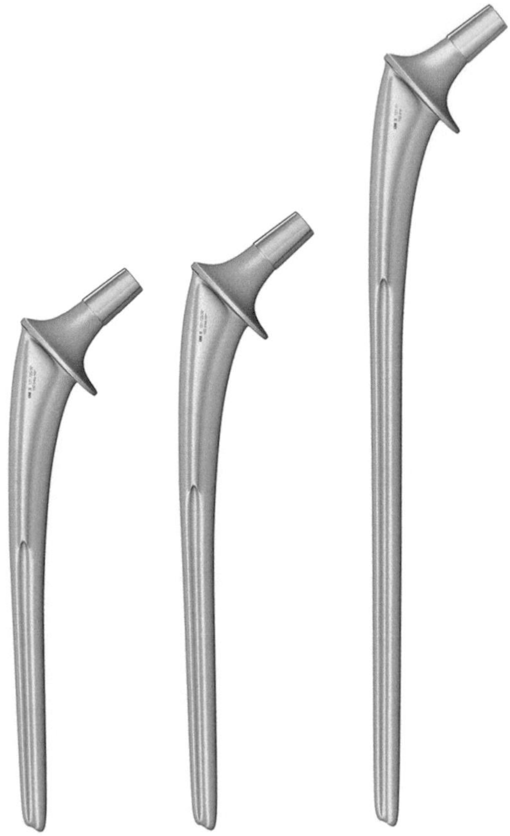

Fig. 5.2 Cemented curved revision stem (SPII stem, Waldemar Link, Hamburg, Germany)

5.1.2 Outcomes

The disadvantage of the cemented revision technique is that the bony prosthesis bed is widened, thinned, and sclerotic as a result of the loosening of the primary prosthesis. This significantly reduces the interdigitation of the cement in the cancellous bone and thus the adhesion of the cement to the bone. For example, Dohmae et al. [2] showed that the strength of the bone–cement interface with respect to shear forces is reduced by 79% in cemented revisions compared to a cemented primary implantation. This explains the relatively high loosening and re-revision rates of cemented revision stems (Table 5.1 and

Table 5.1 Outcomes of the nonmodular cemented revision stems

Author	Cases (*n*)	Follow-up (years)	Revision (%)	Subsidence (%)	Loosening (%)	Dislocation (%)	Infection (%)	Fracture (%)
Estok [7]	38	11.7	10.5		21	2.6	2.6	2.6
Haentjens [8]	16	5	0	0		43.7	12.5	25
Iorio [9]	107	7.7	7.5		12	5	0.9	
Izquierdo [10]	148	10	3.4		8.8		2.7	
Katz [11]	79	10	5.4		16.3	6.3	4.2	
Katz [12]	81	10	5.4		16.3	25.9	2.5	
Kershaw [13]	191	6.2	9.4	25	8.4	16.2	1.1	6.8
Meding [14]	34	2.5	6	38	6	2.9		17.6
Mulroy [15]	43	15.1	16.3		26	4.6		
Pierson [16]	29	8.5	10.3	3.4	14	14	3.4	
Raut [17]	399	7.4	6		8	1.7	0.5	0.8
Gramkow [18]	84	11.4	22		19			4.9
Haydon [19]	97	10.3	13		9	3.1		2.1
Howie [20]	219	6			7	13.7	3.2	1.4
So [6]	34	11.3	0		13	11.7		2.9
Te Stroet [5]	92	10.7	15.2		5.4	13.0	14.1	3.3

CRI calcar replacement implant, *tt* trans-trochanteric, *pl* posterolateral, *p* posterior

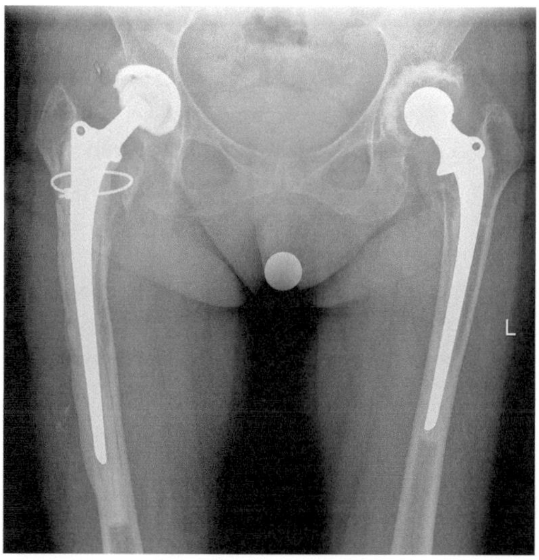

Fig. 5.3 Cemented revision stem on the right 2 years after implantation with radiologically visible loosening in a Paprosky IIIB type bone defect; cemented total hip endoprosthesis on the left

Fig. 5.3). This is significantly higher than for cementless revision components, 4.8 times higher in a review by Wirtz and Niethard [3]. The Swedish Prosthesis Register also shows a significantly higher long-term loosening rate for cemented revision stems than for cementless revision stems (Link MP) [4]. However, Te Stroet et al. [5] and So et al. [6] showed for 92 and 34 stem revisions, respectively, that satisfactory outcomes with 10-year survival rates of 92% can be achieved in cases of low loss of bone stock and a modern third-generation cementing technique. The decisive factor here is that sufficient interdigitation of the cement could take place because only minimal bone loss had occurred and sufficient cancellous bone remained. However, it should be remembered that the cemented revision technique can lead to further bone loss if it fails again, which is contrary to the goal of revision surgery to prevent further bone loss or to rebuild the existing bone loss. Thus, the preoperative analysis of the radiograph and intraoperative assessment of the remaining bone after removal of the old prosthesis and, if necessary, the old cement is critical for the decision to use cemented fixation techniques for the new stem.

5.2 Cement-in-Cement Revision

This surgical technique requires a fully intact cement mantle (at least below the lesser trochanter). Thus, this technique is often used when a cemented stem is removed from the intact cement mantle, for example, to gain better access to the cup during a separate cup replacement or to change the offset of the stem [21]. Usually, a thinner and sometimes shorter cemented stem is cemented into the old cement mantle [22]. Greenwald et al. [23] and Weinrauch et al. [24] showed that the shear strength at a new cement–old cement interface is 84–94% of that of a solid cement block when this contact surface is fully cured and there are no traces of blood. This shear strength is greatest when the new cement is poured into the old cement mantle soon after mixing. This is attributed to the increased availability of free monomer, which increases polymerization with the existing cement mantle [22, 23]. However, a blood film on the cement–cement interface leads to a reduction in the shear strength to 37% [23]. In the acute shear and tensile tests carried out by Li et al. [25], interference by blood and bone debris on the interface resulted in an 80–85% reduction in the load-bearing capacity. Thus, blood and bone debris should be avoided as far as possible when using this technique, although this cannot always be guaranteed.

Rasping the old cement mantle helps to clean the surface, may expose any residual activators/monomers, and provide a better surface for physical bonding of the cement layers [22]. Holsgrove et al. [26] found a positive effect for roughening the old cement mantle on the shear strength in biomechanical tests of different cement combinations prepared for this technique. Furthermore, they found better shear strength for the Simplex cement with tobramycin compared to PALACOS cement with gentamycin as a filling cement for the old cement mantle. However, in biomechanical tests Rudol et al. [27] found that the effect of curing seems to be more important than the roughening of the old cement mantle and that the latter seems to be helpful only for the retention of viscous fluids (probably via the drying process during the roughening process). However, roughening should not lead to damage and cracking of the old cement mantle. Treatment of the old prosthesis bed with ultrasonic cement removal does not have any positive effect on the shear strength at the cement–cement interface [28]. Rosenstein et al. [29] could show that with the correct technique the shear strength was 30% higher at the cement–cement interface than at the cement–bone interface. The aging of the original cement mantle does not seem to have a negative effect on the shear strength of the interface [30].

5.2.1 Surgical Technique

The first step in the procedure with this cement-in-cement technique is to remove the cement around the shoulder of the prosthetic stem that is to be replaced (Fig. 5.4). After removal of the implant, the integrity of the cement mantle is checked. Any loose cement fragments above the lesser trochanter are removed, and the femoral neck is osteotomized by a further 2–3 mm as necessary. The old prosthesis bed can now be roughened with a burr or rasp (Fig. 5.4). As already mentioned, it is important, with or without roughening, to ensure that the prosthesis bed is as clean as possible and absolutely dry before cementing in the new stem, for example, by temporarily applying surgical swabs. A trial prosthesis can be used for a trial fitting after which the prosthesis bed is cleaned and dried again. The fresh cement is mixed under vacuum, then quickly injected into the cement mantle in a retrograde manner with a thin cement gun, and pressurized (Fig. 5.5). A thinner and possibly shorter (preferably smoothly polished) stem of the same shape as the old one is then inserted and held in position until the cement has set [22].

A cement-in-cement revision does not come into question if there is a connective tissue layer at the bone–cement interface below the trochanter minor, if the cement mantle below the trochanter minor is loose, or if there is a bone defect [22, 31].

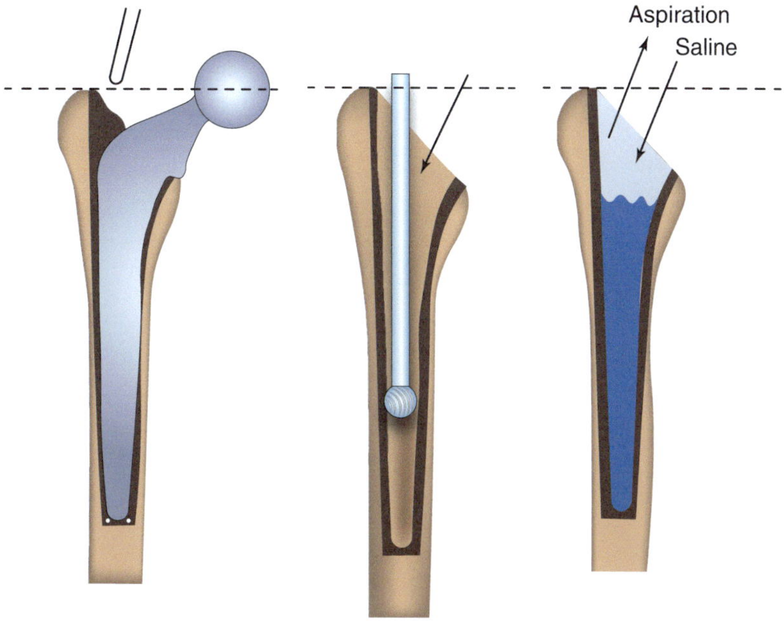

Fig. 5.4 Left: Removal of the cement around the shoulder of the prosthetic stem. Center: Roughening of the old cement mantle with a ball rasp. Right: Cleaning and drying of the old cement bed

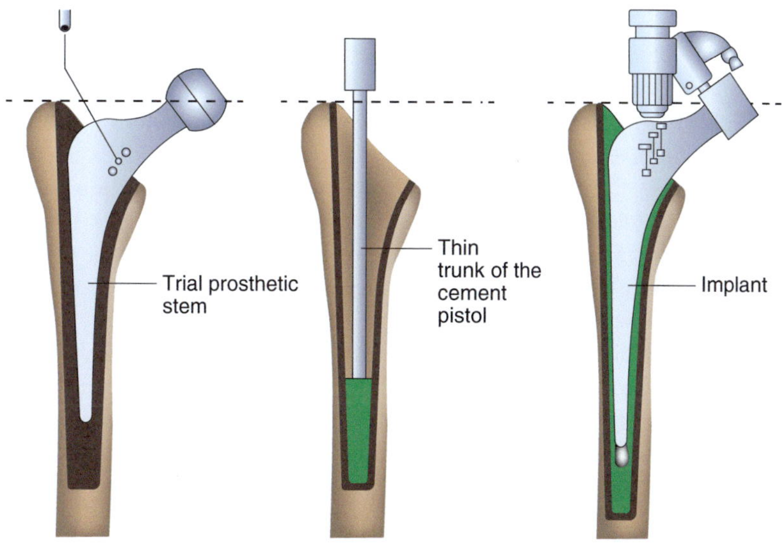

Fig. 5.5 Left: Use of the trial stem for trial positioning. Middle: Retrograde filling of the prosthesis bed with cement. Right: Insertion of the new stem

5.2.2 Outcomes

In the few studies published to date, the results and the survival rate of this surgical technique have been consistently good provided that the indication is correctly defined (Table 5.2). Lieberman et al. [32] report on 19 revised femoral endoprostheses with no loosening during a follow-up period of 59 months, and Archibald et al. [33] describe 7 cases without loosening during an observation period of 3 years. McCallum et al. [34] also found no component loosening in 15 patients after a follow-up of up to 2 years, in which they used a so-called ultrasound cement removal system (Ultra-Drive) to gradually enlarge the existing cement mantle so that the explanted prosthesis stem could be re-cemented. Marcos et al. [35] also reported no aseptic

Table 5.2 Outcomes of the cement-in-cement revision

Author	Hips	Follow-up (years)	Revisions aseptic loosening (%)	Periprosthetic fracture (%)	Perforation (%)
Archibald [33]	7	3.0	0		
Lieberman [32]	19	4.9	0		
McCallum [34]	15	<2	0		
Young [38]	36	4.1 (1–7)	5.5		
Goto [39]	44	5.1 (2–10.1)	0	20.4	2.3
Marcos [35]	37	3.8	0		
Duncan [31]	136	8 (5–15)	8/0	0.7	1.5
Te Stroet [40]	125	6 (5–7)	8/0		
Stefanovich-Lawbzary [41]	44	5.3	4.8		
Mounsey [42]	28	5.8 (2.1–10.3)	0	3.5	3.5
Okuzu [43]	62	10.8 (5–	4.8/3.2		
Cnudde [36]	1179	4.5	2.3	0.7	
Sandiford [37]	24	6.8 (5.3–20)	0		
Amanatullah [44]	63	5.5	21/2		
Kumar [45]	79	1.3 (1–3.8)	6.3/0	1.3	1.3
Woodbridge [46]	166	8.1 (5–11.7)	9.6/0	1.8	
Berg [47]	50	5.1	6/0		

loosening in 37 aseptic cement-in-cement revisions after an average of 46 months. Duncan et al. [31] reported 136 cement-in-cement revisions with an average follow-up period of 8 years (5–15 years) that were performed at Exeter between 1989 and 1999. Of these, 102 were the first revision (75%), 24 were the second revision (17.6%), 4 were the third (2.9%), and one was the fifth (0.7%) revision. In addition, 5 (3.7%) were the second revision in a two-stage septic revision. During the follow-up period, none of the stems had to be changed due to loosening and the survival rate was 92.0%. Subsequent publications confirmed these earlier favorable outcomes (Table 5.2). Cnudde et al. [36] analyzed 1179 cement-in-cement revisions from the Swedish Prosthesis Registry with an Exeter (Stryker, Kalamazoo, MG, USA) or Lubinus stem (Waldemar Link, Norderstedt, Germany) between January 1999 and December 2015 and found better outcomes for the smooth polished Exeter stem compared to the Lubinus stem with a rougher surface structure. Sandiford et al. [37] documented 24 patients with multiple cement-in-cement revisions, as a result of acetabular cup changes, and found no aseptic loosening after 81.7 months (64–240 months) of follow-up.

5.3 Impaction Bone Grafting

One possibility to counteract the problem of poor bone stock in cemented stem revision is the so-called impaction grafting technique, in which the bone defect is reconstructed with homologous cancellous bone chips before the stem (usually of normal length) is cemented into the bone bed. This technique, first described in 1987 by the group in Exeter, England, creates a new endosteal bony bed of compressed homologous bone chips for the new cemented stem [48]. Thus, a three-layer composite of implant, cement, and bone is formed in the femur. This technique has the advantage that the bone stock is remodeled, a desirable feature if further revisions become necessary [48, 49]. The creation of a stable bone graft site is critical to the success of this technically demanding technique. Unstable graft sites would collapse and subside and graft integration and/or bony incorporation with the host bone would not occur.

An impacted bone graft behaves like an aggregate and its properties as such can be described using the Mohr–Coulomb equation:

$\boldsymbol{\tau = I + \sigma \tan\varphi}$where τ is the shear strength of the aggregate, I is the constant for the interlocking or cohesion of the particles, σ is the normal stress, and φ is the angle of internal friction of the particles making up the aggregate. This mathematical expression indicates that the resistance to shear stress is proportional to the interlocking of the bone particles and the force compressing the aggregate. Since most of the forces in the femur act along the axis of the implant and only minor hoop stresses contribute to normal stress, a high degree of interlocking of the particles is required to achieve the necessary shear strength of the aggregate. This explains the importance of interlocking between the bone particles [50].

Remodeling takes place in the first few weeks after surgery because of the gradual increase in weight bearing and force exerted on the aggregate; incremental incorporation with the host bone takes place during the course of the following months [51, 52]. Thus, histologically, a mix of graft and osteoneogenesis with remodeling (new bone trabecula) was observed 2 years after surgery [53]. Since this incorporation seems to be decisive for the durability of the entire construct, many investigators demand a very long period of partial weight bearing on the operated leg of 4–6 months [52].

There are two different opinions regarding the optimal bone particle size. The group from Nijmegen favors larger bone chips at least 4.5 mm in size, as they led to an up to 25% greater stability in vitro for the acetabulum and femur [54–56]. The second school of thought prefers a broadly graded mixture of chips of different sizes as, compared to a random mixture, this allows higher shear strength to be achieved. The ideal mixture is a combination of larger chips around 4 mm and smaller particles that fill the spaces between the larger ones [57]. When the prosthesis is implanted in the new bone bed, the cementation process results in the formation of a solid bone layer at the graft–cement interface, which increases the constant **I** in the Mohr–Coulomb equation; this suggests that particle size is not so critical for shear strength of the implant complex [58]. Furthermore, there is a lack of comparative clinical studies with different particle sizes.

However, there is agreement on the importance of washing the bone chips to improve shear strength [59]. This involves rinsing out the intramedullary fat and fluid, thereby reducing the lubrication between the particles and increasing their frictional resistance. Secondly, the removal of the fat before compaction of the graft chips leads to a better compression of the graft and thus to a better interdigitation of the particles [59, 60]. In clinical applications, a statistically significant reduction in stem subsidence was observed when washed bone chips were used as opposed to unwashed chips [60]. In addition, washing removes most of the bone marrow from the bone and thus the immunologically active cells. This reduces the immunological burden for the patient and minimizes the risk of disease transmission [61–63]. It is also important to remove cartilage from the source of the bone—the femoral head—prior to fragmentation (better still in advance of the first stage of processing, directly after harvesting). This is because the elastic properties of the cartilage impair the impaction of the chips and their interdigitation [64].

The amount of graft required also appears to play a role. The greater the amount of bone graft required, the poorer the remodeling process appears to be and the higher the risk of subsidence [65]. Van der Donk et al. [66] and Linder et al. [67] found necrotic areas in the graft during histologic studies of graft samples from larger grafts between 2 and 10 years after surgery.

5.3.1 Surgical Technique

After removal of the old prosthesis stem and, if necessary, the old cement mantle, a cement stopper is first inserted into the stem. This must be firmly seated in order to withstand the pressures created by the impaction of the bone graft and not move distally during that procedure. In aseptic situations, correctly positioned old cement or an old cement stopper can be left distal to the planned new stem [68]. These serve as a kind of distal barrier or stopper for the new cement. The defatted bone chips are inserted into the femoral shaft with either conical rods of increasing size or initially with cylindrical rods (Fig. 5.6). The allograft chips are then impacted in the femoral

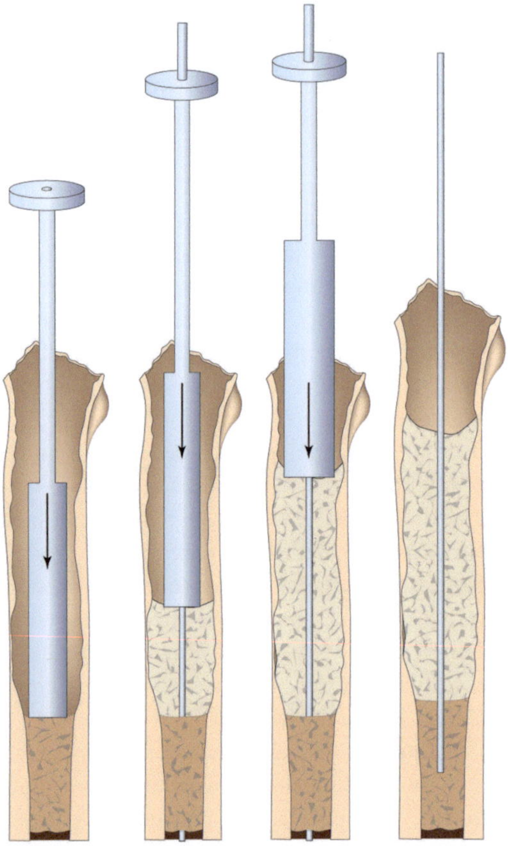

Fig. 5.6 Stepwise introduction of the bone chips with cylindrical rods of increasing size

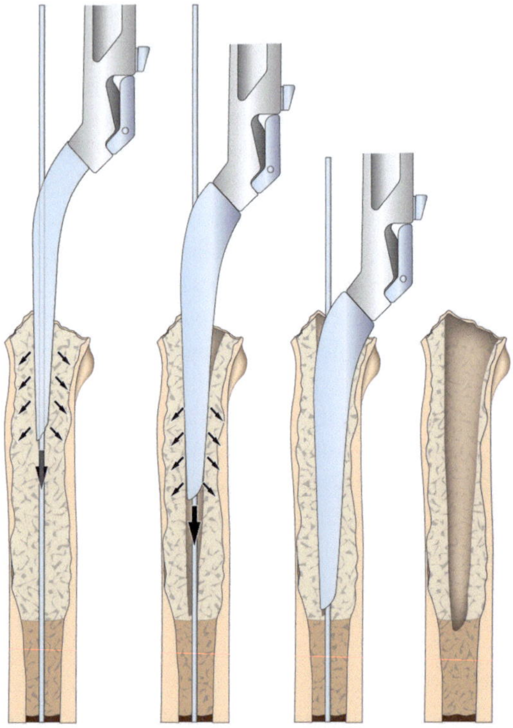

Fig. 5.7 Stepwise insertion of trial prostheses of increasing size, creating the new prosthesis bed (right) into which the new stem is cemented

canal by means of a trial prosthesis of the same size as the stem to be implanted later, which is driven in using a centralizing guidewire [69] (Fig. 5.7). Alternatively, a trial prosthesis of larger size is driven into the cancellous bone graft (Fig. 5.7). The guidewire helps to prevent misalignment of the new prosthesis bed and thus of the prosthesis. The insertion of the trial prosthesis is repeated several times, with the stiffness of the graft increasing logarithmically until about the 30th impaction, but not after that [64]. Alternatively, stem rasps of increasing size may be used, although some authors prefer to use a final rasp or trial prosthesis that is one size larger than the prosthesis to be implanted, so that a sufficiently thick cement mantle of 2 mm can be created during stem cementation [70]. With the final trial prosthesis or rasp, a trial repositioning can be performed before the stem is cemented into place in order to test the mobility and stability of the hip joint. Initially, the technique was performed without special instruments and the impaction was carried out with trial prostheses 2 sizes larger than the final implant. The Exeter group introduced the first cannulated instruments in 1991 and the second generation of instruments in 1998, thereby improving outcomes and reducing complications [71, 72].

The impaction process requires experience. The quality of the impaction determines the durability of the prosthesis and thus the success of the method. On the one hand, the impaction must be sufficiently forceful; on the other hand, excessive impaction can lead to intraoperative fractures [50, 69]. In this respect, the rate of intraoperative fractures has been reported to be between 5 and 24% [68] (Tables 5.3 and 5.4). The new stem is then cemented into this newly created stable graft bed with low-viscosity cement using the vacuum cementing technique (Fig. 5.7) [69]. In contrast to conventional stem cementing, the cement

Table 5.3 Outcomes of the impaction grafting technique with a smooth polished stem

Author	*N*	Follow-up	Fracture (%)	Subsidence	Loosening (%)	Dislocation (%)
Gie [48]	58	30 Mo	7	79%	5	5
Elting [86]	67	31 Mo	5	48%	5	3
Eldridge [55]	79	13 Mo		23% 11% >10 mm	10	
Flugsrud [87]	10	52 Mo	0	80%	0	
Knight [88]	31	31 Mo	16	50%	0	13
Lind [89]	87	42 Mo	2	2%	0	6
Masterson [80]	35		17	20%		6
Meding [14]	34	30 Mo	24	44%	6	3
Mikhail [90]	43	>60 Mo	5	86%	3	8
Pekkarinen [85]	36	1–72 Mo	25	86%	6	3
	21	1–72 Mo	33	90%	5	14
	11	1–72 Mo	64	100%	9	0
van Biezen [91]	21	60 Mo	10	81%	0	5
Francés [82]	54	60 (19–152) Mo	14.8	38.9% 13% >10 mm	18.5	3.7
Wraighte [77]	75	10.5 Yr (6.3–14.1 Yr)	9.3	6.6% >10 mm		4
Garcia-Cimbrelo [75]	81	10.4 (5–17) Yr	50.6	70.4% 14.8% >10 mm		
Lamberton [71]	540	6.7 (2–15) ja	19.8	2.2% >10 mm	2	4.1
Ten Have [65]	31	10–14.7 Yr	12.9	67.7% 12.9% >10 mm	22.6	3.2
Garvin [76]	69	10.6 (2–19) Yr	8.6		2	2.8
te Stroet [52]	208	10.6 Yr (4.7–20.9 Yr)	12.1	10.1%	5.8	5.8
Wilson [72]	116 318 271	14.7 (9.8–28.3) Yr	12.1 22.0 5.5	43.9% 6.9% >10 mm 38.4% 8.5% >10 mm 25.8% 1.1% >10 mm	1.7 1.3 0.4	

Mo month, *Yr* year

Table 5.4 Outcomes of the impaction grafting technique with an alternative stem design with a collar and differently roughened finishes

Author	*N*	Follow-up [Mo]	Fracture (%)	Subsidence	Loosening (%)	Dislocation (%)
Boldt [92]	79	48	1.2	9%	1.2	10
				3% >10 mm		
Fetzer [93]	39	67	12	4%	0	12
Hostner [60]	24	3		0.19%		
Karrholm [94]	22	30		0.4%	0	
Leopold [78]	29	63	24	8%	12	4
Piccaluga [95]	59	56.7 (24–144) Mo	18.7	3.5% >10 mm	7	5

should be injected into the shaft in a less viscous state (i.e., earlier) with a cement gun and the shaft should be backfilled to achieve better cement penetration into the neoendosteum of compressed bone graft [68].

Overall, this technique is technically challenging, often time-consuming, and involves a significant learning curve [68, 73, 74]. This is probably why it is only performed in very few centers worldwide.

5.3.2 Outcomes

Numerous publications report satisfactory loosening rates and/or survival rates of over 90% after 10 years [52, 65, 71, 74–77] (Table 5.3). In accordance with the principle of fixation, the stem is seen to subside into the cement to a significant degree in the initial phase [78] (Tables 5.3 and 5.4). This subsidence is usually not progressive, has been explained by a cold flow of the cement, and therefore has no clinical consequences [68]. In fact, the originators of the technique claimed that the subsidence of the smooth, collarless, double-conical stem would improve graft incorporation and integration by increasing the compressive forces of the stem on the bone graft as it sinks [48, 79]. However, contrary to these theoretical considerations, subsidence-induced fractures have been described in the cement mantle [80]. Furthermore, van Doorn et al. [81] found no correlation between the extent of the subsidence and the radiological changes in the proximal bone in radiosteriometric analyses. The authors concluded that osteoinductive properties of growth factors in the graft, in addition to the osteoconductive properties of the bone matrix, are at least as important in the process of graft remodeling as the compression forces exerted by the subsidence of the stem [81]. But there is also subsidence of the whole construct by compression or resorption of the graft [82]. As long as it is not progressive, it also has very little clinical relevance. A progressive subsidence (>10 mm) was reported in 11% of cases in Eldridge et al. [55] and 13% of cases in Francés et al. [82] and was associated with a significantly higher failure and revision rate. The authors also found a significant relationship between graft resorption and revision [82].

Wraighte et al. [77] found a significant relationship between the size of the preoperative bone defect and the postoperative degree of subsidence. Francés et al. [82] found the quality or thickness of the cement mantle to be another significant factor influencing the revision rate. An inadequate cement mantle (less than 2 mm), particularly distally, was associated with a significantly higher failure and revision rate. In addition, Francés et al. [82] found a clear correlation between revision and misalignment of the stem. In contrast to the technique as originally described, Francés et al. [82] used neither a cannulated impactor nor a distal centralizer for the stem, thus underlining their true importance for this technique.

A major issue associated with impaction grafting concerns intraoperative and postoperative periprosthetic fractures. Studies have reported rates of between 5 and 24% (up to 50.1% if perforations are included) for intraoperative fractures and between 1.8 and 20% for postoperative fractures [68, 75, 82] (Tables 5.3 and 5.4). Furthermore, the use of longer cemented stems (≥220 mm length) does not significantly reduce fracture risk [83]. Fractures are increasingly common with larger bone defects (i.e., higher defect type) [68]. Periprosthetic infections between 3 and 6% and dislocations between 0 and 13% have also been reported as complications [68] (Tables 5.3 and 5.4). Nonunion of the greater trochanter occurs after trans-trochanteric access in 33–50% of cases, so this form of access is not recommended for impaction grafting [68]. Transfemoral access is also not recommended for impaction grafting, because this compromises the femoral graft site and the presence of cement in the osteotomy makes healing less reliable [68].

Overall, the outcome of impaction grafting depends on the extent of the bone defect. Garcia-Cimbrelo et al. [75], for example, demonstrated that a survival rate of 100% after 14 years was achieved for Endoklinik type 2 bone defects, 81.2% for type 3 defects, and 70.8% for type 4 defects. The average subsidence was 2.3 ± 3.7 mm for type 2 defects, 4.3 ± 7.2 mm for type 3 defects, and 9.6 ± 10.8 mm for type 4 defects. Progressive subsidence was significantly more frequent in type 4 defects. The clinical outcomes regarding pain, function, limping, and range of motion were also significantly worse in type 4 defects than in the other types. Intraoperative fractures and perforations of the femur were seen in 30% of cases for type 2 defects, 42.5% for type 3 defects, and 95% for type 4 defects. In summary, I believe that the technique of impaction grafting in cavitary defects with sufficiently stable cortical bone (Paprosky type I and type II or Endoklinik classification types 1 to 3) is effective with reproducibly good outcomes, assuming a corresponding level of experience for the surgeon [65, 69, 75, 84]. With segmental defects and thin cortical bone (Paprosky type IIIA and type IIIB with thin cortical bone and Paprosky type IV or Endoklinik classification type 4), the outcomes are no longer reproducibly good and there is also a significantly increased risk of fracture [65, 75, 85]. In cases of segmental defects, some authors advocate the use of a metal mesh that is bound around the femur for stabilization [52, 65]. The disadvantage of this technique is the necessity to denude the femur of the muscles before these meshes can be attached.

References

1. Crawford SA, Siney PD, Wroblewsky BM. Revision of failed total hip arthroplasty with a proximal femoral modular cemented stem. J Bone Joint Surg Br. 2000;82-B:684–8.
2. Dohmae Y, Bechthold JE, Sherman RE, Puno RM, Gustilo RB. Reduction in cement-bone interface shear strength between primary and revision arthroplasty. Clin Orthop Relat Res. 1988;(236):214–220.
3. Wirtz DC, Niethard FU. Ursachen, Diagnostik und Therapie der aseptischen Hüftendoprothesenlockerung—eine Standortbestimmung. Z Orthop. 1997;135:270–80.
4. Weiss RJ, Stark A, Kärrholm J. A modular cementless stem vs. cemented long-stem prostheses in revision surgery of the hip. A population-based study from the Swedish Arthroplasty Register. Acta Orthop. 2011;82:136–42.
5. Te Stroet MAJ, Rijnen WHC, Gardeniers WM, Van Kampen A, Scheures BW. Medium-term follow-up of 92 femoral component revisions using a third-generation cementing technique. Acta Orthop. 2016;87:106–12.
6. So K, Kuroda Y, Matsuda S, Akiyama H. Revision total hip replacement with a cemented long femoral component: minimum 9-year follow-up results. Arch Orthop Trauma Surg. 2013;133:869–74.
7. Estok II DM, Harris WH. Long-term results of cemented femoral revision surgery using second-generation techniques. Clin Orthop Relat Res. 1994;(299):180–202.
8. Haentjens P, De Boeck H, Opdecam P. Proximal femoral replacement prosthesis for salvage of failed hip arthroplasty. Acta Orthop Scand. 1996;67:37–42.
9. Iorio R, Eftekhar NS, Kobayashi S, Greisamer RP. Cemented revision of failed total hip arthroplasty. Clin Orthop Relat Res. 1995;(316):121–130.
10. Izquierdo RJ, Northmore-Ball MD. Long-term results of revision hip arthroplasty. J Bone Joint Surg Br. 1994;76-B:34–9.
11. Katz RP, Callaghan JJ, Sullivan PM, Johnston RC. Results of cemented femoral revision total hip arthroplasty using improved cementing techniques. Clin Orthop Relat Res. 1995;(319):178–183.
12. Katz RP, Callaghan JJ, Sullivan PM, Johnston RC. Long-term results of revision total hip arthroplasty with improved cementing technique. J Bone Joint Surg Br. 1997;79-A:322–6.
13. Kershaw CJ, Atkins RM, Dodd CAF, Bulstrode CJK. Revision total hip arthroplasty for aseptic failure. J Bone Joint Surg Br. 1991;73-B:564–8.
14. Meding JB, Ritter MA, Keating EM, et al. Impaction bone-grafting before insertion of a femoral stem with cement in revision total hip arthroplasty: a minimum two-year follow-up study. J Bone Joint Surg Am. 1997;79-A:1834–41.
15. Mulroy WF, Harris WH. Revision total hip arthroplasty with use of so-called second generation cementing techniques for aseptic loosening of the femoral component. J Bone Joint Surg Am. 1996;78-A:325–30.
16. Pierson JL, Harris WH. Cemented revision for femoral osteolysis in cemented arthroplasties. J Bone Joint Surg Br. 1994;76-B:40–4.
17. Raut VV, Siney PD, Wroblewski BM. Outcome of revision for mechanical stem failure using the cemented Charnley's stem. A study of 399 cases. J Arthroplasty. 2006;11:405–10.
18. Gramkow J, Jensen TH, Varmarken JE, Retpen JB. Long-term results after cemented revision of the femoral component in total hip arthroplasty. J Arthroplasty. 2001;16:777–83.
19. Haydon CM, Mehin R, Burnett S, Rorabeck CH, Bourne RB, McCalden RW, Mac Donald SJ. Revision total hip arthroplasty with use of a cemented femoral component. Results at a mean of ten years. J Bone Joint Surg Am. 2004;86-A:1179–85.
20. Howie DW, Wimhurst JA, McGee MA, Carbone TA, Badaruddin BS. Revision total hip replacement using cemented collarless double-taper femoral components. J Bone Joint Surg Br. 2007;89-B:879–86.
21. Cross M, Broström M. Cement mantle retention: filling the hole. Orthopedics. 2009;32.
22. Holt G, Hook S, Hubble M. Revision total hip arthroplasty: the femoral side using cemented implants. Int Orthop. 2011;35:267–73.
23. Greenwald AS, Narten NC, Wilde AH. Points in the technique of recementing in the revision of an implant arthroplasty. J Bone Joint Surg Br. 1978; 60-B:107–10.
24. Weinrauch PC, Bell C, Wilson L, Goss B, Lutton C, Crawford RW. Shear properties of bilinear polymethylmethacrylate cement mantles in revision hip arthroplasty. J Arthroplasty. 2007;22:394–403.
25. Li PLS, Ingle PJ, Dowell JK. Cement-within-cement revision hip arthroplasty; should it be done? J Bone Joint Surg Br. 1996;78-B:809–11.

26. Holsgrove TP, Pentlow A, Spencer RF, Miles AW. Cement brand and preparation effects cement-in-cement mantle shear strength. Hip Int. 2015;25:67–71.
27. Rudol G, Wilcox R, Jin Z, Tsiridis E. The effect of surface finish and interstitial fluid on the cement-in-cement interface in revision surgery of the hip. J Bone Joint Surg Br. 2011;93-B:188–93.
28. Liddle A, Webb M, Clement N, Green S, Liddle J, German M, Holland J. Ultrasonic cement removal in cement-in-cement revision total hip arthroplasty. What is the effect on the final cement-in-cement bond? Bone Joint Res. 2019;8:246–52.
29. Rosenstein A, MacDonald W, Iliadis A, McLandy-Smith P. Revision of cemented fixation and cement-bone interface strength. Proc Inst Mech Eng H. 1992;206:47–9.
30. Keeling P, Lennon AB, Kenny PJ, O'Reilly P, Prendergast PJ. The mechanical effect of the existing cement mantle on the in-cement femoral revision. Clin Biomech (Bristol, Avon). 2012;27:673–9.
31. Duncan WW, Hubble MJW, Howell JR, Whitehouse SL, Timperley AJ, Gie FA. Revision of the femoral stem using a cement-in-cement technique: a five- to 15-year review. J Bone Joint Surg Br. 2009;91-B:577–82.
32. Lieberman JR, Moeckel BH, Evans BG, Salvati EA, Ranawat CS. Cement-within-cement revision hip arthroplasty. J Bone Joint Surg Br. 1993;75-B:869–71.
33. Archibald DAA, Protheroe K, Stother IG, Campbell A. A simple technique for acetabular revision: brief report. J Bone Joint Surg Br. 1985;70-B:838.
34. McCallum JD, Hozack WJ. Recementing a femoral component into a stable cement mantle using ultrasonic tools. Clin Orthop Relat Res. 1995;(319):232–237.
35. Marcos L, Buttaro M, Comba F, Piccaluga F. Femoral cement within cement technique in carefully selected aseptic revision arthroplasties. Int Orthop. 2009;33:633–7.
36. Cnudde PHJ, Kärrholm J, Rolfson O, Timperley AJ, Mohaddes M. Cement-in-cement revision of the femoral stem. Analysis of 1179 first-time revisions in the Swedish Hip Arthroplasty Register. Bone Joint J. 2017;99-B(4 Suppl B):27–32.
37. Sandiford NA, Jameson SS, Wilson MJ, Hubble MJ, Timperley AJ, Howell JR. Cement-in-cement femoral component revision in the multiply revised total hip arthroplasty: results with a minimum follow-up of five years. Bone Joint J. 2017;99-B:199–203.
38. Young J, Vallsmshetla VR, Lawrence T. The polished tri-tapered stem for cement-in-cement revision arthroplasty, a reliable and reproducible technique? Hip Int. 2008;18:272–7.
39. Goto K, Kawanabe K, Akiyama H, Horimoto T, Nakamura T. Clinical and radiological evaluation of revision hip arthroplasty using the cement-in-cement technique. J Bone Joint Surg Br. 2008;90-B: 1013–8.
40. Te Stroet MA, Moret-Wever SG, de Kam DC, Gardeniers JW, Schreurs BW. Cement-in-cement femoral revisions using a specially designed polished short revision stem; 24 consecutive stems followed for five to seven years. Hip Int. 2014;24:428–33.
41. Stefanovich-Lawbuary NS, Parry MC, Whitehous MR, Blom AW. Cement in cement revision of the femoral component using a collarless triple taper: a midterm clinical and radiographic assessment. J Arthroplasty. 2014;29:2002–6.
42. Mounsey EJ, Williams DH, Howell JR, Hubble MJ. Revision of hemiarthroplasty to total hip arthroplasty using the cement-in-cement technique. Bone Joint J. 2015;97-B:1623–7.
43. Okuzu Y, Goto K, So K, Kuroda Y, Marsuda S. Mid- and long-term results of femoral component revision using the cement-in-cement technique: average 10.8-year follow-up study. J Orthop Sci. 2016;21: 810–4.
44. Amanatullah DF, Pallante GD, Floccari LV, Vasileiadis GI, Trousdale RT. Revision total hip arthroplasty using the cement-in-cement technique. Orthopedics. 2017;40:e348–51.
45. Kumar A, Porter M, Shah N, Gaba C, Siney P. Outcomes of cement in cement revision, in revision total hip arthroplasty. Open Access Maced J Med Sci. 2019;15(7):4059–65.
46. Woodbridge AB, Hubble MJ, Whitehouse SL, Wilson MJ, Howell JR, Timperley AJ. The Exeter short revision stem for cement-in-cement femoral revision: a five to twelve year review. J Arthroplasty. 2019;34:S297–301.
47. Berg AJ, Hoyle A, Yates E, Chougle A, Mohan R. Cement-in-cement revision with the Exeter short revision stem: a review of 50 consecutive hips. J Clin Orthop Trauma. 2020;11:47–55.
48. Gie GA, Liner L, Ling RS, et al. Contained morselized allograft in revision total hp arthroplasty. Surgical technique. Orthop Clin North Am. 1993;24:717–25.
49. Nelissen RG, Bauer TW, Weidenhielm LR, et al. Revision hip arthroplasty with the use of cement and impaction grafting: histological analysis of four cases. J Bone Joint Surg Am. 1995;77-A:412–22.
50. Board TN, Rooney P, Kearney JN, Kay PR. Impaction allografting in revision total hip replacement. J Bone Joint Surg Br. 2006;88-B:852–7.
51. Wang JS, Aspenberg P. Load-bearing increases new bone formation in impacted and morselized allografts. Clin Orthop Relat Res. 2000;(378):274–281.
52. Te Stroet MAJ, Rijen WHC, Gardeniers JWM, van Kampen A, Schreurs BW. The outcome of femoral component revision arthroplasty with impaction allograft bone grafting and a cemented polished Exeter stem. A prospective cohort study of 208 revision arthroplasties with a mean follow-up of ten years. Bone Joint J. 2015;5:771–9.
53. Ullmark G, Obrant KJ. Histology of impacted bone-graft incorporation. J Arthroplasty. 2002;17:150–7.
54. Bolder SB, Schreurs BW, Verdonschot N, et al. Particle size of bone graft and method of impaction affect initial stability of cemented cups. Human cadaveric and synthetic pelvic specimen studies. Acta Orthop Scand. 2003;74:652–7.

55. Eldridge JDJ, Hubble K, Nelson K, Smith EJ, Learmonth ID. The effect of bone chip size on initial stability following femoral impaction grafting. J Bone Joint Surg Br. 1997;79-B(Suppl III):364.
56. Wallace IW, Ammon PR, Day R, Lee DA, Beaver RJ. Does size matter? An investigation into the effects of particle size on impaction grafting in vitro. J Bone Joint Surg Br. 1997;79-B(Suppl III):366.
57. Brewster NT, Gillespie WJ, Howie CR, et al. Mechanical considerations in impaction bone grafting. J Bone Joint Surg Br. 1999;81-B:118–24.
58. Craig RF. Soil mechanics. 7th ed. London: Son Press; 2004.
59. Dunlop DG, Brewster NT, Madabhushi SP, et al. Techniques to improve the shear strength of impacted bone graft: the effect of particle size and washing of the graft. J Bone Joint Surg Am. 2003;85-A:639–46.
60. Hostner J, Hultmark P, Karrholm J, Malchau H, Tveit M. Impaction technique and graft treatment in revisions of the femoral component: laboratory studies and clinical validation. J Arthroplasty. 2001;16: 76–82.
61. Bos GD, Goldberg VM, Gordon NH et al. The long-term fate of fresh and frozen orthotopic bone allografts in genetically defined rats. Clin Orthop Relat Res. 1985;(197):245–254.
62. Burchardt H. The biology of bone graft repair. Clin Orthop Relat Res. 1983;(174):28–42.
63. Czitrom AA, Axelrod T, Fernandes B. Antigen presenting cells and bone allotransplantation. Clin Orthop Relat Res. 1985;(197):27–31.
64. Bavedekar A, Cornu O, Godits B, et al. Stiffness and compactness of morselized graft during impaction: an in vitro study with human femoral heads. Acta Orthop Scand. 2001;72:470–6.
65. Ten Have BL, Brower RW, van Biezen FC, Verhaar JA. Femoral revision surgery with impaction bone grafting. 31 hips followed prospectively for 10 to 15 years. J Bone Joint Surg Br. 2012;94-B:615–8.
66. Van der Donk S, Buma P, Slooff TJ, Gardeniers JW, Schreurs BW. Incorporation of morselized bone grafts: a study of 24 acetabular biopsy specimens. Clin Orthop Relat Res. 2002;(396):131–141.
67. Linder L. Cancellous impaction grafting in the human femur: histological and radiographic observations in 6 autopsy femurs and 8 biopsies. Acta Orthop Scand. 2000;71:543–52.
68. Morgan HA, McCallister W, Cho MS, Casnelli MT, Leopold SS. Impaction allografting for femoral component revision. Clinical update. Clin Orthop Relat Res. 2004;420:160–8.
69. Gehrke T, Gebsuer M, Kendoff D. Femoral stem impaction grafting: extending the role of cement. Bone Joint J. 2013;95-B(11 Suppl A):92–4.
70. Masterson EL, Masri BA, Duncan CP, et al. The cement mantle in femoral impaction allografting: a comparison of three systems from four centres. J Bone Joint Surg Br. 1997;79-B:908–13.
71. Lamberton TD, Kenny PJ, Whitehous SL, Timperley AJ, Gie GA. Femoral impaction grafting in revision total hip arthroplasty: a follow-up of 540 hips. J Arthroplasty. 2011;26:1154–60.
72. Wilson MJ, Hook S, Whitehaous SL, Timperley AJ, Gie GA. Femoral impaction bone grafting in revision hip arthroplasty: 705 cases from the originating centre. Bone Joint J. 2016;98-B:1611–9.
73. Ornstein E, Atroshi I, Fenzén H, et al. Early complications after one hundred and forty-four consecutive hip revisions with impacted morselized allograft bone and cement. J Bone Joint Surg Am. 2002;84-A:1323–8.
74. Ornstein E, Linder L, Ranstam J, Lewold S, Eisler T, Torper M. Femoral impaction bone grating with the Exeter stem—the Swedish experience. Survivorship analysis of 1305 revisions performed between 1989 and 2002. J Bone Joint Surg Br. 2009;91-B:441–6.
75. Garcia-Cimbrelo E, Garcia-Rey E, Cruz-Paros A. The extent of the bone defect affects the outcome of femoral reconstruction in revision surgery with impaction grafting: a five- to 17-year follow-up study. J Bone Joint Surg Br. 2011;93-B:1457–64.
76. Garvin KL, Konigsberg BS, Ommen ND, Lyden ER. What is the long-term survival of impaction allografting of the femur? Clin Orthop Relat Res. 2013;471:3901–11.
77. Wraighte PJ, Howard PW. Femoral impaction bone allografting with an Exeter cemented collarless, polished, tapered stem in revision hip replacement. A mean follow-up of 10.5 years. J Bone Joint Surg Br. 2008;90-B:1000–4.
78. Leopold SS, Berger RA, Rosenberg AG, Joacobs JJ, Qugley LR, Galante J, et al. Impaction allografting with cement for revision of the femoral component: a minimum 4-year follow-up study with use of a precoated femoral stem. J Bone Joint Surg Am. 1999;81-A:1092.
79. Ling RS, Timperley AJ, Linder L. Histology of cancellous impaction grafting in the femur: a case report. J Bone Joint Surg Br. 1993;75-B:693–6.
80. Masterton EL, Busch CA, Duncan CP, Drabu K. Impaction allografting on the proximal femur using a Charnley-type stem: a cement mantle analysis. J Arthroplasty. 1999;14:59–63.
81. Van Doorn WJ, Ten HB, van Biezen FC, ,et al: Migration of the femoral stem after impaction bone grafting: first results of an ongoing, randomised study of the Exeter and elite plus femoral stems using radiostereometric analysis. J Bone Joint Surg Br 2002;84-B:825–831.
82. Francés A, Moro E, Cebrian JL, Marco F, Garcia-López S, López-Durán L. Reconstruction of bone defects with impacted allograft in femoral stem revision surgery. Int Orthop. 2007;31:457–63.
83. Sierra RJ, Charity J, Tsiridis E, Timperley JA, Gie GA. The use of long cemented stems for femoral impaction grafting in revision total hip arthroplasty. J Bone Joint Surg Am. 2008;90-A:1330–6.
84. Maurer SG, Baitner AC, Di Cesare PE. Reconstruction of the failed femoral component and proximal femoral bone loss in revision hip surgery. J Am Acad Orthop Surg. 2000;8:354–63.

85. Pekkarinen J, Alho A, Lepisto J, et al. Impaction bone grafting in revision hip surgery: a high incidence of complications. J Bone Joint Surg Br. 2000;82-B:103–7.
86. Elting JJ, Mikhail WE, Zicat BA, et al. Preliminary report of impaction grafting for exchange femoral arthroplasty. Clin Orthop Relat Res. 1995;(319):159–167.
87. Flugsrud GB, Ovre S, Grogaard B, et al. Cemented femoral impaction bone grafting for severe osteolysis in revision hip arthroplasty: good results at 4-year follow-up of 10 patients. Arch Orthop Trauma Surg. 2000;120:386–9.
88. Knight JL, Helming C. Collarless polished tapered impaction grafting of the femur during revision total hip arthroplasty: pitfalls of the surgical technique and follow-up of 31 cases. J Arthroplasty. 2000;15:159–65.
89. Lind M, Krarup N, Mikkelsen S, et al. Exchange impaction allografting for femoral revision hip arthroplasty: results in 87 cases after 3.6 years follow-up. J Arthroplasty. 2002;17:158–64.
90. Mikhail WE, Wretenberg PF, Weidenhielm LR, et al. Complex cemented revision using polished stem and morselized allograft: minimum 5-years follow-up. Arch Orthop Trauma Surg. 1999;119:288–91.
91. Van Biezen FC, Ten HB, Verhaar JA. Impaction bone-grafting of severely defective femora in revision total hip surgery: 21 hips followed for 41-85 months. Acta Orthop Scand. 2000;71:135–42.
92. Boldt JG, Dilawari P, Agarwal S, et al. Revision total hip arthroplasty using impaction bone grafting with cemented nonpolished stems and Charnley cps. J Arthroplasty. 2001;16:943–52.
93. Fetzer GB, Callaghan JJ, Templeton JE, et al. Impaction allografting with cement for extensive femoral bone loss in revision hip surgery: a 4- to 8-year follow-up study. J Arthroplasty. 2001;16:195–202.
94. Karrholm J, Hulmark P, Carlsson L, et al. Subsidence of a non-polished stem in revision of the hip using impaction allograft. Evaluation with radiostereometry and dual-energy X-ray absorptiometry. J Bone Joint Surg Br. 1999;81-B:135–42.
95. Piccaluga F, Gonzáles Della Valle A, Encinas Fernández JC, Pusso R. Revision of the femoral prosthesis with impaction allografting and a Charnley stem. A 2- to 12 year. J Bone Joint Surg Br. 2002;84-B:544–9.

6 Cementless Revision Stems

Contents

6.1 **Nonmodular Cementless Revision Stems for Proximal Fixation** 35
6.1.1 Surgical Technique 36
6.1.2 Outcomes 37

6.2 **Cementless Proximal-Fixing Modular Revision Stems** 37
6.2.1 Surgical Technique 40
6.2.2 Outcomes 41

6.3 **Cementless Nonmodular Revision Stems for Distal Fixation** 44
6.3.1 Extensively Porous-Coated Stems 44
6.3.2 Corundum-Blasted, Tapered Titanium Stems 47
6.3.3 Cementless Distal Fixation Modular Revision Stems 51

References 69

The different cementless revision stems can be grouped as proximal and distal fixation stems, each of which is available either as a monoblock or as modular version (Fig. 4.1).

6.1 Nonmodular Cementless Revision Stems for Proximal Fixation

The nonmodular, cementless revision stems for proximal fixation are mainly the so-called "proximally porous-coated stems" or "calcar replacement stems". These are long stems made of cobalt–chromium (historical) or titanium (e.g., Mallory-Head Calcar Monoblock Prosthesis, Biomet, Warsaw IN, USA) (Fig. 6.1). They are coarsely structured proximally and are available in straight (e.g., Mallory-Head, Biomet, Warsaw, IN, USA) or curved form.

Four different, often synergistically acting concepts have been designed to achieve proximal fixation of these stem systems:

Firstly, a proximal medial cortical support is created via a collar (e.g., CORAIL Revision Stem, DePuy Synthes, Warsaw, IN, USA) or, in the case of the so-called calcar prostheses, directly via the proximal platform of the prosthesis fitting onto the medial and posteromedial bone of the proximal femur (Figs. 6.1 and 6.2).

Secondly, fixation is achieved by the conical shape of the proximal third of the prosthesis.

B. Fink, *Femoral Revision Arthroplasty*, https://doi.org/10.1007/978-3-030-84821-7_6

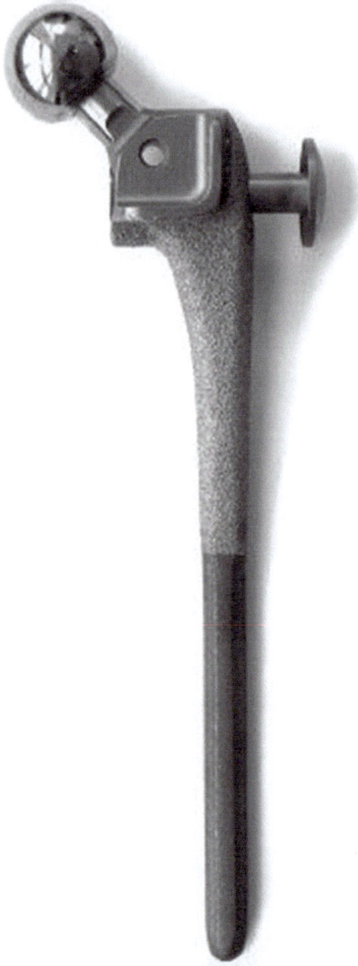

Fig. 6.1 Cementless nonmodular revision stem with proximal fixation Mallory-Head Monoblock (Biomet, Warsaw, IN, USA)

Thirdly, the cylindrical shape in the distal region of the prosthesis (in the case of the calcar prostheses) stabilizes the system, and

Fourthly, in the case of the calcar prostheses, further proximal fixation can be achieved using the trochanter plate or grip, which generates a compressive force on the trochanter (Fig. 6.1).

The proximal fixation follows the theoretical consideration of proximal forces being exerted on the femur. The goal here is to avoid distal force transmission, which would result in stress shielding. Some stem systems have a proximal or full-length, hydroxyapatite coating (e.g., CORAIL Revision stem, DePuy Synthes, Warsaw, IN), which is intended to accelerate and improve osteointegration (Fig. 6.2).

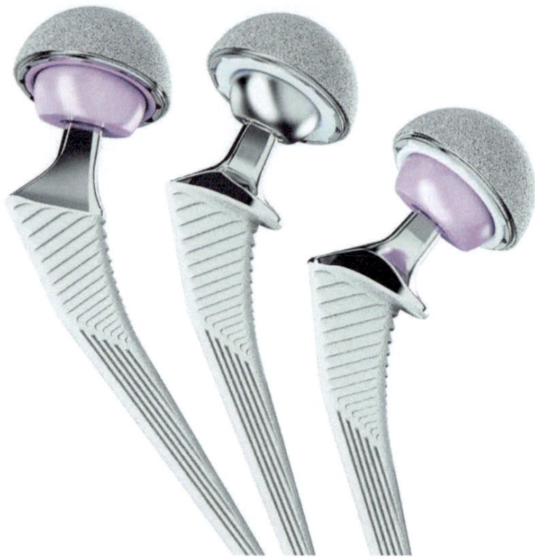

Fig. 6.2 Cementless nonmodular revision stem with proximal fixation Corail (DePuy Synthes, Warsaw, IN, USA) made of titanium with hydroxyapatite coating

6.1.1 Surgical Technique

The implantation of these stem systems is performed using either longer rasps, which are used in the same way as for primary stems, or the medullary canal is first reamed distally and then proximal rasps are employed (Fig. 6.3a, b). With the calcar prosthesis, the medial proximal bone is first resected to create the proximal prosthesis support (Fig. 6.4). Subsequently, distal reaming is carried out with a flexible cylindrical medullary reamer or broach that is 0.5 mm to 1 mm larger than the intended prosthesis size (thickness of the distal section of the prosthesis) when fixed proximally (Fig. 6.4b). The proximal fixation bed is then prepared with a rasp, which can then also be used as a trial stem for trial reduction (Fig. 6.4c). The final step is the implantation of the actual prosthesis itself.

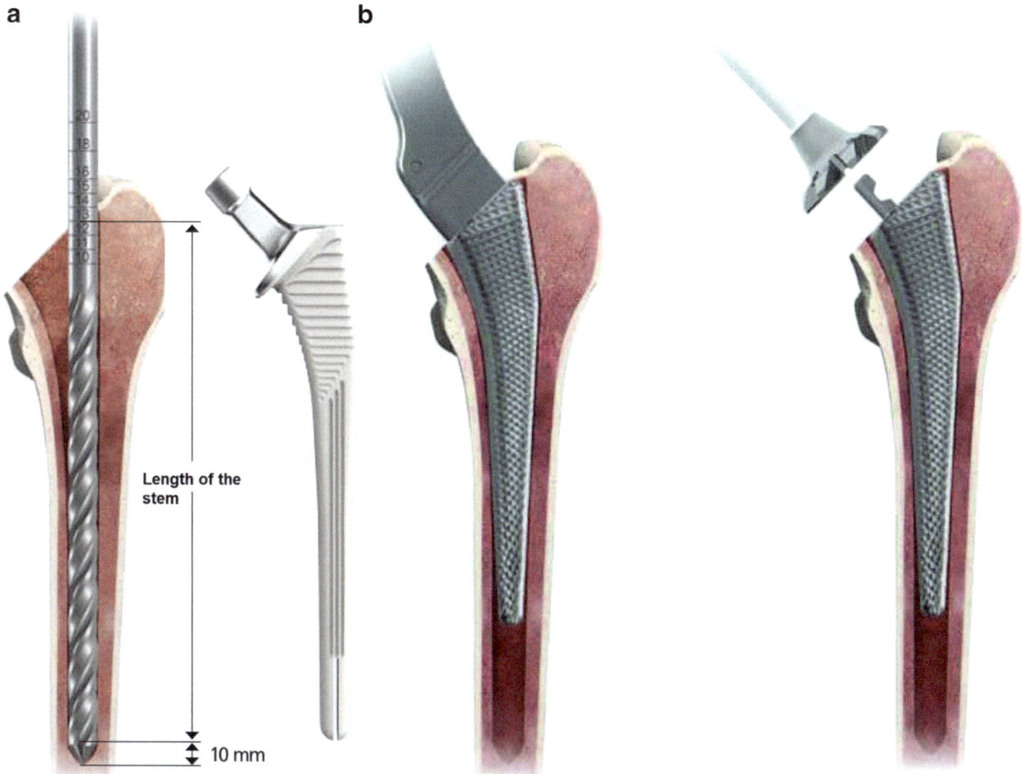

Fig. 6.3 Preparation of the fixation bed for the CORAIL revision stem (DePuy Synthes, Warsaw, IN, USA). (**a**) Reaming of the medullary canal with a rigid reamer. (**b**) Preparation of the proximal fixation bed with rasps and the proximal collar seating with a router

6.1.2 Outcomes

A sufficiently stable bone stock is required for the preparation of the prosthesis bed and fixation of the new stem in the proximal femur. Thus, cavitary defects in the proximal femur are more suitable for these stems than segmental ones. Some authors have used strut grafts in the proximal femur to reconstruct smaller segmental defects and for additional fixation of the stem [1–4]. Nevertheless, the fixation quality in this region does not appear to be consistently good because the stability and fixation of the stem are sought in proximal bone weakened by the loosening of the old stem. Due to the loosening process, this bone is often thin, sclerotic, distended, and deficient and sometimes has a poor blood supply. As a result, these stem systems have been reported to have high rates of loosening and subsidence, especially in femurs with segmental and diaphyseal defects (Table 6.1). Probably because of the difficulty of achieving reproducibly good long-term results with the proximally coated calcar replacement systems, these have been largely withdrawn from the market in recent years and replaced by fully porous-coated, distal fixation systems (e.g., Mallory-Head System by Arcos One-Piece, Zimmer Biomet, Warsaw, IN, USA).

6.2 Cementless Proximal-Fixing Modular Revision Stems

Because monoblock implants do not always allow optimal fitting of the prosthesis to the proximal femur, cementless, proximally

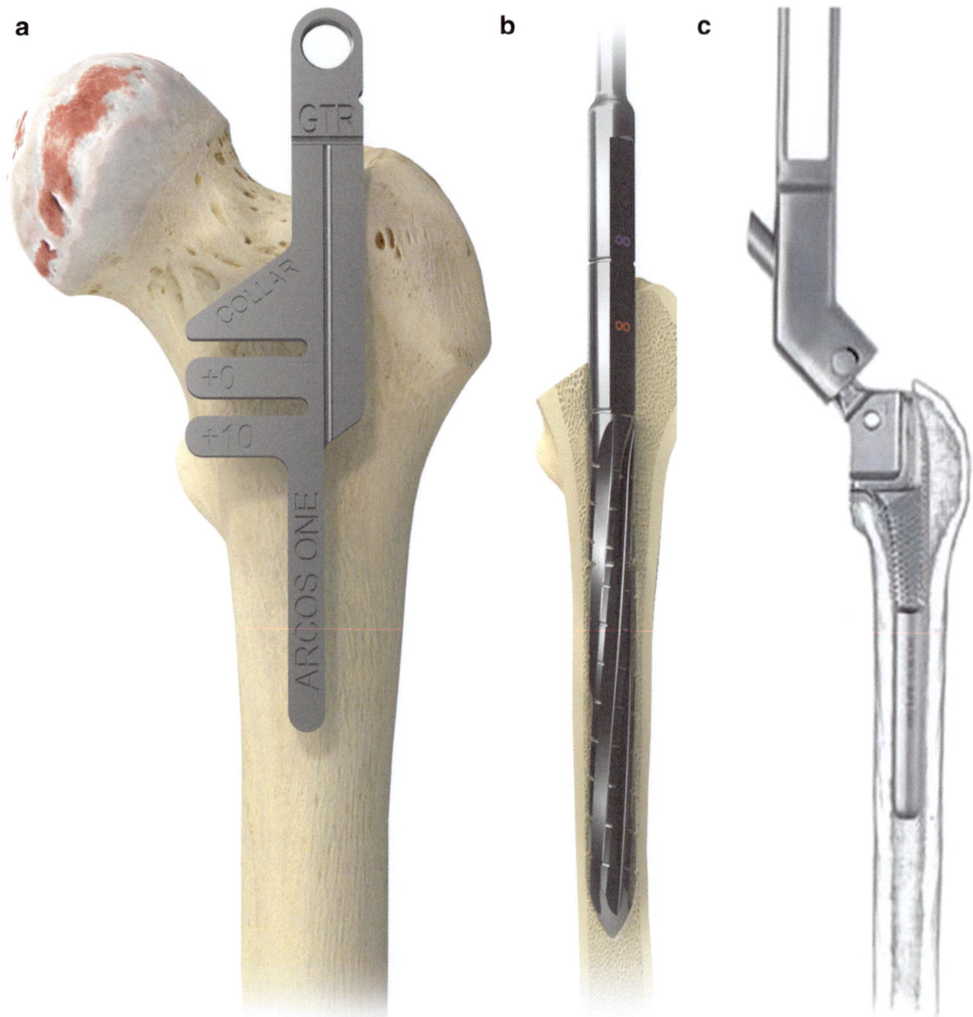

Fig. 6.4 Preparation of the fixation bed for a proximally coated calcar prosthesis stem. (**a**) Proximal medial resection of the femoral bone to support the calcar prosthesis (from the Arcos surgical technique brochure (Zimmer Biomet, Warsaw, IN, USA) to illustrate this surgical procedure). (**b**) Reaming of the diaphysis of the femur with a cylindrical reamer (from the Arcos surgical technique brochure (Zimmer Biomet, Warsaw, IN, USA) to illustrate this surgical procedure). (**c**) Preparation of the proximal fixation bed with a rasp

porous-coated modular stems for proximal fixation were introduced by Konstantin Sivash in 1967 [15]. Further developments of this stem system include the S-ROM stem (DePuy, Warsaw, IL) (Fig. 6.5) or the Mallory-Head Modular Calcar Revision System (Biomet, Warsaw, IL) (Fig. 6.6) and their successors as Broach and Calcar Proximal Bodies variants of the Arcos Modular Femoral Revision System with a distal slotted component (Zimmer Biomet, Warsaw, IN, USA) (Fig. 6.7). This improved the principle of "maximum fit and fill" for proximal stem fixation by individually adapting the proximal stem component to the femoral anatomy. Modularity allows the proximal fixation of the stem via the sleeves in the S-ROM prosthesis to be carried out separately from the setting of the biomechanical parameters (leg length or height of the prosthesis head, version of the proximal femur and offset) and adjusted independently of each other. The

Table 6.1 Outcomes of nonmodular cementless stems (proximally porous-coated); defect classification according to Paprosky (except AAOS); p = posterior, al = anterolateral, pl = posterolateral, tt = trans-trochanteric, tg = transgluteal

Author	Cases, *n*	Prosthesis	Defect, Mostly	Follow-up (years)	Approach	Revision (%)	Subsidence (%)	Loosening (%)	Dislocation (%)	Infection (%)	Fracture (%)
Berry [5]	375	Various	I–IIIA	4.7		20.8%	55%	15.7%		4%	26%
Buoncristiani [6]	66	APR		4.7	p	6%	3%	3%			15.1%
Head [1]	177	Mallory-Head	I–IIIA	2.8	al, strut grafts	3.3%					
Head [2]	177	Mallory-Head	I–IIIA	3	al, strut grafts	3%	2.8%				
Head [3]	304	Mallory-Head	I–IIIA	10–13	Strut grafts	3%	0.3%	0%	1%		0%
Head [4]	1179	Mallory-Head	I–IIIA	6.2	al, strut grafts	1%			0.6%		0.1%
Hussamy [7]	41	BIAS		5	tt	0%	32%		7%	0%	12.2%
Gosens [8]	48	Mallory-Head	I, II	6.1	tg	0%			8.3%		
Kim [9]	36	IPS + strut graft	IIC–IIIB	6.5	Pl	3%	3%	8.3%		6%	
Malkani [10]	69	Osteonics	I, II	2.8	tg, al, p, tt	8.7%	57%	20%	2.%		46%
Mulliken [11]	52	Mallory-Head	I–IIIA	4.6	tg	10%	10%	24%			38.5%
Peters [12]	49	BIAS	I–III AAOS	5.4	tg, tt	4%	57%	4%	4.1%	2%	22.4%
Woolson [13]	25	Harris-Galante	I, II	5.5	tt, p, tg	20%	48%	40%			24%
Wood [14]	20	CORAIL	I–IIIA	1		0%	0%	0%	5%	5%	5%

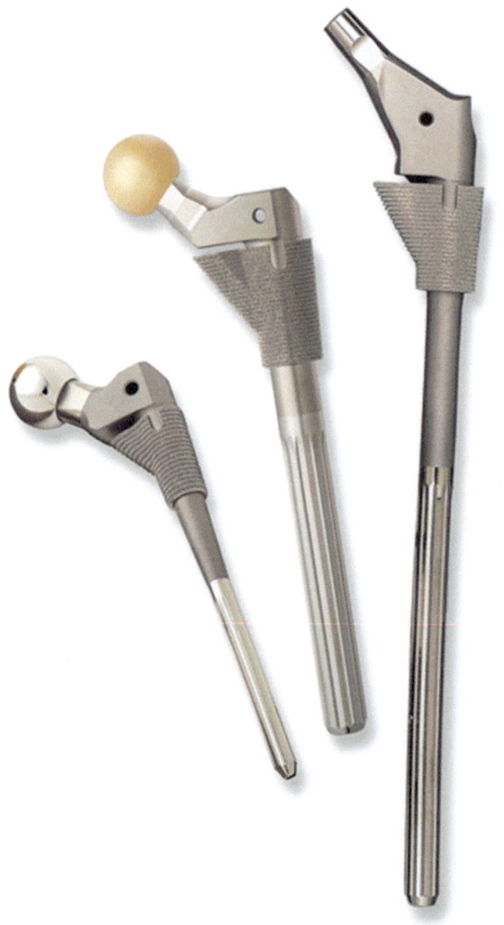

Fig. 6.5 Modular proximal fixation revision stem S-ROM (DePuy Synthes, Warsaw, IN, USA)

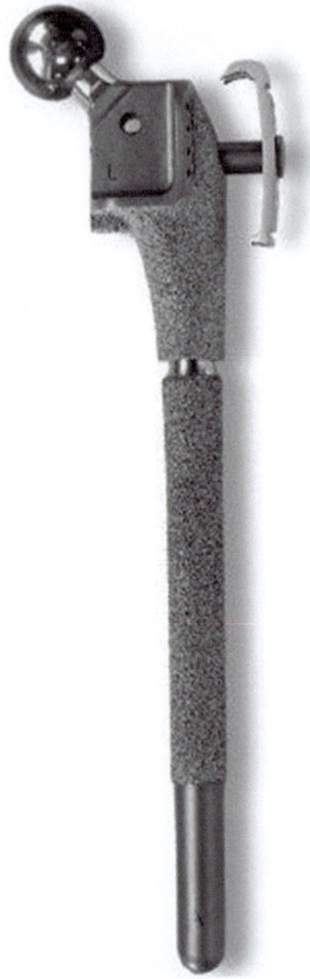

Fig. 6.6 Mallory-Head Modular Calcar Revision System (Biomet, Warsaw, IN, USA)

proximal sleeves are available as porous-coated and hydroxyapatite-coated versions.

6.2.1 Surgical Technique

In the case of these modular revision stems with proximal fixation, the distal femoral diaphysis is first reamed, depending on the system, either first with a flexible medullary reamer (Fig. 6.8) and then with a rigid reamer, or directly with the latter tool (Fig. 6.9a). Depending on the system and bone quality, the shaft is reamed either to the same thickness of the implant or usually 0.5 mm or 1 mm greater than the diameter of the distal component of the intended stem (Fig. 6.9a) [16, 17].

The proximal fixation bed of the stem is then prepared with a proximal reaming or rasp system (depending on the stem). For the S-ROM prosthesis, the conical portion of the sleeve is first prepared proximally with a conical reamer and then the fit for the medial sleeve extension is prepared using a reaming template guide (Fig. 6.9b, c). The selected trial sleeve is then placed in position (Fig. 6.9d), and the central trial stem is implanted through it (Fig. 6.9e). After the trial fitting with the assembled trial prosthesis, either the final components that have been assembled on the operating table (e.g., the Arcos Broach version) or the final sleeve for the S-ROM

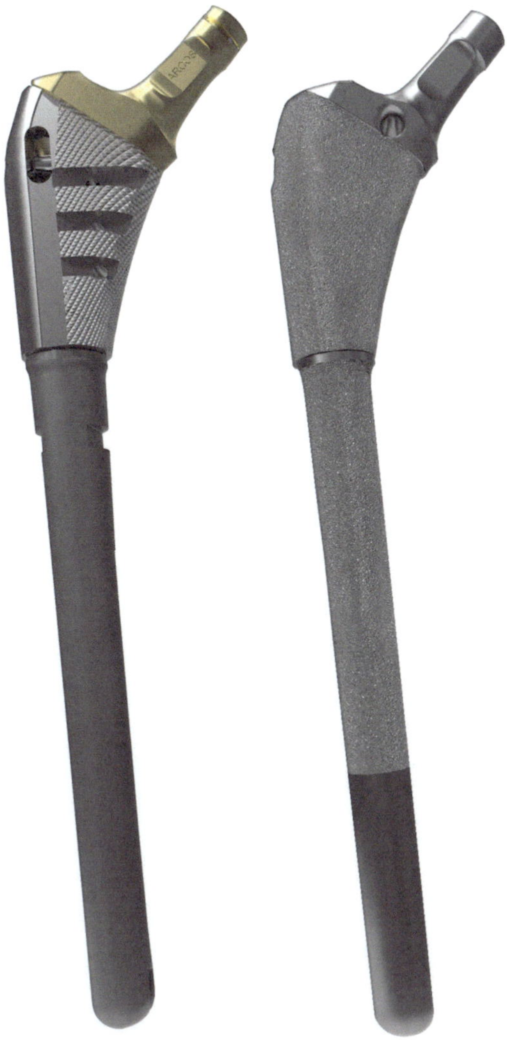

Fig. 6.7 Trial prosthesis and actual prosthesis of the modular Arcos system (Zimmer Biomet, Warsaw, IN, USA) with proximal fixation

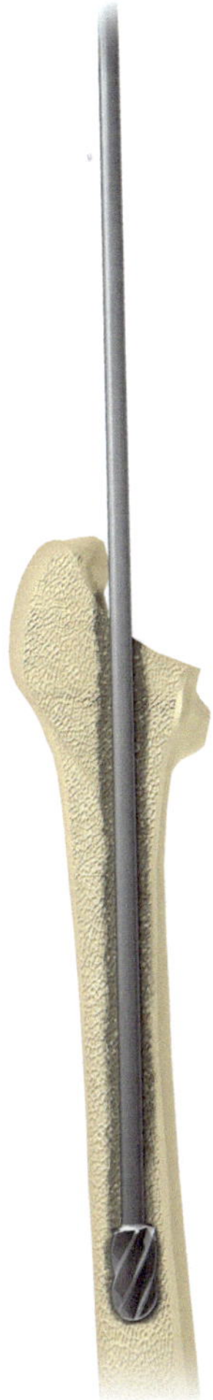

Fig. 6.8 Reaming of the distal femoral diaphysis with a flexible medullary reamer for the proximal fixation version

prosthesis is implanted (Fig. 6.9g). In the latter, the central trial stem can now be guided through the sleeve before the final central S-ROM stem is implanted (Fig. 6.9g, h).

6.2.2 Outcomes

The individual fitting of the modular prosthesis to the proximal bone allows a reproducibly better proximal fixation of the modular prostheses than is possible with the fully porous-coated monoblock prostheses. As a result, the loosening and subsidence rates are reduced with these modular proximal fixation revision stems compared to nonmodular stems (Table 6.2). Li et al. [31] showed that in Paprosky type IIIA and IIIB defects, the modular proximal S-ROM prosthesis had significantly better 5-year survival rates (89.5%) than the monoblock revision prosthesis SLR-Plus (Smith & Nephew, Baar, Switzerland), which exhibited a rate of 42.1%. In a further development, the sleeves of the S-ROM prosthesis are now also available with a hydroxyapatite coating [16]. Bolognesi et al. [18] were able to show that the probability of bone integration in

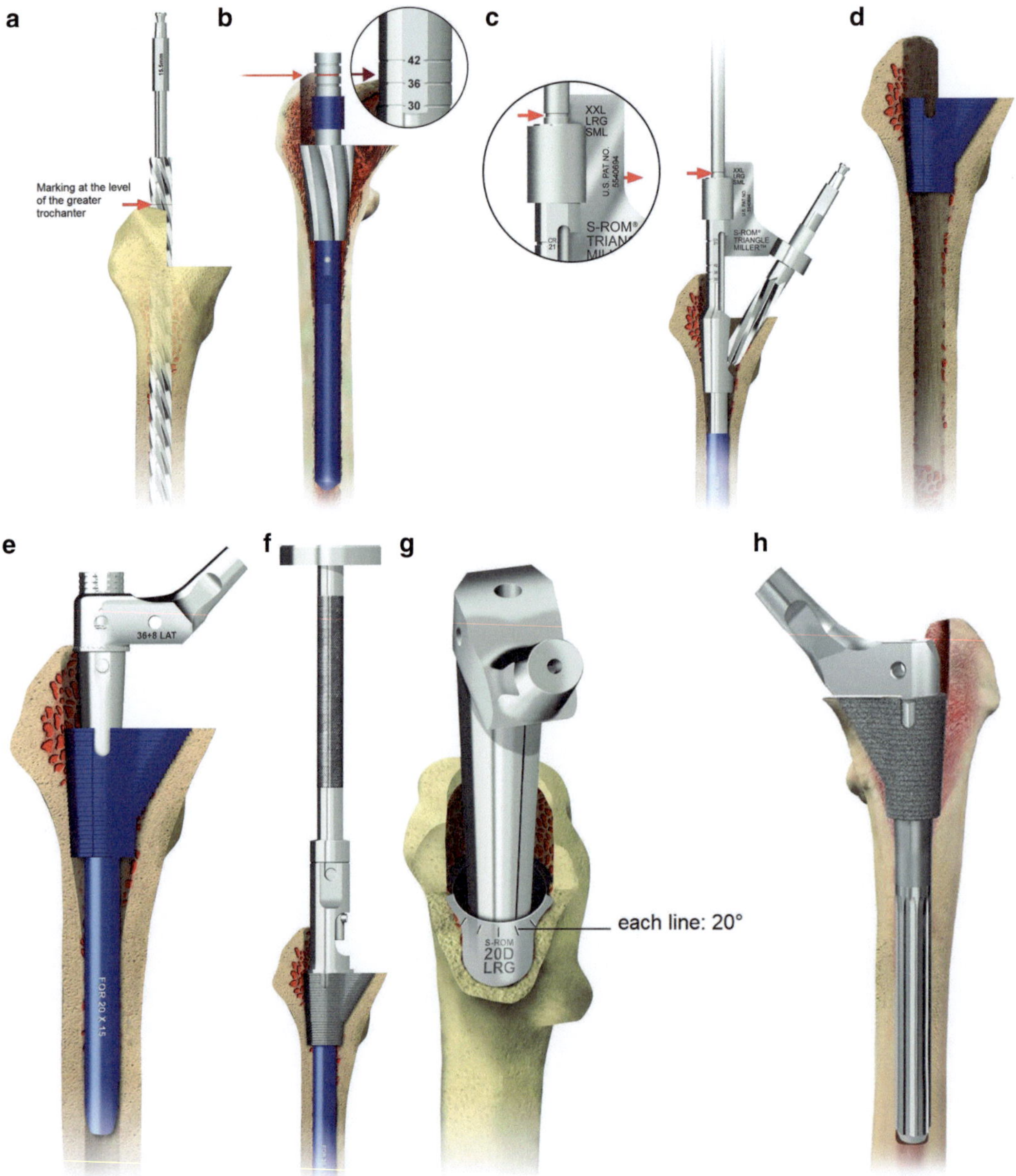

Fig. 6.9 Preparation of the fixation bed and implantation of the modular proximal fixation S-ROM stem system (DePuy Synthes, Warsaw, IN, USA). (**a**) Reaming the distal femoral diaphysis with the rigid reamer. (**b**) Reaming the proximal femur for the conical sleeve portion with a conical reamer. (**c**) Reaming for the proximal medial spout of the sleeve through the attached reaming template. (**d**) Implantation of the trial sleeve. (**e**) Implantation of the trial stem through the trial sleeve. (**f**) Implantation of the selected final sleeve. (**g**) Implantation of the selected final stem through the final sleeve. (**e**) Implantation of the trial stem through the trial sleeve. (**f**) Implantation of the selected final sleeve. (**g**) Implantation of the selected final stem through the original sleeve. (**h**) Implanted S-ROM stem

Paprosky type III defects was 2.6 times higher with the hydroxyapatite-coated sleeves than with the porous-coated titanium sleeves. There was no difference in the case of Paprosky type I and II defects. Park and Lim [26] also found no difference in survival and loosening rates

Table 6.2 Outcomes of the modular proximal fixation revision stem S-ROM (DePuy Synthes, Warsaw, IN); p = posterolateral, tt = trans-trochanteric, tg = transgluteal, ef = end-ofemoral, tf = transfemoral, ts = trochanteric slide, vs = vastus slide; Paprosky defect classification (except AAOS)

Author	Cases, *N*	Defect, Mostly	Follow-up (years)	Approach	Revision (%)	Subsidence (%)	Loosening (%)	Dislocation (%)	Infection (%)	Fracture (%)
Bolognesi [18]	43	I–IIIB	4	p + tt	5%	1.9%	1.9%	3.8%		25.6%
Bono [19]	62	II + III AAOS	5.9	p	14%	6.4%	6.4%			0%
Cameron [20]	62		3.9		16.1%			1.6%	4.8%	4.8%
Cameron [21]	157		2		6.4%	3.2%	1.3%	4.5%	3.2%	7%
Chandler [22]	30		1.8	tt + allogr	10%			16.7%	3.3%	
Chandler [23]	52		3	ts, vs + allogr	25%		9.6%	23.1%	6%	28%
Christie [24]	129	I-IIIA	6.2		0.8%	2.9%	2.9%			0%
Imbuldeniya [16]	221	I-IIIA	12.9	p + tg	7.8%		1%	7.3%	2%	10.5%
McCarthy [25]	67	II-IV	8	Pl, tf			9%		10%	
Moreta [17]	51	I-IIIA	5.7	tg, pl			0%	5.9%	7.8%	5.9%
Park [26]	28	I-IIIA	9.8	pl	11%	17.8%	11%	3.6%		28.6%
Piao [27]	21	II-IIIA			4.8%		0%	0%	0%	28.6%
Smith [28]	66		3.4	p	3%		7.6%	7.6%	3%	27.3%
Walter [29]	62	I, II	6	tg	1.6%	3.2%	5%	2%	2%	2%
Wei-Li [30]	21	I-III	4.5	pl	0%		19.1%	0%		9.5%

between porous-coated and hydroxyapatite-coated sleeves in Paprosky type I and II defects. Overall, type I and II defects show significantly better survival rates than Paprosky type III defects [18, 26]. In their study, Bolognesi et al. [18] found a 2.7 times lower probability of bony integration of the proximal sleeves in Paprosky type III defects than in type I or II defects. If these stems are to be used in cases of type III defects, the distended and deficient proximal femur requires a residual bone quality that is still good enough for press-fit fixation of the sleeves without an increased risk of fracture [18]. This cannot be reliably assessed pre- and intraoperatively. Some authors report frequently occurring femoral fractures with these proximal-fixing modular revision prostheses, particularly in cases of type III defects [18, 23, 27, 28]. Thus, the main indication for proximally fixed modular revision stems is femurs with Paprosky I and II type bone defects [17, 18, 26, 27]. Transfemoral approaches result in inadequate rotational stability of the proximal fixation stems, and therefore, these stems should not be used in a transfemoral scenario [32]. A disadvantage of these modular prostheses is the possibility of micromovement at the stem–sleeve transition and the resulting corrosion and fretting [19, 24]. Furthermore, thigh pain has been described for between 6.2 and 18% of cases and is related to the thickness of the stem [16, 21, 23, 24, 29, 30]. Stems of more than 17 mm diameter in their cylindrical distal portion are more prone to thigh pain [17, 29]. The introduction of a longitudinal slit in the distal component has made it less rigid, and this has reduced the frequency of thigh pain [33].

The combination of a modular proximally bulky segment and a slotted or curved distal component with rough structuring of both components was designed to achieve a combination of distal and proximal fixation that would improve overall fixation and reduce the incidence of stress shielding and thigh pain [34]. A variant of the Arcos stem (Zimmer Biomet, Warsaw, IN, USA) as a further development of the modular Mallory-Head stem produced relatively good short-term outcomes (Table 6.3).

6.3 Cementless Nonmodular Revision Stems for Distal Fixation

Cementless nonmodular, distally fixing revision stems use a different fixation principle. They bridge the proximal femur, which is weakened and often widened due to loosening, and are fixed in the diaphysis of the femur, often below the old prosthesis bed in the isthmus of the femur. This group of stems can be divided into the so-called "extensively porous-coated stems" and the corundum-blasted tapered titanium stems.

6.3.1 Extensively Porous-Coated Stems

The "extensively porous-coated stems" are long, distally cylindrical, straight stems with a complete coarse porous surface structure made of cobalt–chromium (e.g., AML or Solution stem, DePuy Synthes, Warsaw, IN, USA (Fig. 6.10)) or, in the newer models, made of titanium alloys (e.g., Arcos One-Piece, Zimmer Biomet, Warsaw, IN, USA (Fig. 6.11) or Echelon stem, Smith & Nephew, Memphis, TN) (Fig. 6.12)). Due to the coarse porous surface, they achieve their fixation in the isthmus of the femur after reaming with medullary reamers, whereby the stem diameter is usually 0.5 mm greater than the last medullary reamer used [37, 38]. Paprosky et al. [39] called this type of fixation "scratch fit", which produces a cylinder-in-cylinder fixation (cylindrical stem in cylindrical fixation bed of the bone) over a fixation distance of 4 to 6 cm in the isthmus of the femur [40]. The rotational stability of the stem is created by the shape and especially by the rough surface over the corresponding length of 4 to 6 cm. Paprosky therefore set the cutoff point for bone defects between type IIIA and IIIB defects at 4 cm (personal communication), since cylindrical revision stems will not function with a scratch-fit fixation zone less than 4 cm fixation distance (Paprosky IIIB defects) and are therefore not indicated [40]. Although Kim et al. [41] achieved satisfactory outcomes with this type of stem with simultaneous use of proximal strut

Table 6.3 Outcomes of the modular proximal-fixing revision stems, Mallory-Head, and Arcos (Zimmer Biomet, Warsaw, IN); al = anterolateral

Author	Cases, *n*	Stem	Follow-up (years)	Approach	Revision (%)	Subsidence (%)	Loosening (%)	Dislocation (%)	Infection (%)	Fracture (%)
Lombardi [35]	123	Mallory-Head	3.7	al	4.9%		0%		4%	0.8%
Pelt [36]	62	Arcos	2.9		14.5%	6.4%	6.8%	4.8%	12.9%	3%

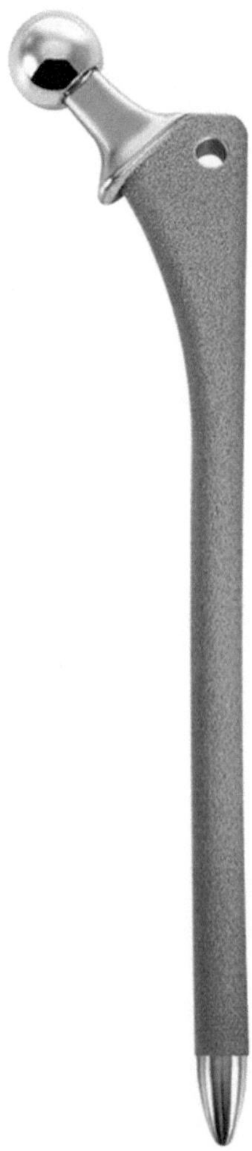

Fig. 6.10 Solution revision stem (DePuy Synthes, Warsaw, IN, USA)

Fig. 6.11 Arcos One-Piece revision stem (Zimmer Biomet, Warsaw, IN, USA)

grafts in Paprosky type IIIB and IV defects, stem systems that involve a distal scratch fit are generally only recommended for type II and IIIA bone defects.

6.3.1.1 Surgical Technique

The fixation bed in the isthmus of the femur is reamed with medullary reamers until good cortical contact over a distance of 4–6 cm is achieved (Fig. 6.13a). When using straight stems, this is done with a straight, cylindrical reamer and, for curved stems, with a flexible medullary reamer. Straight stems are more commonly used for Paprosky I and II defects and curved stems are more commonly used for Paprosky type III defects, because straight stems, when used for type III defects, carry the risk of anterior perforation of the femoral cortex and unintentional fractures. Reaming is carried out until good endosteal cortical contact is achieved. The relationship between the diameter of the reamer and the thickness of the stem to be implanted depends on the extent of the bone defect. For Paprosky I defects, reaming tends to be 0.5 mm greater than the distal diameter of the stem, as this can generate a more proximal fixation. For Paprosky II defects, reaming tends to be carried out to the same diameter as the distal

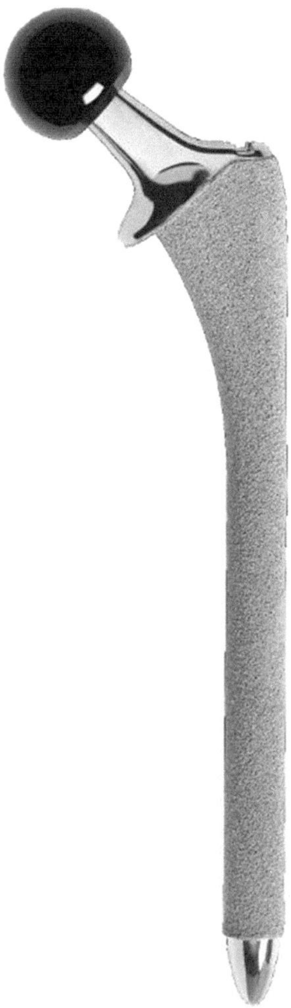

Fig. 6.12 Echelon revision stem (Smith & Nephew, Memphis, TN, USA)

diameter of the stem, and for Paprosky III defects, for the classic distal scratch fit, reaming is 0.5 mm less than the distal diameter of the stem to be implanted.

In cases of Paprosky type I and II defects, the proximal femur must still be prepared for fitting the prosthesis (Fig. 6.13b). Rasps are used for this purpose. If necessary, bone may have to be removed proximally using a high-speed milling device, for example, before using the rasps. The rasps can then also be used as trial prostheses for trial reduction. The final stem is implanted once satisfactory trial reduction has been achieved (Fig. 6.13c).

6.3.1.2 Outcomes

Reproducible good results can be achieved with this technique (Table 6.4). A disadvantage of these types of stems is their rigidity and the resulting stress shielding of the proximal femur bone, which is observed in 18–33% of cases with cobalt–chromium stems and occurs mainly in osteoporotic bone [1, 13, 37, 43, 48, 51, 52]. Their rough surface coating makes it difficult to remove these stems when it becomes necessary (e.g., in case of periprosthetic infection) [13, 37]. A further problem with these stems is the frequently reported thigh pain, which was observed in 31% of cases in Paprosky et al. [39] and in 36% of cases in Moreland and Bernstein [51]. In Ahmet et al. [42], thigh pain was seen in 10% of cases. This is also attributed to the rigid properties of the cobalt–chromium stems. This phenomenon is observed less frequently for the current titanium stems. Mahoney et al. [55] reported thigh pain in only 2.5% of cases with a more flexible, completely hydroxylapatite-coated titanium stem.

6.3.2 Corundum-Blasted, Tapered Titanium Stems

Another principle of distal stem fixation is the press-fit principle, which was first introduced by Heinz Wagner in 1986 for his Wagner SL stem [56] (Figs. 6.14 and 6.15). In this method, a tapered distal stem (2 degrees for the Wagner SL stem) is driven into a conical prosthesis bed that has been formed with reamers. This results in a cone-in-cone fixation and provides axial stability. The eight longitudinal ribs or splines of the Wagner SL stem cut into the cortex of the femur and create rotational stability of the prosthesis anchorage (Fig. 6.16). Other conical, nonmodular revision stems developed later follow this principle, such as the Redapt (Smith & Nephew, Memphis, TN, USA), which is characterized by a greater taper angle of 3 degrees (Fig. 6.17).

6.3.2.1 Surgical Technique

The distal fixation bed of the stem is reamed with a conical reamer until a solid cortical contact and

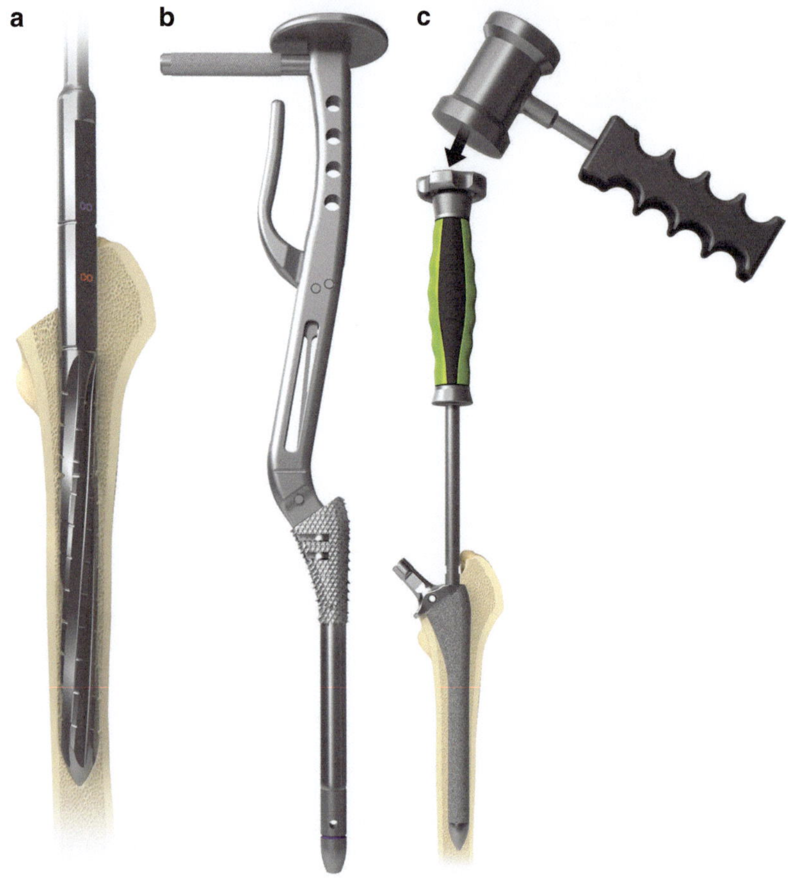

Fig. 6.13 Preparation of the fixation bed and implantation of a fully porous-coated revision stem with scratch fit using the example of a Arcos One-Piece revision stem (Zimmer Biomet, Warsaw, IN, USA). (**a**) Reaming of the fixation bed in the femur with a rigid cylindrical reamer. (**b**) Rasping the proximal femur. (**c**) Implantation of the stem

a conical fixation bed are obtained (Fig. 6.18a, b). Initially, the thinner reamers can be inserted using a machine. However, the final reaming steps to create the conical fixation bed should be performed manually with the T handle attachment in order to reduce the risk of fracture. The proximal marks on the reamer indicate the length of the prosthesis to be implanted (Fig. 6.18c). Shorter prostheses should be implanted if possible in order to reduce the risk of unintentional fractures that can occur when implanting long straight stems into the curved femur. Shorter thicker stems are therefore preferable to longer thinner ones and during the bed preparation it should be determined whether the next larger reamer can still be inserted.

The trial prosthesis is then inserted. This can be assembled in a modular fashion, consisting of the distal component with the thickness of the last reamer and the proximal component, the length of which is read off the last reamer at the level of the greater trochanter (Fig. 6.18d, e). After satisfactory trial reduction, the final prosthesis of the corresponding thickness and length is implanted (Fig. 6.18f, g).

6.3.2.2 Outcomes

The challenge with nonmodular tapered revision prostheses with distal fixation is to achieve all of the various goals of stem revision in one step (i.e., at implantation of the stem). These goals are namely the firm distal fixation of the new prosthesis and the correct adjustment of leg length, antetorsion, and offset. The creation of a solid cone-in-cone fixation is technically not easy to achieve using an endofemoral approach. It is not uncommon to implant long and too thin stems that only achieve a three-point fixation instead of a cone-in-cone fixation. This then resulted in high rates of subsidence of the Wagner SL stem

Table 6.4 Outcomes of cementless nonmodular stems (extensively porous-coated); *2 = New England Baptist, Custom P-10, AML; ** = Paprosky III + IV defects only, graft = strut graft; p = posterior, pl = posterolateral, tt = trans-trochanteric, tf = transfemoral, eto = extended trochanteric osteotomy; subsidence >5 mm

Author	Stem	Cases, *n*	Follow-up (years)	Approach	Revision (%)	Subsidence (%)	Loosening (%)	Dislocation (%)	Infection (%)	Fracture (%)
Ahmet [42]	Echelon	70	7.8	tg + eto			1.4%	2.8%	0%	
Aribindi [43]	Solution	71	5.8	p + tf	4.2%		0%	6%		1.4%
Chen [44]	Solution	42	3.6	pl + eto	7%	0%	0%	11%	2.4%	
Ding [45]	Solution + graft	44**								
Engh [46]	AML	21	6.3	p	0%		0%	4.8%	0%	9.5%
Engh [37]	AML	204	4.5	p + eto	4.9%		4%			0.5%
Glassman [47]	AML	154	9.2 (5–15)		4.5%		6.6%	0.6%	0.6%	
Krishnamurthy [48]	AML	297	8.3 (5–13)	pl	1.7%		2.4%	2.6%	0.7%	
Lawrence [49]	*2	83	9 (5–13)	p	10%		11%	3.6%	1.2%	2.4%
Lawrence [38]	AML + Solution	174	7.4	tg + tt	5.7%		1.1%	3.4%	2.9%	0.6%
Kim [41]	Solution + graft	130	16.1	p + eto	9%		9%	3%	5%	3%
Miner [50]	Solution	166	3.9	eto	10.2%		0.6%	10%	2.4%	10.8%
Moreland [51]	AML + Solution	175	5 (2–10)	tt	4%	12.6%	1.7%	2.9%	0.6%	0.6%
Moreland [52]	AML	137	9.3 (5–16)	tt	7%		4%	4.4%	3.6%	1.5%
Paprosky [39]	AML + Solution	170	13.2 (10–16)	p	3.5%	16%	4.1%	7.1%	1.8%	14.7%
Paprosky [53]	Solution	193	5	p + tf	0%			9%	3%	5%
Sugimura [54]	AML	32	4 (2–6.5)		3.1%	28.1%	0%			3.1%
Weeden [40]	Solution	170	14.2 (11–16)	P, tf	3.5%	16%	4.1%	7.1%	1.8%	14.7%

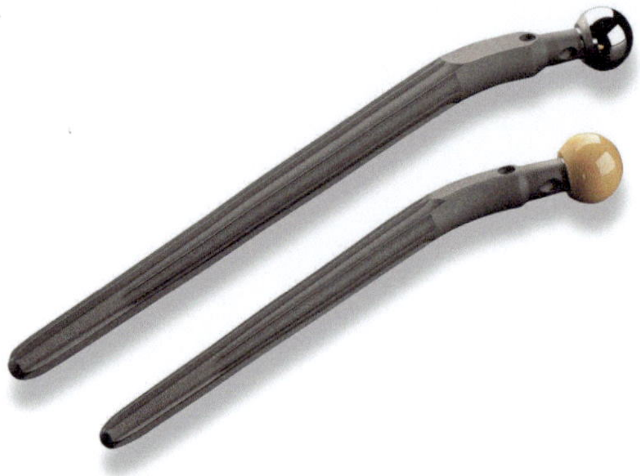

Fig. 6.14 The older version of the Wagner stem (Sulzer, Winterthur, Switzerland)

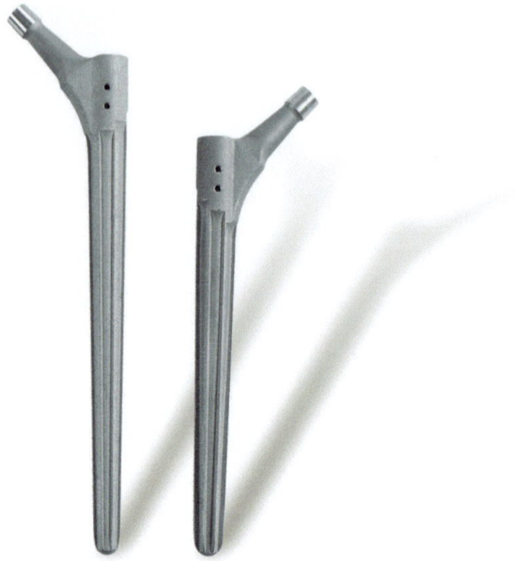

Fig. 6.15 Current Wagner SL revision stem (Zimmer Biomet, Winterthur, Switzerland)

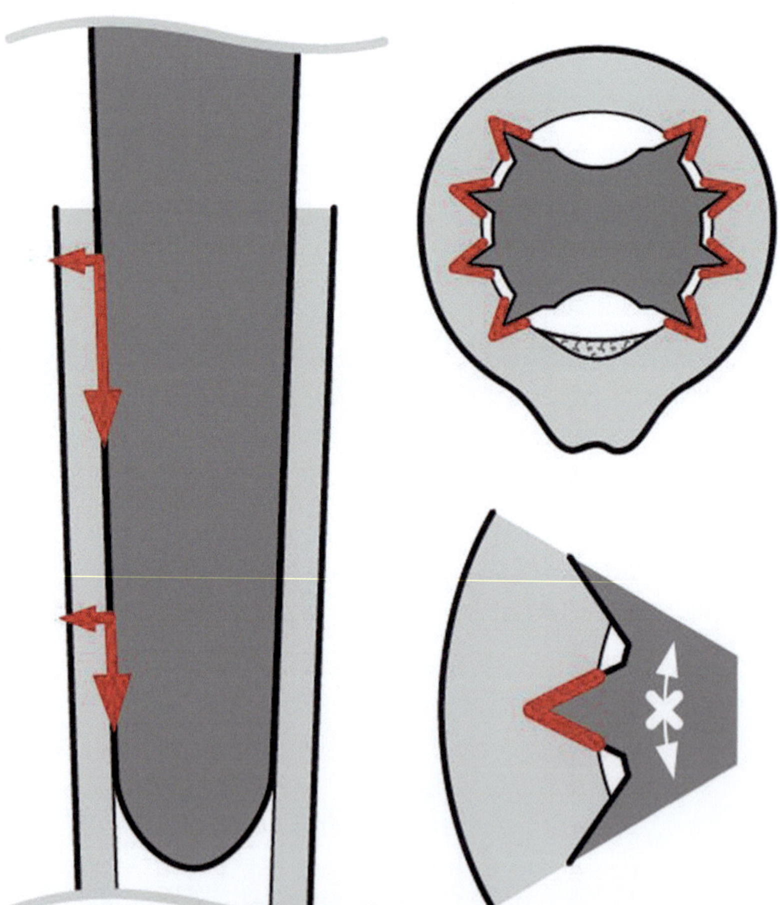

Fig. 6.16 Principle of conical fixation of the stem in the isthmus of the femur with the stem splines cutting into the cortex (with permission of Zimmer Biomet, Winterthur, Switzerland)

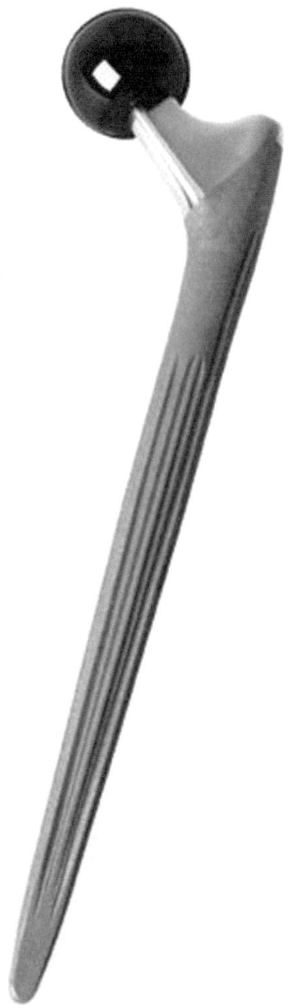

Fig. 6.17 Redapt revision stem (Smith & Nephew, Memphis, TN, USA)

(Table 6.5). In addition, the first two generations of the Wagner stem had a femoral shaft neck angle of 145 degrees due to the manufacturing process, which caused a reduction in the offset to 36 mm. The occurrence of subsidence and the reduced offset again led to double-digit rates of dislocation (Table 6.5). The current generation of Wagner SL stems has a femoral shaft neck angle of 135 degrees with an improved offset of 42–46 mm (depending on the stem size). The challenge remains, however, to achieve the various goals of the revision with the one step of implanting the final component. Other stems follow the principle of the Wagner stem, but like the Redapt stem (Smith & Nephew, London, UK), they have a different taper of 3 degrees. This also produces reproducibly good results (Table 6.6).

6.3.3 Cementless Distal Fixation Modular Revision Stems

Modular distal fixation revision stems consist of two (the distal fixation component and the proximal component) or three stem parts (an additional intermediate piece) and a locking screw or nut (Figs. 6.19a, b and 6.20). The advantage of the modularity of distally fixing stems is that the goals of revision surgery are separated from each other and can be achieved independently of each other. The distal component is used first to obtain secure distal fixation of the stem and then the proximal trial component is used to set the correct leg length and the correct, freely adjustable antetorsion and, if necessary, offset (Fig. 6.21a). If a satisfactory fitting has been achieved during the trial reduction, the modular components are then assembled in situ (Fig. 6.21b). Restrepo et al. [84] were able to reconstruct leg length within 5 mm in 77% of cases and offset within 2 mm in 65% of cases using the modular distal fixation revision stem Restoration (Stryker, Kalamazoo, MG, USA).

These stem systems have straight distal components, straight distal components with a slight bend or kink, and curved distal components (Figs. 6.20, 6.22, 6.23, 6.24, 6.25, and 6.26). In addition to distal conical fixation, some stem systems also enable fixation via a scratch fit (cylinder-in-cylinder fixation), such as the Arcos system, the ZMR system (Zimmer Biomet, Warsaw, IN, USA), or Restoration (Stryker, Kalamazoo, MG, USA) (Figs. 6.24, 6.25, and 6.26).

The same principles of conical fixation or scratch fit as described for nonmodular revision systems (e.g., Wagner SL Stem (Zimmer Biomet, Winterthur, Switzerland) for conical fixation or

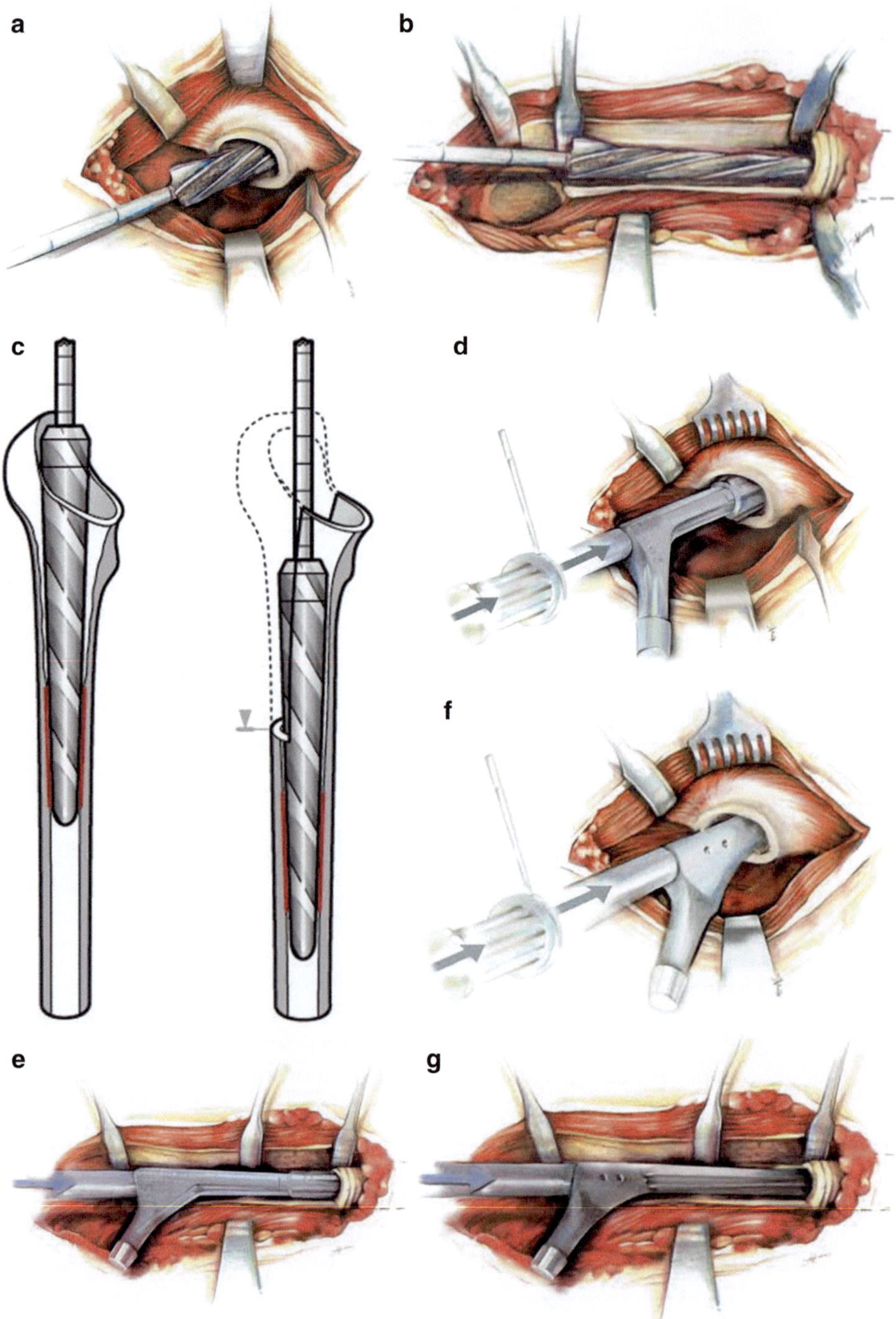

Fig. 6.18 Preparation of the fixation bed and implantation of a conical, distally fixing monoblock prosthesis using the Wagner SL revision stem as an example (Zimmer Biomet, Winterthur, Switzerland). (**a**) Endofemoral introduction of the conical reamers and preparation of the fixation bed. (**b**) Transfemoral introduction of the conical reamers and preparation of the fixation bed. (**c**) Reading the expected prosthesis length on the marking of the reamer. (**d**) Endofemoral fitting of the modular trial prosthesis. (**e**) Transfemoral fitting of the modular trial prosthesis. (**f**) Endofemoral implantation of the final Wagner SL stem. (**g**) Transfemoral implantation of the final Wagner SL stem

Table 6.5 Outcomes of the nonmodular distally fixed Wagner SL revision stem (Zimmer Biomet, Winterthur, Switzerland); tg = transgluteal, tf = transfemoral, tt = trans-trochanteric, a = anterior, al = anterolateral, ve = ventral; subsidence >5 mm, * = subsidence greater than 10 mm

Author	Cases, *n*	Follow-up (years)	Approach	Revision (%)	Subsidence (%)	Loosening (%)	Dislocation (%)	Infection (%)	Fracture (%)
Baktir [57]	64	14.4	p + tf	6.2%	29.7%	1.6%	9.3%	6.2%	3.1%
Bircher [58]	99	5	tg, tf	6.1%	6.1%*		4%	0%	
Böhm [59]	128	5.4	tf, tg, tt, ve	4.7%	34.1%	3.1%	5%	2.3%	4.7%
Böhm [60]	129	4.8	tf, tg, tt, a	4.6%	34.1%		5.4%	2.3%	4.6%
Böhm [47]	129	8.1	tf, tg, tt, a	4.6%	34.1%	0%	5.4%	2.3%	5.4%
Boisgard [61]	52	3.7		3.9%	0%*		4.3%		
Ferruzzi [62]	350	6.8		0.6%	11.4%	0.6%*	4%		
Gutiérrez del Alalmo [63]	79	8.4	tg, tf, tt	6.3%	20.3% 1.3%*	1.3%	13.9%	2.5%	10.1%
Grünig [64]	40	3.9	l, tf, tg	10%	47.5% 20%*	10%	5%	2.5%	22.5%
Hartwig [65]	37	2.3	tf, tg	2.7%	18.9%	2.7%		2.7%	
Hellman [66]	68	3.5	p + tf	23.5%	3.0%	4.4%	7.4%	11.7%	4.4%
Isacson [67]	43	2.1	tf	19.6%	27.9%*	0%	20.9%		
Kolstad [68]	31	3	tf	16.1%	19.3%*		16.1%	3.2%	
Lyu [69]	22	7.1		9.1%	13.6%*		4.5%		
Mandellos [70]	93	4.2		0%	0%*	0%	4.3%		
Mantelos [71]	95	9		2.1%	1.1%*		5.3%		
Regis [72]	41	13.9	al + tf	12.2%	19.5%*	3.4%	12.2%	4.9%	17.7%
Sandiford [73]	104	2.6	p + tf	3%	6%	0%	5%	3%	1%
Singh [74]	53	5.5	p + tf	2%	4.2%		5.6%	13.2%	0%
Wagner [56]	20	< 3	p + tf	0%		0%			
Wagner [75]	38	< 3	p + tf	5.3%	5.3%	0%	0%	0%	0%
Wagner [76]	150	2–7	p + tf	2.6%	6%	0%	2%	1.3%	0%
Warren [77]	17	0.5–1.5	tf	0 %	23%	0%	17.6%		17%
Weber [78]	38	5.4	tf, tt, tg, al	5.3%	21% 12.5%*	5.3%	13.2%	10.5%	31.6%
Wehrli [79]	25	< 4	p + tf	4%	0% *	4%	16%	0%	4%
Wilkes [80]	24	1.5	tf	8.3 %	12.5%	0%	12%		12%
Zang [81]	40	15.7	p + tt	15%	25%	5%	5%	5%	25%

Table 6.6 Outcomes of the distally fixed revision stem Redapt (Smith & Nephew, London, UK) as monoblock or monoblock with proximal modular sleeve; ef = endofemoral, tg = transgluteal, tf = transfemoral, tt = trans-trochanteric, a = anterior, al = anterolateral, ve = ventral; subsidence >5 mm, * = subsidence greater than 10 mm

Author	Cases, *n*	Follow-up (years)	Approach	Revision (%)	Subsidence (%)	Loosening (%)	Dislocation (%)	Infection (%)	Fracture (%)
Ngu [82]	23	5.9	p	0	4	0	4%		0
Gabor [83]	157	1	ef, tf	3.7 %	11,0.8%	0	1.9%	0.6%	3.8%

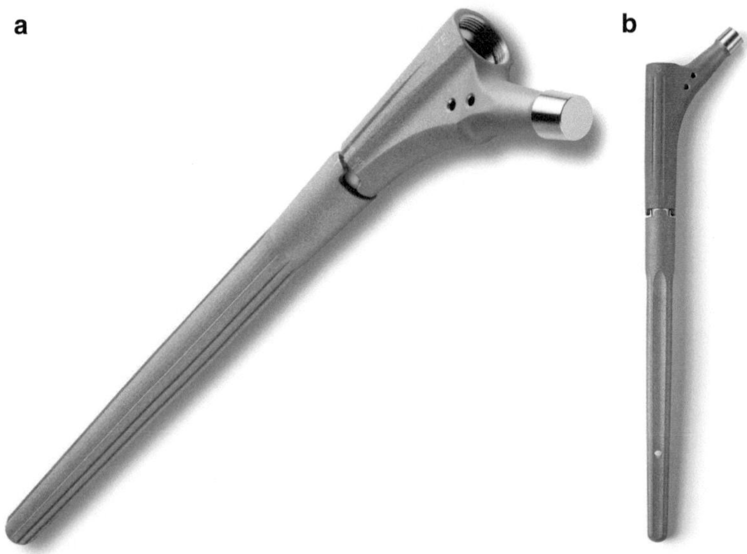

Fig. 6.19 Conical, distally fixing, modular Revitan stem revision stem (Zimmer Biomet, Winterthur, Switzerland); Revitan Straight (**a**); and Revitan Curved (**b**)

Solution stem (DePuy Synthes, Warsaw, IN, USA) and Arcos One-Piece (Zimmer Biomet, Warsaw, IN, USA) for scratch fit) also apply to the modular, distally fixed stem systems. Thus, the high subsidence rates of the PMF-R stem (the modular evolution of the Wagner SL stem) reported in Kessler et al. [85] and McInnis et al. [86] can be explained by the fact that, almost exclusively, only three-point fixation was achieved, a result that should definitely be avoided (see section "Outcomes").

We carried out a cadaver study and were able to show that for modular curved stem systems with distal cone-in-cone fixation, different fixation principles can be realized with both endofemoral and transfemoral implantation techniques [87]. The transfemorally implanted Revitan Curved stem (Zimmer, Winterthur, Switzerland) had a press-fit distal fixation (Fig. 6.18c) and thus a different fixation principle to that of the endofemorally implanted curved stem, which achieved its primary stability with a three-surface fixation (Fig. 6.27a, b) (see Chap. 7). In the latter case, the two lower contact surfaces that were responsible for fixation of the stem were formed by 3 of the 4 splines of the octagonal surface cutting into the bone, while the upper contact surface was merely a close contact of the stem with the bone [87]. If these fixation principles are taken into consideration and correctly implemented during the implantation of such stems, low rates of stem loosening and subsidence can be achieved (see "Outcomes"). We have also shown that a 3 cm press-fit distal fixation in the isthmus of the femur is sufficient for transfemorally implanted Revitan Curved stems [88, 89].

There are differences in the characteristics of the various distal fixation modular revision stems,

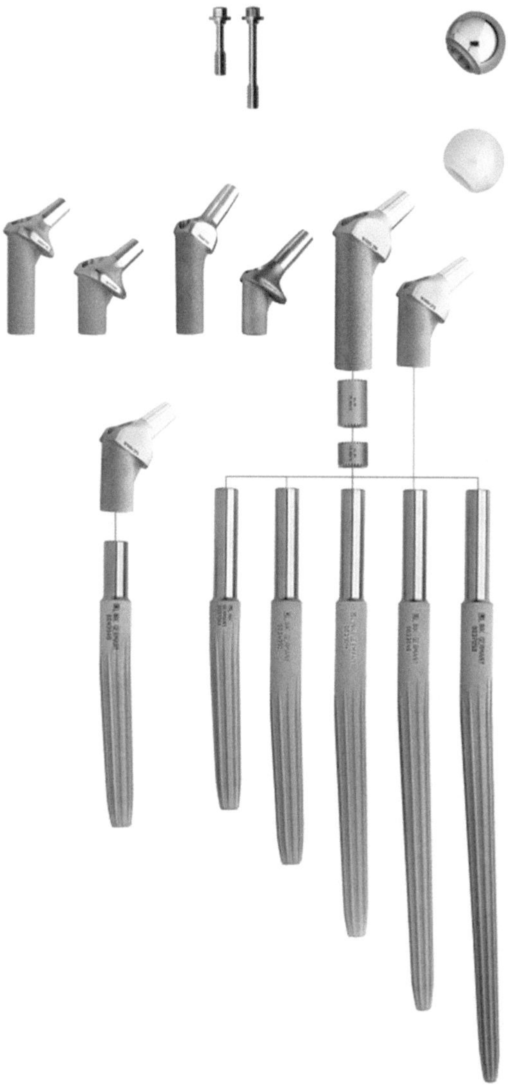

Fig. 6.20 Link MP revision stem system (Waldemar Link, Hamburg, Germany). The distal components have a bend or kink of 3 degrees

which must be taken into account in order to achieve reproducible outcomes (see Chap. 7). The different lengths of the fixation zones required in the isthmus of the femur can also be explained by the differences in stem design and modes of implantation. Firstly, the taper of the stems is different. This ranges from 1.5 degrees (MUTARS revision stem, implantcast, Buxtehude, Germany) (Fig. 6.28) to 3.5 degrees (ZMR stem, Zimmer Biomet, Warsaw, IN, USA) (Fig. 6.29). In addition, some stems are implanted directly after reaming the medullary canal using flexible medullary reamers (e.g., MRP stem, Peter Brehm, Weisendorf, Germany) (Fig. 6.23). In others, the fixation bed is prepared conically, similar to the monoblock prostheses, using conical reamers (e.g., Revitan straight, Arcos, ZMR, Zimmer Biomet, Warsaw, IN, USA, or Reclaim, DePuy Synthes, Warsaw, IN, USA) or rasps (Revitan Curved, Zimmer) to achieve cone-in-cone fixation (Fig. 6.16) A common feature of all distally fixed stems is that sufficient bone contact over a large area must be achieved with stems that are as thick as possible, and the necessity for corrective osteotomies to achieve this goal must be reviewed in the course of the preoperative planning. The reasons for a subsidence of these stems range from the choice of stems that are too thin with insufficient bone contact, to a three-point fixation that usually fails completely.

Some stems allow additional distal locking, although this is only necessary and useful when the isthmus of the femur is deficient and a firm distal fixation is not otherwise assured [90]. In addition to the Revitan Curved (Zimmer Biomet, Winterthur, Switzerland) (Fig. 6.19b), the MRP stem (Peter Brehm, Weisendorf, Germany) (Fig. 6.23), and the MUTARS RS stem (implantcast, Buxtehude, Germany), examples are the Prevision stem (Aesculap, Tuttlingen, Germany) and the Reef stem (DePuy Synthes, Warsaw, IN, USA). In this case, distal locking screws are utilized as a salvage procedure for additional stability in femurs with a deficient isthmus, where the distal fixation distance is less than 3 to 4 cm (depending on the stem used). The locking screws help to temporarily improve stem fixation until biological osteointegration has occurred to the point where this additional stability is no longer required (Fig. 6.29a–c). However, if there is insufficient prosthesis–bone contact and/or osteointegration, these locking screws will become stressed and eventually break. A different

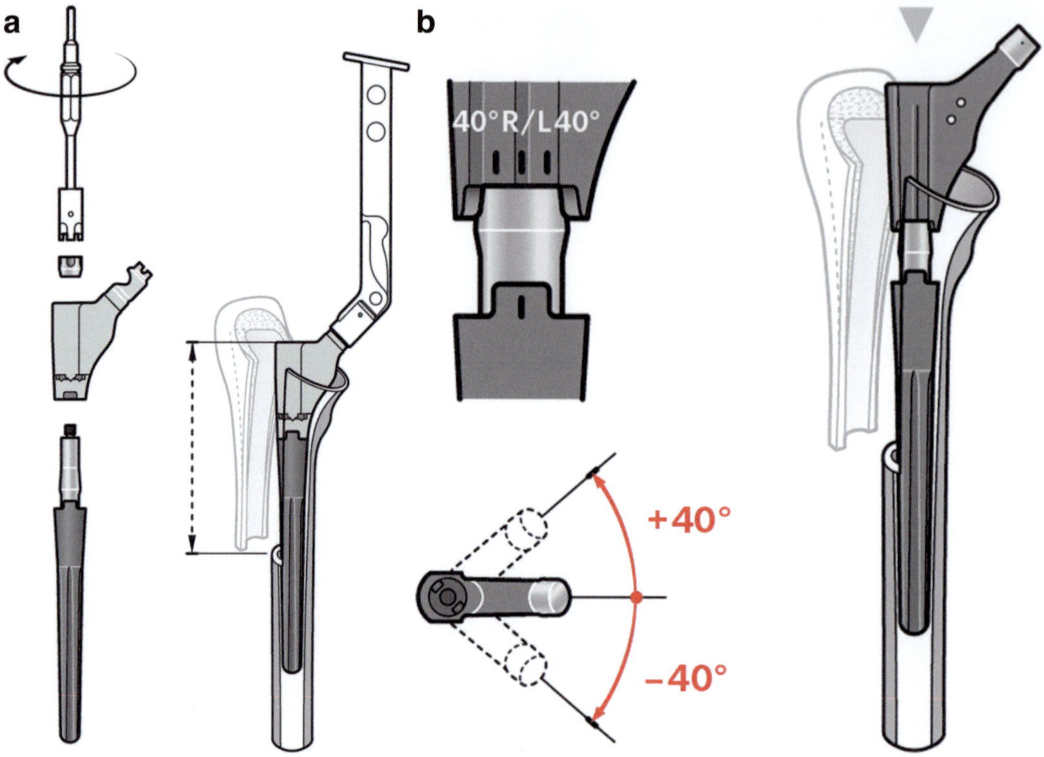

Fig. 6.21 Principle of implantation of a modular, distally fixing stem using the Revitan straight stem as an example (Zimmer Biomet, Winterthur, Switzerland). (**a**) Placing the proximal trial prosthesis on the final distal component that has already been implanted. (**b**) In situ installation of the final proximal component on the final distal component after satisfactory trial fitting

locking concept is used for the cylindrical curved, coarse-structured Arcos version, in which additional locking screws are inserted over the entire length of the distal stem component to improve its stability (Fig. 6.26).

6.3.3.1 Surgical Technique

Since this book focuses on modular distal fixation revision stems, a separate chapter (Chap. 11) is devoted to the surgical techniques used for these stems. However, here we would like to mention the correct procedures for working with the modularity of such revision prostheses and briefly describe the surgical principles using one of these revision systems as an example (here Reclaim, DePuy Synthes, Warsaw, IN, USA). First, the fixation bed is prepared distally in the femur (depending on the type of fixation using a cylindrical or conical reamer (here conical) (Fig. 6.30a) or a cylindrical medullary reamer, followed by a conical rasp for the Revitan Curved component). The distal component is then inserted into this fixation bed so that it is firmly seated (Fig. 6.30b). The proximal component may require some space to be created by means of routing, and this should be guided carefully by hand to avoid unintentional fractures of the trochanter (Fig. 6.30c). A proximal trial component is then placed on the distal component to carry out a trial reduction. If testing is satisfactory, the final proximal component is implanted (Fig. 6.30d). The two components are then joined together in situ (Fig. 6.30e).

If the advantages of modularity are to be fully exploited, this makes it necessary to assemble the components in the patient, or, to put it another

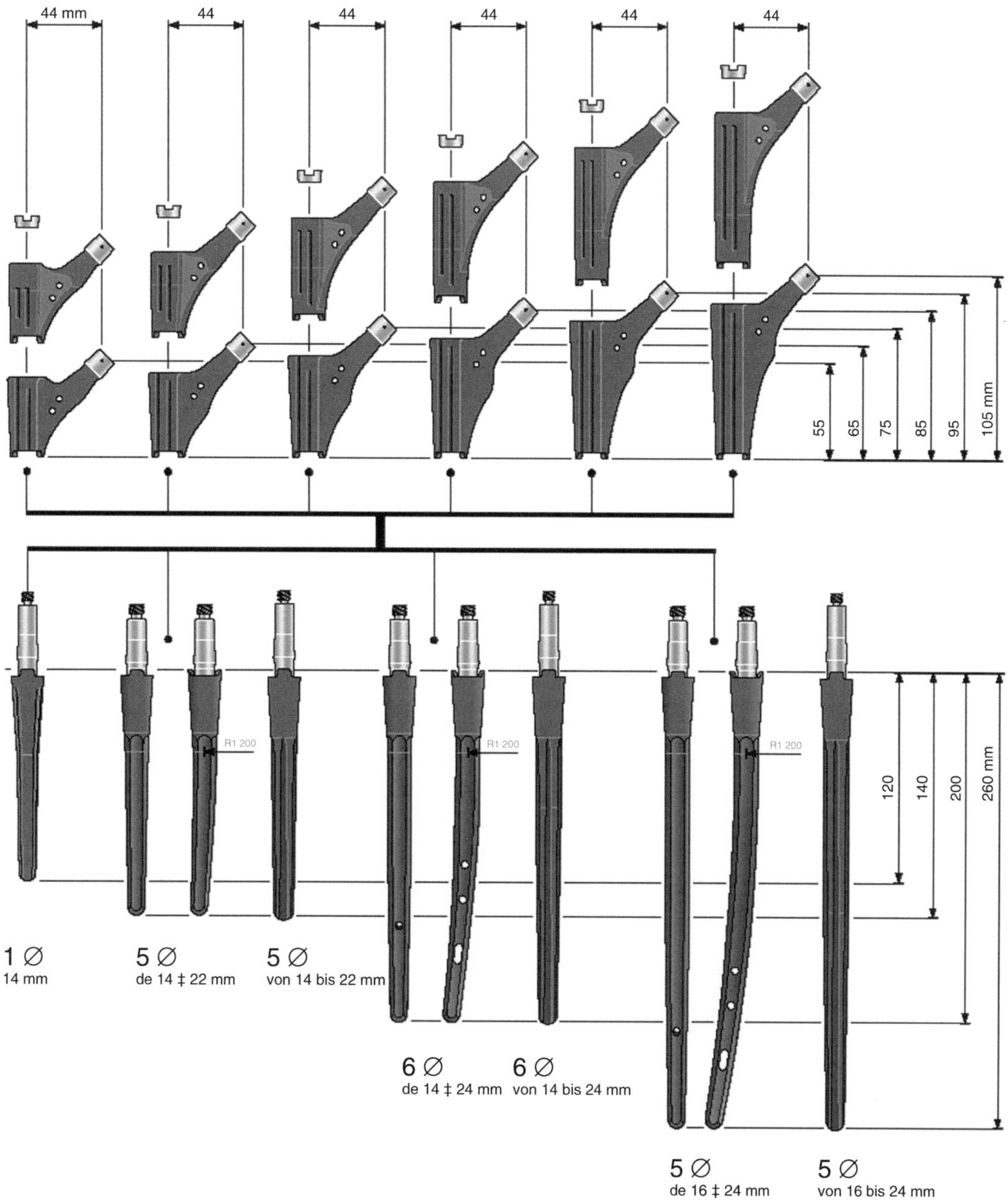

Fig. 6.22 Conical, distally fixing, modular Revitan stem revision system (Zimmer Biomet, Winterthur, Switzerland)

way, this excludes the tabletop mounting of the modular components (i.e., on the operating table). Tabletop mounting should not therefore be used with modular revision stems because it turns a modular revision stem into a nonmodular revision stem, for which one pays a substantial purchase price. In addition, the advantages of modularity are lost through tabletop mounting. Moreover, unintentional fractures of the greater trochanter may occur during endofemoral procedures because the prosthesis was assembled on the operating table. The distal fit of the prosthesis

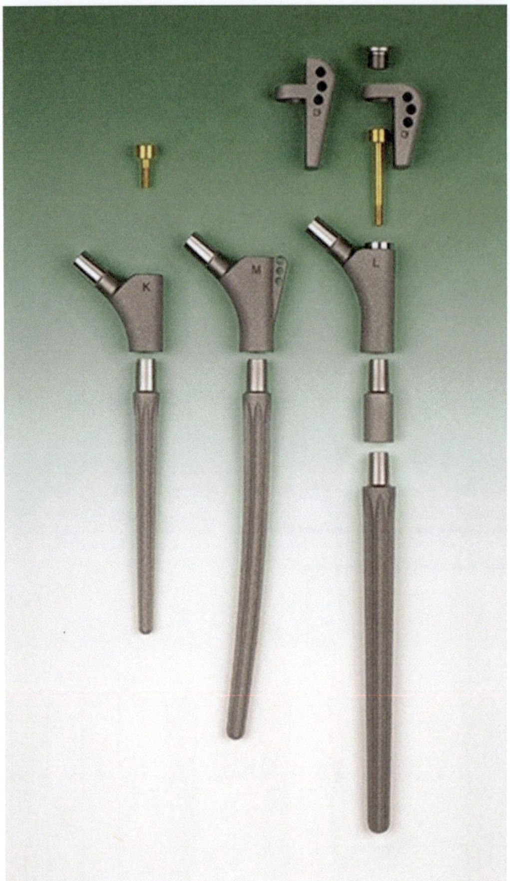

Fig. 6.23 Modular revision system MRP (Peter Brehm, Weisendorf, Germany)

may also be affected. The reamers or rasps are usually only used to prepare the distal regions, and the site for the proximal component is not necessarily prepared in the same way. When the trial prosthesis or, later, the final components have been assembled on the operating table and then implanted, an area of bone may be present proximally at the trochanter that can then be subjected to pressure by the proximal component or even compromise the insertion of the prosthesis and thus its distal fit. This bone, although it is usually only slightly troublesome, must be removed, for example, with a hollow reamer, after the final distal component has been positioned, so that the proximal trial component (and later the final component) can be positioned without hindrance.

6.3.3.2 Outcomes

Reproducibly satisfactory outcomes can be achieved with modular, distally fixing conical revision stems (Tables 6.7, 6.8, 6.9, and 6.10). In a comparative analysis, both nonmodular cylindrical extensively coated cobalt–chromium stems and cylindrical modular revision stems fixed by scratch fit performed less well than modular conical revision stems with a cone-in-cone fixation. In a retrospective comparison of 61 conical and 44 cylindrical stems with Paprosky type III and IV defects, whereby the conical stems group included more type IIIB and IV defects (51%) than the group of cylindrical stems (20%), the conical stems showed significantly lower re-revision rates (4.9% vs. 22.7%) and less failure of osteointegration (1.6% vs. 15.9%) [93]. When Richards et al. [134] compared 105 cylindrical extensively porous-coated cobalt–chromium stems to 95 conical titanium stems, with significantly more type IIIB and IV defects in the conical stem group, they found significantly better clinical scores in the latter group with less frequent thigh pain, a lower fracture rate, and better bone regeneration of the proximal femur. The latter is due to the lower modulus of elasticity of the titanium stems, which are therefore less rigid and have no tendency to induce stress shielding, unlike the cobalt–chromium stems. In our own studies, it has been shown that even on average there is proximal bone remodeling with modular, distally fixed titanium revision stems [123, 135]. The transfemorally implanted stems showed significantly greater proximal femoral bone gains due to callus formation compared to endofemorally implanted stems [123]. The analysis of factors influencing bone regeneration showed that it was only affected by the type of preoperative bone defect and the preoperative cortical thickness, not by the thickness or length of the stem [135].

However, the outcome of the use of such stems depends on the correct implementation of the surgical techniques. McInnis et al. [86] reported poor outcomes with the modular, distally fixed conical titanium stem (PFMR, Sulzer AG, Winterthur, Switzerland), which is the precursor of the current Revitan system. They implanted 70

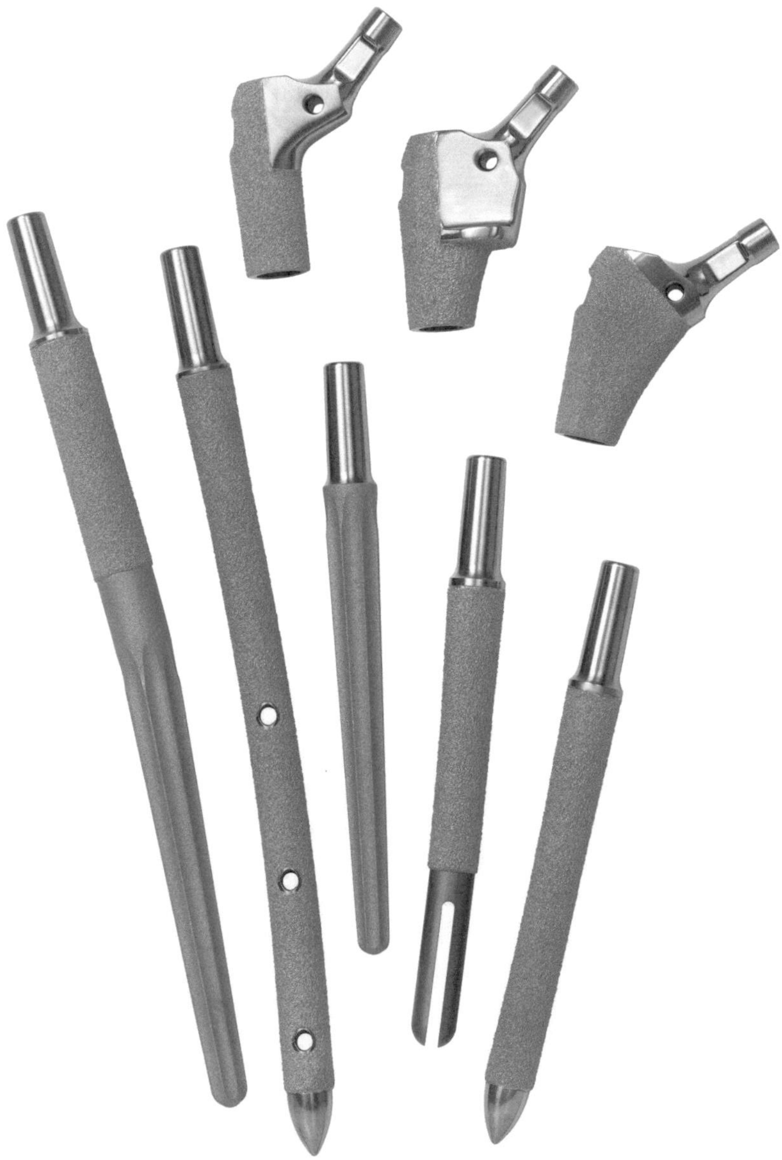

Fig. 6.24 Modular revision system Arcos, (Zimmer Biomet, Warsaw, IN, USA)

stems using purely endofemoral approaches and reported periprosthetic fracture in 24.2% of cases, subsidence of the stem in 55.7%, and loosening of the stem in 12.8% of cases. The authors concluded that this was due to the exclusive use of an endofemoral approach. In a separate study, we examined 116 Revitan Curved stems (Zimmer Biomet, Winterthur, Switzerland) with a minimum follow-up of 5.3 years and an average follow-up of 7.5 years, all of which had been implanted according to the following, clearly defined concept [123]:

- Preoperative planning determined, among other things, the indication for the transfemoral approach (77 cases).
- The modular components were always assembled in situ.
- The revision stems were chosen to be as short as possible with fixation at the tip of the stem

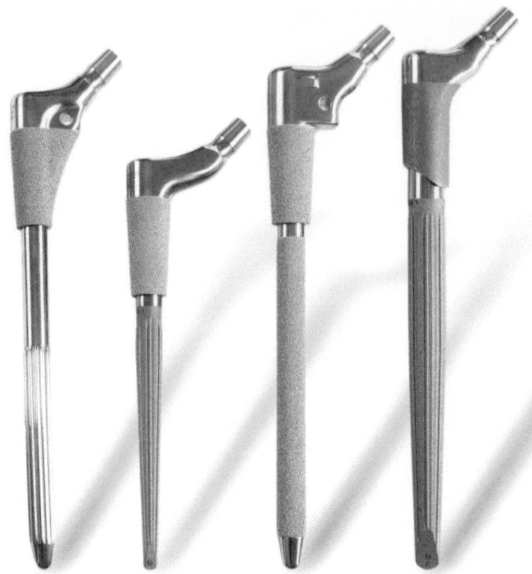

Fig. 6.25 Modular revision system ZMR (Zimmer Biomet, Warsaw, IN, USA)

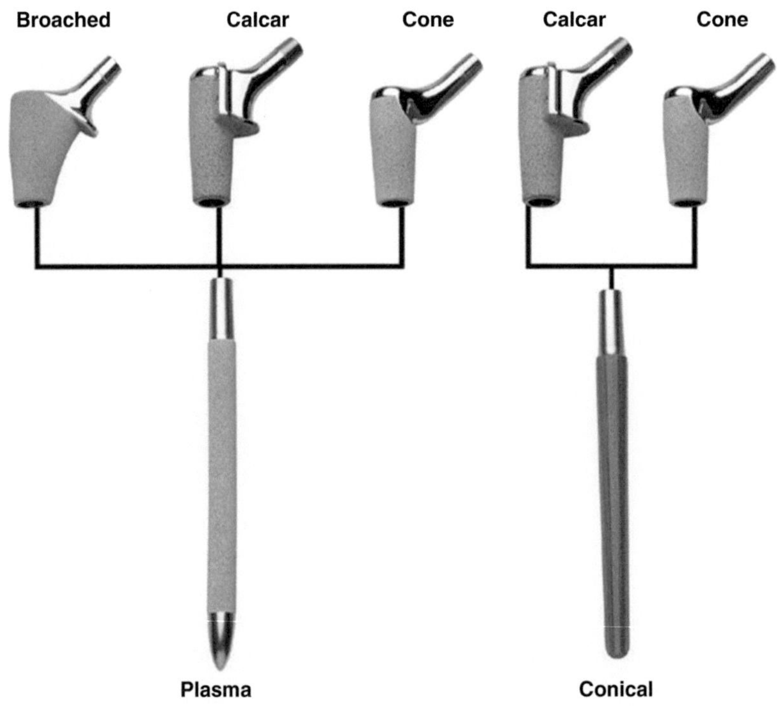

Fig. 6.26 Modular revision system Restoration (Stryker, Kalamazoo, MG, USA)

in the isthmus of the femur provided the isthmus was intact.

- In the case of Paprosky IIIB and IV type defects with a fixation zone of less than 3 cm in the isthmus of the femur, additional distal locking was implemented.

With this clear concept, we achieved a survival rate of 95.7% after 9 years for all stem-related revisions and a survival rate of 100% for aseptic loosening alone (Fig. 6.31). Revision of the stem because of periprosthetic infections was necessary in 2.3% of cases. A subsidence of the stem of more than 5 mm was seen in 2.9% and a dislocation in 4.3%. There were no periprosthetic fractures (0%). The Harris hip score increased from 46.7 ± 16.0 preoperatively to 88.2 ± 13.5 5 years after surgery.

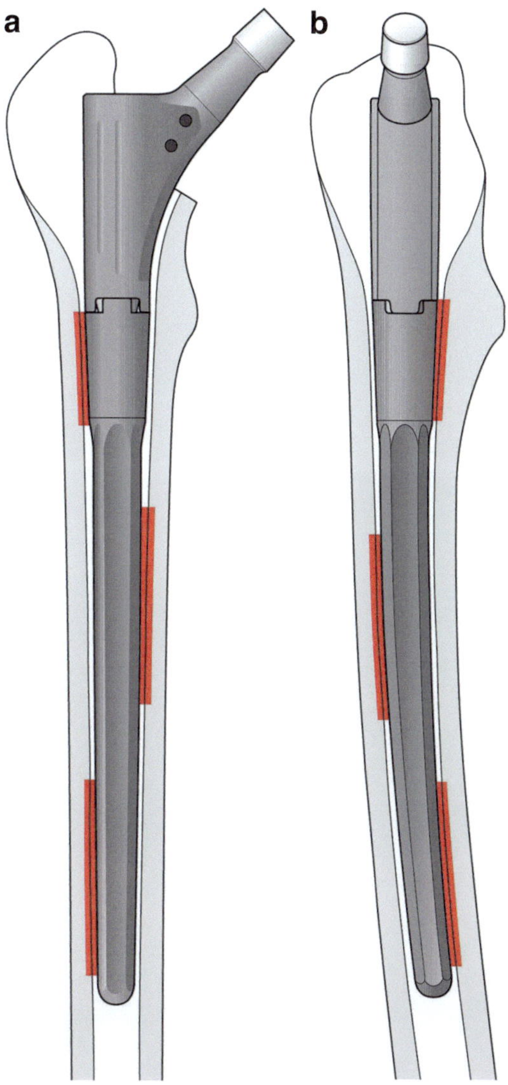

Fig. 6.27 (**a**, **b**) Principle of three-surface fixation with an endofemorally implanted cementless curved revision stem (with permission of Zimmer Biomet, Winterthur, Switzerland). (**a**) a.p. view, (**b**) side view

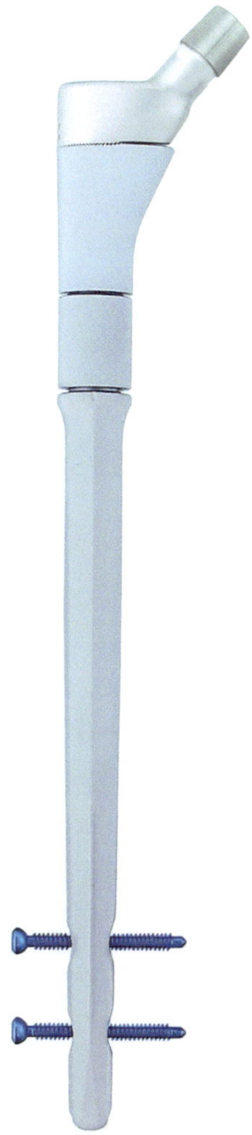

Fig. 6.28 Modular revision system MUTARS, RS (implantcast, Buxtehude, Germany)

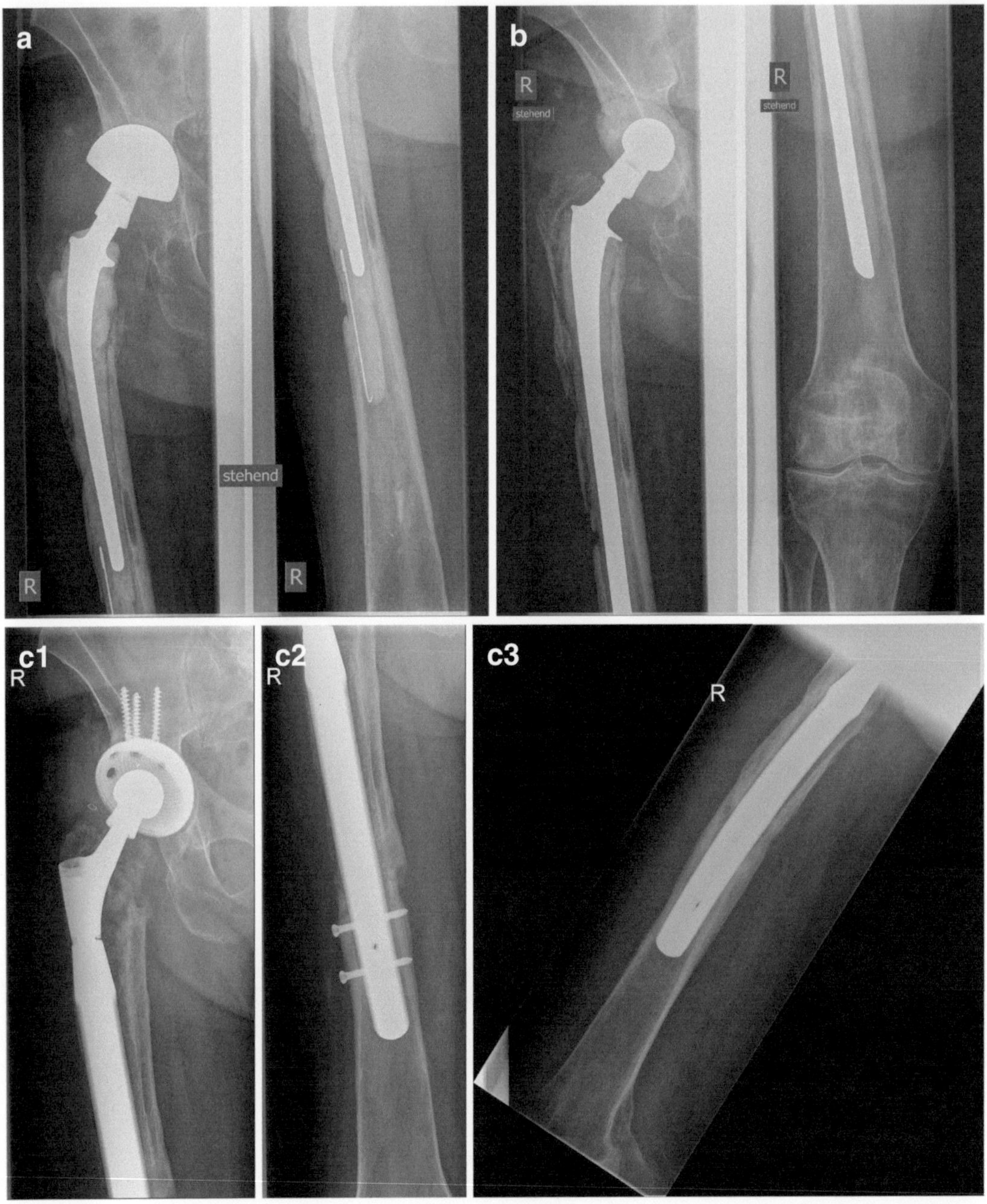

Fig. 6.29 (**a**) Periprosthetic infection after multiple extramural prosthesis revisions with cemented stem and a dual-mobility head with a Paprosky IIIB type bone defect. (**b**) Interim prosthesis after transfemoral prosthesis removal; a long cement-coated stem is used as an interim prosthesis in two-stage septic revision. (**c1–3**) Radiographs 12 months after surgery after reimplantation of a modular revision stem Revitan Curved with distal locking and Allofit-S Press-fit cup (Zimmer Biomet, Winterthur, Switzerland)

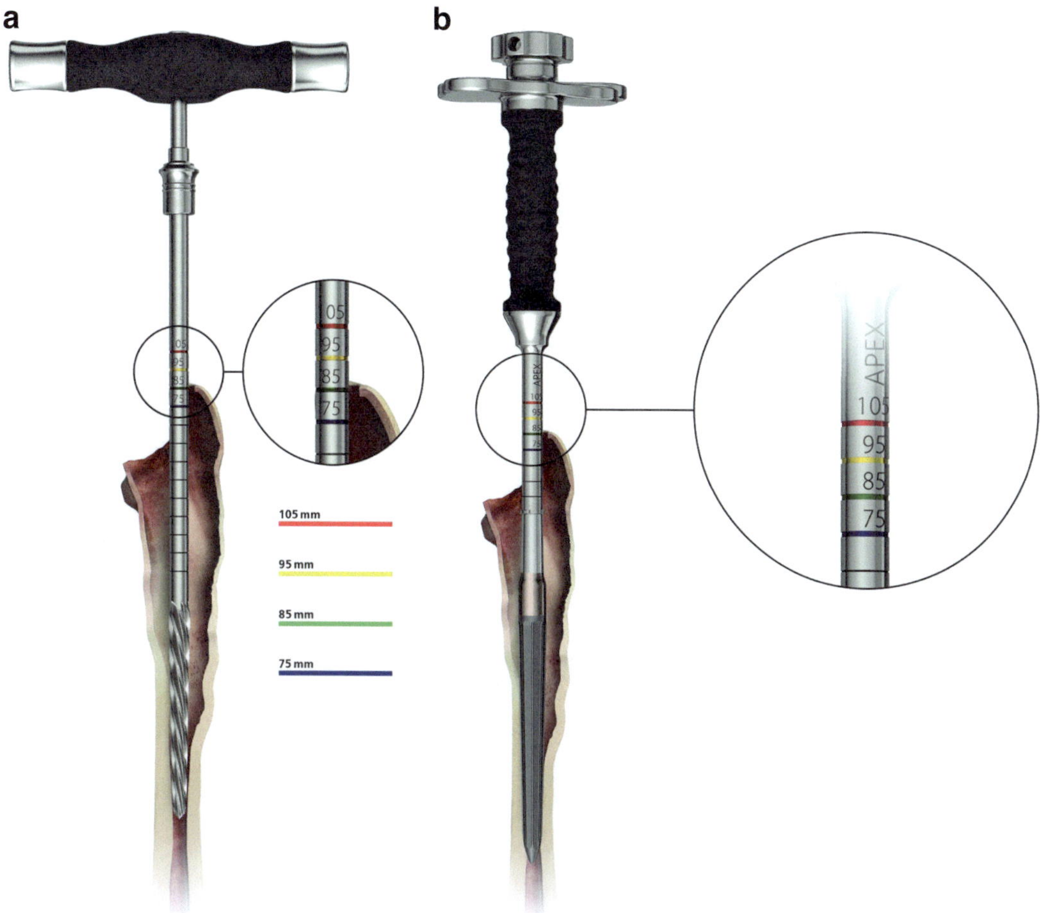

Fig. 6.30 Principle of preparation of the distal fixation bed and implantation of a distally fixed modular revision stem using the example of the modular Reclaim Stem (DePuy Synthes, Warsaw, IN, USA). (**a**) Preparation of the distal fixation bed using a conical reamer. (**b**) Implantation of the distal stem component in the prepared distal fixation bed. (**c**) Creating room for the proximal component by reaming. (**d**) Implantation of the proximal component. (**e**) Connecting the two components in situ

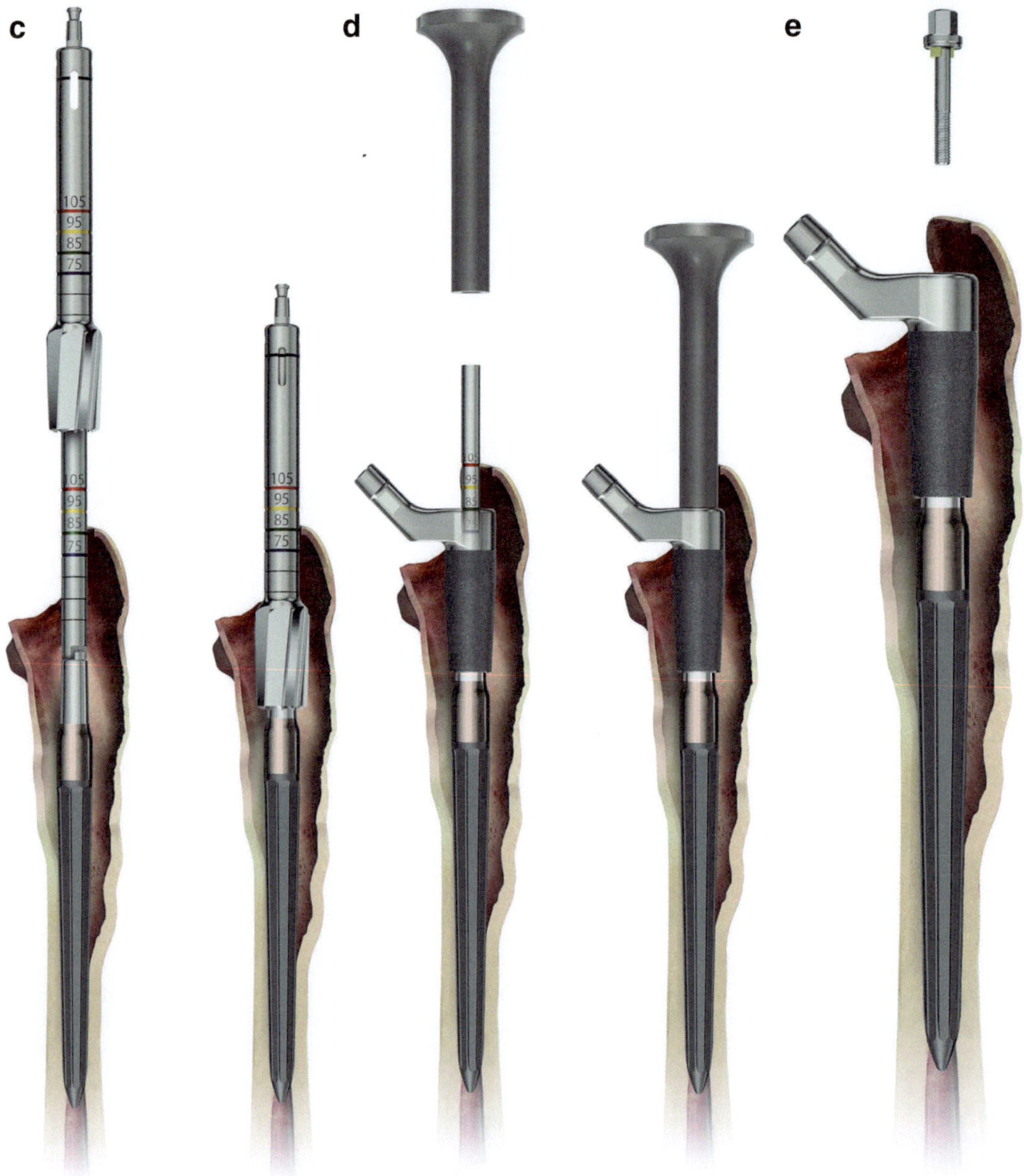

Fig. 6.30 (continued)

Table 6.7 Modular distal cylindrical porous-coated stems; al = anterolateral, p = posterior, tf = transfemoral, ef = endofemoral, ts = trochanteric slide; * = only Paprosky type III + IV defects; subsidence >5 mm, ** > 10 mm

Author	Stem	*N*	Follow-up (years)	Approach	Revision (%)	Subsidence (%)	Loosening (%)	Dislocation (%)	Infection (%)	Fracture (%)
Lakstein [91]	ZMR	72	7	tf, ts	5.5	11	2.8	4.2	2.8	2.8
Jibodh [92]	ZMR	54	7	p, tf		0	0	9		7
RTHASG [93]	ZMR	44*	5		22.7	9.1**				11.4

Table 6.8 Modular distal conical straight stems; al = anterolateral, p = posterior, tf = transfemoral, ef = endofemoral, ts = trochanteric slide, * = only Paprosky type III + IV defects; subsidence >5 mm

Author	Stem	*N*	Follow-up [years]	Approach	Revision (%)	Subsidence (%)	Loosening (%)	Dislocation (%)	Infection (%)	Fracture (%)
Holt [94]	Restoration	46	3.5	p, tf			0	7		2.2
Desai [95]	Restoration	52	3.8	ef, tf	5.7			5.7	3.8	15.3
Dzaja [96]	Restoration	55*	2.7	tf	4	3	2	5	3	4
Restrepo [84]	Restoration	122	4	al, tf	8	2	0	3	2	2
Stimac [97]	Restoration	86	4.3	p	11.6		0	2.3	4.6	4.6
Palumbo [98]	Restoration	18*	4.5	ef, tf	5.5	11.1	5.5		5.5	
Riesgo [99]	Restoration	161	5.9	p	14.9		2	4.3	6.2	
Smith [100]	Restoration	115	>2	p, tf	13	6	0.9	0.9	3.4	5
Picado [101]	Restoration	41	5.1	tg, tf	17	12.2	4.8	7.3	4.9	7.3
Park [102]	Lima-Lto	62	4.2	p, tf	4.8	6.5	0	5	2	12.9
Kessler [85]	PFMR	50	1	tg		24				
McInnis [86]	PFMR	70	3.9	p, (efo*)	4.3	55.7	12.8	10	2.9	24.2
Ovesen [103]	ZMR	125	4.2	p, tf	3.2	8				5.6
Canella [104]	ZMR	30	2	p, tf		0		3.3	6.6	0
Munro [105]	ZMR	109	3.1		6	5.5	0		0.9	
Van Houwelingen [106]	ZMR	48*	7	tg, p, tf	10.4	12.5	0	10	0 / 25	16
RTHASG [93]	ZMR + restoration	61*	5		4.9	8.2**				13.1
Rieger [107]	Revitan straight	70	4.3	tf	6	14.7	1.5	8.6	0	3
Wronka [108]	Revitan straight	47	4.7	p, tf	4.2	6.3	4.2	4.2	0	0

Table 6.9 Modular revision stems, straight with kink; al = anterolateral, p = posterior, tf = transfemoral, ef = endofemoral, ts = trochanteric slide, l = lateral; subsidence >5 mm

Author	Stem	*N*	Follow-up (years)	Approach	Revision (%)	Subsidence (%)	Loosening (%)	Dislocation (%)	Infection (%)	Fracture (%)
Kwong [109]	Link MP	143	3.3	ef, tf	2.8		0	2.1	4.9	2.1
Murphy [110]	Link MP	35	3.6	ef, tf	2.9			17.1		
Tamvakopoulos [111]	Link MP	40	5.7	l, tf	7.5	5	0	12.5	10	0
Rodriguez [112]	Link MP	93	3.2	p, tf	5	3		1.1	1	5.4
Rodriguez [113]	Link MP	64	6.2	p, tf		3.1		4.7		3.1
Schofer [114]	Link MP	81	1.4	p, l	4.9	23	1.3	14.8	6.2	9.8
Weiss [115]	Link MP	63	6	ef, tf	10	15	2	19	3.3	2.2
Skyttä [116]	Link MP	408	9		19.1		3	6.4	2.2	1.5
Klauser [117]	Link MP	63	8.5	p	4.7			3.2	1.6	17
Wang [118]	Link MP	58	4.3	ef, (tf)	3.5	9	2	3	1.7	17
Amanatullalh [119]	Link MP	92	6.4	ef, tf	4.3	7	1	19	7	12
Zhang [120]	Link MP	246	5.7			1.6*		2	2.8	11.7
Wronka [108]	Link MP	57	4.7	p tf	3.5	3.5	1.7	1.7	1.7	1.7
Hashem [121]	Link MP	132	4.4	p,(tf)	22		0.8	8	5.5	5
Hancock [122]	Reclaim	48	1	al, p. tf	8.3	8	2.1	4.2	10.4	

Table 6.10 Modular curved stems; al = anterolateral, p = posterior, tf = transfemoral, ef = endofemoral, ts = trochanteric slide; subsidence >5 mm

Author	Stem	N	Follow-up (years)	Approach	Revision (%)	Subsidence (%)	Loosening (%)	Dislocation (%)	Infection (%)	Fracture (%)
Fink [88]	Revitan curved	68	2.6	tf	4.4%	5.9%	2.9%	4.4%	0%	0%
Fink [89]	Revitan curved	120	3.2	p, tf	1.7%	7.5%	1.7%	4.2%	0%	0%
Fink [123]	Revitan curved	116	7.5 (5–9)	p, tf	4.3%	2.9%	0%	4.3%	2.3%	0%
Köster [124]	Profemur R	73	6.2	tg, tf	4.1%	2.7%	2.7%	1.3%	1.3%	9.5%
Artiaco [125]	Profemur R	35	4.7	ef	5.7%	17.1%	11.4%	0%	5.7%	5.7%
Pattyn [126]	Profemur R	68	5.2	p, tf	7.3%	1.4%	1.4%	4.4%	1.4%	11.7%
Wirtz [127]	MRP	142	2.3	ef, tf	4.9%	4%	1.4%	11.3%	1.4%	1.4%
Schuh [128]	MRP	79	4	ef, tf	3.8%	2.5%	0%	5.1%	2.5%	6.3%
Schuh [129]	MRP	130	2.9	ef, tf	4.6%	0.8%	0.8%	3.8%	2.3%	1.5%
Mumme [130]	MRP	48	4.7	tg	2.1%	2.1%	2.1%	12.5%	2.1%	2.1%
Wimmer [131]	MRP	243	4.4		4.5%	2.1%	2.4%	6.1%	1.6%	5.3%
Wirtz [132]	MRP	163	5–16		6.1%	4.3%	4.9%	12.3%	2.5%	7.3%
Hoberg [133]	MRP	89	4.6	lat	6.8%	0%		2.2%	3.3%	

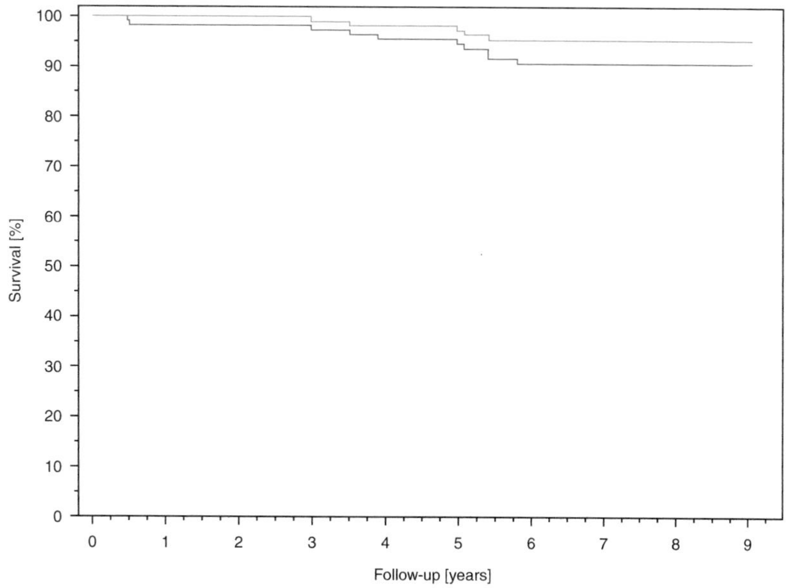

Fig. 6.31 Kaplan–Maier curve of the survival of 116 modular curved revision stems Revitan Curved (Zimmer Biomet, Winterthur, Switzerland). Green curve = stem-related revisions, blue curve = revision for all reasons

References

1. Head WC, Wagner RA, Emerson RH, Malinin T. Restoration of femoral bone stock in revision total hip arthroplasty. Orthop Clin North Am. 1993;24:697–703.
2. Head WC, Wagner RA, Emerson RH, Malinin TI. Revision total hip arthroplasty in the deficient femur with a proximal load-bearing prosthesis. Clin Orthop Relat Res. 1994;298:119–26.
3. Head WC, Malinin TI, Emerson RH, Mallory TH. Restoration of bone stock in revision surgery of the femur. Int Orthop. 2000;24:9–14.
4. Head WC, Emerson RH, Higgins LL. A titanium cementless calcar replacement prosthesis in revision surgery of the femur. 13-year experience. J Arthroplasty. 2001;16:183–7.
5. Berry DJ, Harmsen WS, Ilstrup D, Lewallen DG, Cabanela ME. Survivorship of uncemented proximally porous-coated femoral components. Clin Orthop Relat Res. 1995;319:168–77.
6. Buoncristiani AM, Dorr LD, Johnson C, Wan Z. Cementless revision of total hip arthroplasty using the anatomic porous replacement revision prosthesis. J Arthroplasty. 1997;12:403–15.
7. Hussamy O, Lachiewicz PF. Revision total hip arthroplasty with the BIAS femoral component. J Bone Joint Surg. 1994;76-A:1137–48.
8. Gosens T, van Langelaan EJ. Clinical and radiological outcome of hydroxyapatite-coated femoral stem in revision hip arthroplasty. Int Orthop. 2005;29:219–23.
9. Kim Y-H. Cementless revision hip arthroplasty using strut allografts and primary cementless proximal porous-coated prosthesis. J Arthroplasty. 2004;19:573–81.
10. Malkani AL, Lewallen DG, Cabanela ME, Wallrichs SL. Femoral component revision using an uncemented, proximally coated, long-stem prosthesis. J Arthroplasty. 1996;11:411–8.
11. Mulliken BD, Rorabeck CH, Bourne RB. Uncemented revision total hip arthroplasty. Clin Orthop Relat Res. 1996;325:156–62.
12. Peters CL, Rivero DP, Kull LR, Jacobs JJ, Rosenberg AG, Galante JO. Revision total hip arthroplasty without cement: subsidence of proximally porous-coated femoral components. J Bone Joint Surg. 1995;77-A:1217–26.
13. Woolson ST, Delaney TJ. Failure of a proximally porous-coated femoral prosthesis in revision total hip arthroplasty. J Arthroplasty. 1995;10(Suppl):S22–8.
14. Wood TJ, Alzahrani M, Marsh JD, Somerville LE, Vasarhelyi EM, Lanting BA. Use of the Corail stem for revision total hip arthroplasty: evaluation of clinical outcomes and cost. J Cancer Chir. 2019;62:78–82.
15. Mehran N, North T, Laker M. Failure of a modular hip implant at the stem-sleeve interface. Orthopedics. 2013;36:e978–81.
16. Imbuldeniya AM, Walter WK, Zicat BA, Walter WL. The S-ROM hydroxyapatite proximally-coated modular femoral stem in revision hip replacement. Results of 397 hips at a minimum ten-year follow-up. Bone Joint J. 2014;96-B:730–6.
17. Moreta J, Uriare I, Foruria X, Lorono A, Agirre U, Jáurequi I, Martinez-de Los Mozos JL. Medium term outcomes of the S-ROM modular femoral stem in revision hip replacement. Eur J Orthop Surg Traumatol. 2018;28:1327–34.

18. Bolognesi MP, Pietrobon R, Clifford PE, Parker VT. Comparison of a hydroxyapatite-coated sleeve and a porous-coated sleeve with a modular revision hip stem. J Bone Joint Surg. 2004;86-A:2720–5.
19. Bono JV, McCarthy JC, Lee J-A, Carangei RJ, Turner RH. Fixation with a modular stem in revision total hip arthroplasty. Instr Course Lect. 2000;49:131–9.
20. Cameron HU. The two- to six-year results with a proximally modular noncemented total hip replacement used in hip revisions. Clin Orthop Relat Res. 1994;298:47–53.
21. Cameron HU. Modulare Schäfte in der Hüftprothesenrevisionschirurgie. Orthopäde. 2001;30:287–93.
22. Chandler H, Clark J, Murphy S, Mc Carthy J, Penenberg B, Danylchuk K, Roehr B. Reconstruction of major segmental loss of the proximal femur in revision total hip arthroplasty. Clin Orthop Relat Res. 1994;298:67–74.
23. Chandler HP, Ayres DK, Tan RC, Anderson LC, Varma AK. Revision total hip replacement using the S-ROM femoral component. Clin Orthop Relat Res. 1995;319:130–40.
24. Christie MJ, DeBoer DK, Tingstad EM, Capps M, Brinson MF, Trick LW. Clinical experience with a modular noncemented femoral component in revision total hip arthroplasty, 4- to 7-year results. J Arthroplasty. 2000;15:840–8.
25. McCarthy JC, Lee J. Complex revision total hip arthroplasty with modular stems at a mean of 14 years. Clin Orthop Relat Res. 2007;465:166–9.
26. Park YS, Lim SJ. Long-term comparison of porous and hydroxyapatite sleeves in femoral revision using the S-ROM modular stem. Hip Int. 2010;20:179–86.
27. Piao S, Zhou YG, Du YQ, Ma HY, Sun JY, Gao ZS, Peng YW, Wu WM. Clinical results in early and mid term of using the S-ROM femoral stem in revision. Zhongguo Gu Shang. 2017;30:322–8.
28. Smith JA, Dunn HK, Manaster BJ. Cementless femoral revision arthroplasty, 2-to 5-year results with a modular titanium alloy stem. J Arthroplasty. 1997;12:194–201.
29. Walter WL, Walter WK, Zicat B. Clinical and radiographic assessment of a modular cementless ingrowth femoral stem system for revision hip arthroplasty. J Arthroplasty. 2006;21:172–8.
30. Wei-Li, Lian YY, Yue Q, Yue WJ, Zhao CB, Meng QG. Revision hip arthroplasties with use of the modular S-ROM prosthesis. Indian J Med Sci. 2011;65:444–51.
31. Li H, Chen F, Wan Z, Chen Q. Comparison of clinical efficacy between modular cementless stem prostheses and coated cementless long-stem prostheses on bone defect in hip revision arthroplasty. Med Sci Monit. 2016;22:670–7.
32. Bhagia UT, Corpe RS, Steflink DE, Young TR, Schnars J. Cementless S_ROM femoral component: effect of stem length on stability after extended proximal osteotomy. J South Orthop Assoc. 2001;10:6–11.
33. Spitzer AI. The S-ROM cementless femoral stem: history and literature review. Orthopedics. 2005;28:S1117–24.
34. Dyreborg K, Petersen MM, Balle SS, Kjersgaard AG, Solgaard S. Observational study of a new modular femoral revision system. World J Orthop. 2020;11:167–76.
35. Lombardi Lombardi AV, Berend KR Jr, Mallory TH, Adams JB. Modular calcar replacement prosthesis with strengthened taper junction in total hip arthroplasty. Surg Technol Int. 2007;16:206–9.
36. Pelt CE, Stagg ML, van Dine C, Anderson MB, Peters CL, Gililland JM. Early outcomes after revision total hip arthroplasty with a modern modular femoral revision stem in 65 consecutive cases. Arthroplasty Today. 2019;5:106–12.
37. Engh CA, Glassman AH, Suthers KE. The case for porous-coated hip implants. The femoral side. Clin Orthop Relat Res. 1990;261:63–81.
38. Lawrence JM, Engh CA, Macalino GE. Revision total hip arthroplasty. Long-term results without cement. Clin Orthop North Am. 1993;24:635–44.
39. Paprosky WG, Greidanus NV, Antoniou J. Minimum 10-year-results of extensively porous-coated stems in revision hip arthroplasty. Clin Orthop. 1999;369:230–42.
40. Weeden SH, Paprosky WG. Minimal 11-year follow-up of extensively porous-coated stems in femoral revision total hip arthroplasty. J Arthroplasty. 2002;17(Suppl):134–7.
41. Kim Y-H, Park J-W, Kim J-S, Rastogi D. High survivorship with cementless stems and cortical strut allografts for large femoral bone defects in revision THA. Clin Orthop Relat Res. 2015;473:2990–3000.
42. Ahmet S, Ismet KO, Mehmet E, Eren Y, Remzi T, Önder Y. Midterm results of the cylindrical fully porous-coated uncemented femoral stem in revision patients with Paprosky I-IIIA femoral defects. J Orthop Surg. 2018;26:1–5.
43. Aribinidi R, Barba M, Solomon MI, Arp P, Paprosky W. Bypass fixation. Orthop Clin North Am. 1998;29:319–29.
44. Chen WM, McAuley JP, Engh CA Jr, Hopper RH Jr, Engh CA. Extended slide trochanteric osteotomy for revision total hip arthroplasty. J Bone Joint Surg. 2000;82-A:1215–9.
45. Ding ZC, Ling TX, Yuan MC, Qin YZ, Mou P, Wang HY, Zhou ZK. Minimum 8-year follow-up of revision THA with severe femoral bone defects using extensively porous-coated stems and cortical strut allografts. BMC Musculoskelet Disord. 2020;21(1):218.
46. Engh CA, Culpepper WJ, Kassapidis E. Revision of loose cementless femoral prostheses to larger porous coated components. Clin Orthop Relat Res. 1998;347:168–78.
47. Böhm P, Bischel O. The use of tapered stems in femoral revision surgery. Clin Orthop. 2004;420:148–59.
48. Krishnamurthy AB, MacDonald SJ, Paprosky WG. 5-to 13-year follow-up study on cementless femo-

ral components in revision surgery. J Arthroplasty. 1997;12:839–47.
49. Lawrence JM, Engh CA, Macalino GE, Lauro GR. Outcome of revision hip arthroplasty done without cement. J Bone Joint Surg. 1994;76-A:965–73.
50. Miner TM, Momberger NG, Chong D, Paprosky WL. The extended trochanteric osteotomy in revision hip arthroplasty. A critical review of 166 cases at mean 3-year, 9-month follow-up. J Arthroplasty. 2001;16(Suppl):188–94.
51. Moreland JR, Bernstein ML. Femoral revision hip arthroplasty with uncemented, porous-coated stems. Clin Orthop Relat Res. 1995;319:141–50.
52. Moreland JR, Moreno MA. Cementless femoral revision arthroplasty of the hip: minimum 5 years follow-up. Clin Orthop Relat Res. 2001;393: 194–201.
53. Paprosky WG, Weeden SH, Bowling JW Jr. Component removal in revision total hip arthroplasty. Clin Orthop Relat Res. 2001;393:181–93.
54. Sugimura T, Tohkura A. THA revision with extensively porous-coated stems. Acta Orthop Scand. 1998;69:11–3.
55. Mahoney OM, Kinsey TL, Asayama I. Durable fixation with a modern fully hydroxyapatite-coated long stem in complex revision total hip arthroplasty. J Arthroplasty. 2010;25:355–62.
56. Wagner H. Revisionsprothese für das Hüftgelenk bei schwerem Knochenverlust. Orthopäde. 1987;16:295–300.
57. Baktir A, Karaaslan F, Gencer K, Karaoglu S. Femoral revision using the Wagner SL revision stem: a single-surgeon experience featuring 11-19 years of follow-up. J Arthroplasty. 2015;30:827–34.
58. Bircher HP, Riede U, Lüem M, Ochsner PE. Der Wert der SL-Revisionsprothese nach Wagner zur Überbrückung großer Femurdefekte. Technik und Resultate. Orthopäde. 2001;30:294–303.
59. Böhm P, Bischel O. Das zementfreie diaphysäre Verankerungsprinzip für den Hüftschaftwechsel bei großen Knochendefekten—Analyse von 12 Jahren Erfahrung mit dem Wagner-Revisionsschaft. Z Orthop. 2001;139:229–39.
60. Böhm P, Bischel O. Femoral revision with the Wagner SL revision stem. Evaluation of one hundred and twenty-nine revisions followed for a mean of 4,8 years. J Bone Joint Surg. 2001;83-A:1023–31.
61. Boisgard S, Moreau PE, Tixier M, Levai JP. Bone reconstruction, leg length discrepancy, and dislocation rate in 52 Wagner revision total hip arthroplasties at 44-month follow-up. Rev Chir Orthop Reparative Appar Mot. 2001;87:147–54.
62. Ferruzzi A, Calderoni P, Gualtieri G. Hip prostheses revisions with LS stem: indications and results. Chir Organi Mov. 2003;88:285–9.
63. Gutiérrez del Alamo J, Garcia-Cimbrelo E, Castellanos V, Gil-Garay E. Radiographic bone regeneration and clinical outcome with the Wagner SL revision stem. A 5-year or 12-year follow-up study. J Arthroplasty. 2007;22:515–24.
64. Grünig R, Morscher E, Ochsner PE. Three- to 7-year results with the uncemented SL femoral revision prosthesis. Arch Orthop Trauma Surg. 1997;116:187–97.
65. Hartwig CH, Böhm P, Czech U, Reize P. The Wagner revision stem in alloarthroplasty of the hip. Arch Orthop Trauma Surg. 1996;115:5–9.
66. Hellmsn MD, Kearns SM, Bohl DD, Haughom BD, Levine BR. Revision total hip arthroplasty with a monoblock splined tapered grit-blasted titanium stem. J Arthroplasty. 2017;32:3698–703.
67. Isacson J, Stark A, Wallensten R. The Wagner revision prosthesis consistently restores femoral bone structure. Int Orthop. 2000;24:139–42.
68. Kolstad K, Adalberth G, Mallmin H, Milbrink J, Sahlstedt B. The Wagner revision stem for severe osteolysis. Acta Orthop Scand. 1996;67:541–4.
69. Lyu SR. Use of Wagner cementless self-locking stems for massive bone loss in hip arthroplasty. J Orthop Surg (Hong Kong). 2003;11:43–7.
70. Mandellos GH, Kotsovolos H, Handes M, et al. Long distal fitting Wagner stem in failed total hip arthroplasty with extensive bone loss. Acta Orthop Trumat Hellencia. 2001;52:285–9.
71. Mantelos G, Koulouvaris P, Kotsovolos H, Xenakis T. Consistent new bone formation in 95 revisions: average 9-year follow-up. Orthopedics. 2008;31:654.
72. Regis D, Sandri A, Bonetti I, Graggion M, Bartolozzi P. Femoral revision with Wagner tapered stem. A ten-to 15 year follow-up study. J Bone Joint Surg Br. 2011;93:1320–6.
73. Sandiford NA, Garbuz DS, Masri BA, Duncan CP. Nonmodular tapered fluted titanium stems osseointegrate reliably at short term in revision THAs. Clin Orthop Relat Res. 2017;475:186–92.
74. Singh SP, Bhalodiya HP. Results of Wagner SL revision stem with impaction bone grafting in revision total hip arthroplasty. Indian J Orthop. 2013;47:357–63.
75. Wagner H. Revisionsprothese für das Hüftgelenk. Orthopäde. 1989;18:438–53.
76. Wagner H, Wagner M. Femur-Revisionsprothese. Z Orthop. 1993;131:574–7.
77. Warren PJ, Thompson P, Flechter MDA. Transfemoral implantation of the Wagner SL stem. The abolition of subsidence and enhancement of osteotomy union rate using Dall-Miles cables. Arch Orthop Trauma Surg. 2002;122:557–60.
78. Weber M, Hempfing A, Orler R, Ganz R. Femoral revision using the Wagner stem: results at 2-9 years. Int Orthop. 2002;26:36–9.
79. Wehrli U. Wagner-Revisionsprothesenschaft. Z Unfallchir Versicherungsmed. 1991;84:216–24.
80. Wilkes RA, Birch J, Pearse MF, Lee M, Atkins RM. The Wagner technique for revision arthroplasty of the hip: a review of 24 cases. J Orthop Rheumatol. 1994;7:196–8.
81. Zang J, Uchiyama K, Moriya M, Fuksuhima K, Takahira N, Takaso M. Long-term outcomes of Wagner self-locking stem with bone allograft for

Paprosky type II and III bone defects in revision total hip arthroplasty: a mean 15.7 year follow-up. J Orthop Surg. 2019;27:1–6.
82. Ngu AWT, Rowan FE, Carli AV, Haddad FS. Single 3° tapered fluted femoral stems demonstrate low subsidence at mid-term follow-up in severe bone deficiency. Ann Transl Med. 2019;7:725.
83. Gabor JA, Padilla A, Feng JE, Schnaser E, Lujes WG, Park KJ, Incova S, Vigdorchil J, Schwarzkopf R. Short-term outcomes with the REDAPT monolithic, tapered, fluted, grit-blasted, forged titanium revision femoral stem. Bone Joint J. 2020;102-B:191–7.
84. Restrepo C, Mashadi M, Parvizi J, Austin MS, Hozack WJ. Modular femoral stems for revision total hip arthroplasty. Clin Orthop Relat Res. 2011;469:476–82.
85. Kessler S, Kinkel S, Kafer W, Puhl W. Revision total hip arthroplasty: how do metaphyseal onset, diaphyseal fill and a three-point-stem-fixation influence the postoperative subsidence of a revision straight-stem? Z Orthop. 2002;140:595–602.
86. McInnis DP, Horne G, Devane PA. Femoral revision with a fluted, tapered, modular stem. Seventy patients followed for a mean of 3.9 years. J Arthroplasty. 2006;21:372–80.
87. Fink B, Hahn M, Fuerst M, Thybaut L, Delling G. Principle of fixation of the cementless modular revision stem Revitan. Unfallchirurg. 2005;108:1029–37.
88. Fink B, Grossmann A, Schubring S, Schulz MS, Fuerst M. A modified transfemoral approach using modular cementless revision stems. Clin Orthop Relat Res. 2007;462:105–14.
89. Fink B, Grossman A, Schubring S, Schulz MS, Fuerst M. Short-term results of hip revisions with a curved cementless modular stem in association with the surgical approach. Arch Orthop Trauma Surg. 2009;129:65–73.
90. Fink B, Grossmann A, Fuerst M. Distal interlocking screws with a modular revision stem for revision total hip arthroplasty in severe bone defects. J Arthroplasty. 2010;25:759–65.
91. Lakstein D, Backstein D, Safir O, Kosashvili Y, Gross AE. Revision total hip arthroplasty with porous-coated modular stem. 5 to 10 years follow-up. Clin Orthop Relat Res. 2010;468: 1310–5.
92. Jibodh SR, Schwarzkopf R, Anthony SG, Malchau H, Dempsey KE, Estik DM II. Revision hip arthroplasty with a modular cementless stem: mid-term follow up. J Arthroplasty. 2013;28:1167–72.
93. Revision Total Hip Arthroplasty Study Group. A comparison of modular tapered versus modular cylindrical stems for complex femoral revisions. J Arthroplasty. 2013;28(8 Suppl):71–3.
94. Holt G, McCaul J, Jones B, Ingram R, Stark A. Outcome after femoral revision using the restoration cone/conical femoral revision stem. Orthopaedics. 2011;34:11.
95. Desai RR, Malkani AI, Hitt KD, et al. Revision total hip arthroplasty using a modular femoral implant in Paprosky III and IV femoral bone loss. J Arthroplasty. 2012;27:1492–8.
96. Dzaja I, Lyons MC, McCalden RW, Naudie DDD, Howard JL. Revision hip arthroplasty using a modular revision system in cases of severe bone loss. J Arthroplasty. 2014;29:1594–7.
97. Stimac JD, Boles J, Parkes N, Della Valle AG, Boettner F, Westrich GH. Revision total hip arthroplasty with modular femoral stems. J Arthroplasty. 2014;29:2167–70.
98. Palumbo BT, Morrison KL, Baumgarten AS, Stein MI, Haidukewych GJ, Bernasek TL. J Arthroplasty. 2013;28:690–4.
99. Riesgo AM, Hochfelder JP, Adler EM, Slover JD, Specht LM, Iorio R. Survivorship and complications of revision total hip arthroplasty with a mid-modular femoral stem. J Arthroplasty. 2015;30:2260–3.
100. Smith MA, Deakin AH, Allen D, Baines J. Midterm outcomes of revision total hip arthroplasty using a modular revision hip system. J Arthroplasty. 2016;31:446–50.
101. Picado CHF, Savarese A, dos Santos Cardamoni V, Sugo AT, Garica FL. Clinical, radiographic, and survivorship analysis of a modular fluted tapered stem in revision hip arthroplasty. J Orthop Surg. 2019;28:1–8.
102. Park YS, Moon YM, Lim SJ. Revision total hip arthroplasty using a fluted and tapered modular distal fixation stem with and without extended trochanteric osteotomy. J Arthroplasty. 2007;22:993–9.
103. Ovesen O, Emmeluth C, Hofbauer C, Overgaard S. Revision total hip arthroplasty using a modular tapered stem with distal fixation. Good short-term results in 125 revisions. J Arthroplasty. 2010;25:348–54.
104. Canella RP, de Alencar PGC, Ganev GG, de Vinceni LF. Revision total hip arthroplasty using a modular cementless distal fixation prosthesis: the ZMR hip system. Clinical and radiographic analysis of 30 cases. Rev Bras Orthop. 2010;45: 279–85.
105. Munro JT, Garbuz DS, Masri BA, Duncan CP. Role and results of tapered fluted modular titanium stems in revision total hip arthroplasty. J Bone Joint Surg Br. 2012;94(11 Suppl A):58–60.
106. van Houwelingen AP, Duncan CP, Masri BA, Greidanus NV, Garbuz DS. High survival of modular tapered stems for proximal femoral bone defects at 5 to 10 years follow-up. Clin Orthop Relat Res. 2013;471:454–62.
107. Rieger B, Ilchmann T, Bollinger L, Stoffel KK, Zwicky L, Clauss M. Mid-term results of revision total hip arthroplasty with an uncemented modular femoral component. Hip Int. 2018;28:84–9.
108. Wronka KS, Cnudde PHJ. Midterm results following uncemented, modular, fully porous coated stem used in revision hip arthroplasty: comparison of two stem systems. J Orthop. 2016;13:298–300.

109. Kwong KL, Miller AJ, Lubinus P. A modular distal fixation option for proximal bone loss in revision total hip arthroplasty: a 2- to 6-year follow-up study. J Arthroplasty. 2003;18(3 Suppl 1):94–7.
110. Murphy SB, Rodriguez J. Revision total hip arthroplasty with proximal bone loss. J Arthroplasty. 2004;19:115–9.
111. Tamvakopoulos GS, Servant CT, Clark G, Ivory JP. Medium-term follow-up series using a modular distal fixation prosthesis to address proximal femoral bone deficiency in revision total hip arthroplasty. A 5- to 9-year follow-up study. Hip Int. 2007;17:143–9.
112. Rodirguez JA, Fada R, Murphy SB, Rasquinha VJ, Ranawat CS. Two-year to five-year follow-up of femoral defects in femoral revision treated with the link MP modular stem. J Arthroplasty. 2009;24:751–8.
113. Rodriguez JA, Deshmukh AJ, Klauser WU, Rasquinha VJ, Lubinus P, Ranawat CS. Patterns of osseointegration and remodeling in femoral revision with bone loss using modular, tapered, fluted, titanium stems. J Arthroplasty. 2011;26:1409–17.
114. Schofer MD, Efe T, Heyse TJ, Timmesfeld N, Velte R, Hinrichs F, Schmitt J. Zementfreier Femurschaftwechsel mit einem modularen Hüftendoprothesenrekonstruktionsschaft. Orthopäde. 2010;39:209–16.
115. Weiss RJ, Stark A, Kärrholm J. A modular cementless stem vs. cemented long-stem prostheses in revision surgery of the hip. A population-based study from the Swedish hip arthroplasty register. Acta Orthop. 2011;82:136–42.
116. Skyttä ET, Eskelinen A, Remes V. Successful femoral reconstruction with a fluted and tapered modular distal fixation stem in revision total hip arthroplasty. Scand J Surg. 2012;101:222–6.
117. Klauser W, Bangert Y, Lubinus P, Kendoff D. Medium-term follow-up of a modular tapered titanium stem in revision total hip arthroplasty: a single-surgeon experience. J Arthroplasty. 2013;28:84–9.
118. Wang L, Dai Z, Wen T, Li M, Hu Y. Three to seven year follow-up of a tapered modular femoral prosthesis in revision total hip arthroplasty. Arch Orthop Trauma Surg. 2013;133:275–81.
119. Ammanatullah DF, Howard JL, Siman H, Trousdale RT, Mabry TM, Berry DJ. Revision total hip arthroplasty in patients with extensive proximal femoral bone loss using a fluted tapered modular femoral component. Bone Joint J. 2015;97-B:312–7.
120. Zhang ZD, Zhuo Q, Zhang QM, Song JL, Yang F, Chen JY. Application of modular cementless femoral stems in complex revision hip arthroplasty. Zhongguo Gu Shang. 2015;28:198–204.
121. Hashem A, Al-Azzawi A, Riyadh H, Mukka S, Syed-Noor A. Cementless, modular, distally fixed stem in hip revision arthroplasty: a single-center study of 132 consecutive hips. Eur J Orthop Surg Traumatol. 2018;28:45–50.
122. Hancock DS, Sharplin PK, Larsen PD, Phillips FT. Early radiological and functional outcomes for a cementless press-fit design modular femoral stem revision system. Hip Int. 2019;29:35–40.
123. Fink B, Urbansky K, Schuster P. Mid term results with the curved modular tapered, fluted titanium Revitan stem in revision hip replacement. Bone Joint J. 2014;96-B(7):889–95.
124. Köster G, Walde TA, Willert H-G. Five- to 10-year results using a noncemented modular revision stem without bone grafting. J Arthroplasty. 2008;23:964–70.
125. Artiaco S, boggio F, Titolo P, Zoccola K, Bianchi P, Bellomo F. Clinical experience in femoral revision with the modular Profemur R stem. Hip Int. 2011;21:39–42.
126. Pattyn C, Mulliez A, Verdonk R, Audenaert E. Revision hip arthroplasty using a cementless modular tapered stem. Int Orthop. 2012;36:35–41.
127. Wirtz DC, Heller KD, Holzwarth U, Siebert C, Pitto RP, Zeiler G, Blencke BA, Forst R. A modular femoral implant for uncemented stem revision in THR. Int Orthop. 2000;24(3):134–8.
128. Schuh A, Werber S, Holzwarth U, Zeiler G. Cementless modular hip revision arthroplasty using the MRP titan revision stem: outcome of 79 hips after an average of 4 years' follow-up. Arch Orthop Trauma Surg. 2004 Jun;124(5):306–9.
129. Schuh A, Holzwarth U, Zeiler G. Titanium modular revision prosthesis stem in revision hip prosthesis. Orthopade. 2004 Jan;33(1):63–7.
130. Mumme T, Müller-Rath AS, Wirtz DC. Zementfreier Femurschaftwechsel in der Moularen Revisions Prothese MRP-Titan-Revisionsschaft. Oper Orthop Traumatol. 2007;19:56–77.
131. Wimmer MD, Randau TM, Deml MC, Ascherl R, Nöth U, Forst R, Gravius N, Wirtz D, Gravius S. Impaction grafting in femur in cementless modular revision total hip arthroplasty: a descriptive outcome analysis of 243 cases with the MRP-titan revision implant. BMC Musculoskel Dis. 2013; 14:19.
132. Wirtz D, Gravius S, Ascherl R, Thorweihe M, Forst R, Noeth U, Maus UM, Wimmer MD, Zeiler G, Deml MC. Uncemented femoral revision arthroplasty using a modular tapered, fluted titanium sem. 5- to- 16-years results in 163 cases. Acta Orthop. 2014;85:562–9.
133. Hoberg M, Konrads C, Engelien J, Oschmann D, Holder M, Walcher M, Rudert M. Outcome of a modular tapered uncemented titanium femoral stem in revision hip arthroplasty. Int Orthop. 2015;39:1709–13.
134. Richards CJ, Duncan CP, Masri BA, Garbuz DS. Femoral revision hip arthroplasty. A comparison of two stem designs. Clin Orthop Relat Res. 2010;468:491–6.
135. Fink B, Grossmann A, Schulz MS. Bone regeneration in the proximal femur following implantation of modular revision stems with distal fixation. Arch Orthop Trauma Surg. 2011;131:465–70.

Principles of Cementless Distal Fixation

7

Contents

7.1 **Scratch Fit (Cylinder-in-Cylinder Fixation)** 75

7.2 **Cone-in-Cylinder Fixation** 76

7.3 **Cone-in-Cone Fixation** 76
7.3.1 Length of Fixation Zone 82
7.3.2 Distal Interlocking 84

References 87

In order to achieve reproducibly good outcomes when using distally fixed revision stems, it is of utmost importance for the surgeon to understand the principles of fixation of the revision stem system they are using and to create the fixation zone for the stem as defined in the preoperative planning.

Generally speaking, there are three different principles of distal fixation:

1. The "scratch fit" (cylinder-in-cylinder fixation).
2. The cone-in-cylinder fixation.
3. The cone-in-cone fixation.

7.1 Scratch Fit (Cylinder-in-Cylinder Fixation)

Probably, the best-known revision stem with a so-called scratch-fit fixation is the Solution stem (DePuy Synthes, Warsaw, IN, USA) developed by Wayne Paprosky. In this case, the fixation bed is prepared in the diaphysis of the femur using a cylindrical medullary reamer or a broach. Rigid, straight broaches tend to be used for straight stems, while a flexible medullary reamer is used for curved stems. Reaming is performed until a distal, solid bone contact of approximately 4–6 cm has been established. For a distal scratch-fit fixation in the isthmus of the femur, a distally cylindrical stem, usually 0.5 mm thicker with a coarse surface structure, is then inserted into the prepared fixation bed (Fig. 7.1). Its surface structure provides the necessary rotational stability. A fixation zone in the isthmus of the femur at least 4 cm long is required for this purpose [1, 2]. This minimum fixation zone of 4 cm for the stem used by Paprosky (Solution, DePuy Synthes, Warsaw, IN, USA) prompted him to set the boundary between the Paprosky IIIA and IIIB defects at the same distance of 4 cm. If there was a fixation zone in the isthmus of at least 4 cm (Paprosky IIIA defect), the Solution stem worked with the scratch-fit fixation, but not if the fixation zone in

B. Fink, *Femoral Revision Arthroplasty*, https://doi.org/10.1007/978-3-030-84821-7_7

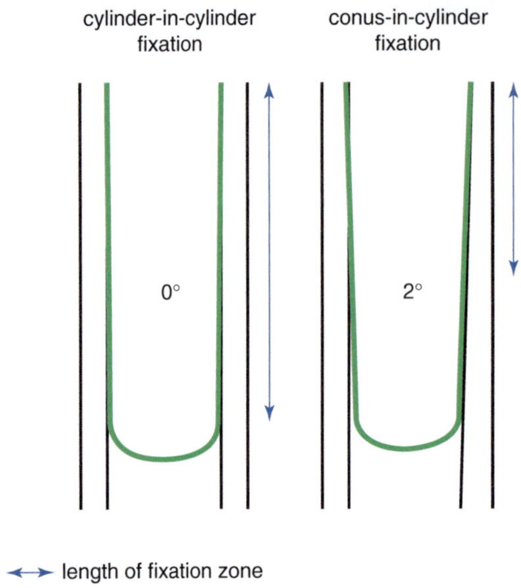

Fig. 7.1 Principle of cylinder-in-cylinder fixation, i.e., scratch fit on the left and cone-in-cylinder fixation on the right with the corresponding lengths of the fixation zone

the isthmus was less than 4 cm (Paprosky IIIB defect) (personal communication). Some modular revision stems follow this fixation principle and have distal components with scratch-fit fixation, such as the Arcos or ZMR system (Zimmer Biomet, Warsaw, IN, USA) and the Restoration stem system (Stryker, Kalamazoo, MI, USA).

7.2 Cone-in-Cylinder Fixation

Here, curved, distally tapered titanium stems are placed in a cylindrically prepared fixation bed of the femur. The fixation bed is prepared with flexible medullary reamers until a firm cortical contact over several centimeters is achieved, and then, a tapered, curved, distally fixing revision stem is inserted. This revision stem has a star shape similar to the tapered straight stems with longitudinal splines that cut into the cortex (Fig. 7.1). Depending on the manufacturer's definition of the stem diameter, a stem that is 2–3 mm thicker than the last medullary reamer is used as the distal stem component. This is recommended for the curved version of the modular MRP stem (Peter Brehm GmbH, Germany), which requires between 7 and 10 cm of bone contact [3, 4]. There is no conical fixation bed prepared in the cortex so the tapered stem must cut into the cylindrical fixation bed as it is being impacted. It is therefore likely that the thickness of the selected stem will be thinner than in the case of a cone-in-cone fixation (see below), as it can be assumed that the stem will not cut so deeply into the cortex if the bed has not been prepared with conical reamers or rasps.

7.3 Cone-in-Cone Fixation

This fixation is based on the fixation principle developed by Heinz Wagner for his revision stem. Conical reamers are used to create a conical fixation bed in the diaphysis of the femur, into which a tapered titanium stem with longitudinal flutes is inserted, cutting into the cortex [5, 6] (Fig. 7.2). In the final stem from Wagner and its direct successor, the Wagner SL revision stem (Zimmer Biomet, Winterthur, Switzerland), the taper is 2°, which creates the axial stability of the stem. The 8 longitudinal splines of the stem create rotational stability by cutting into the cortex (Fig. 7.3). The

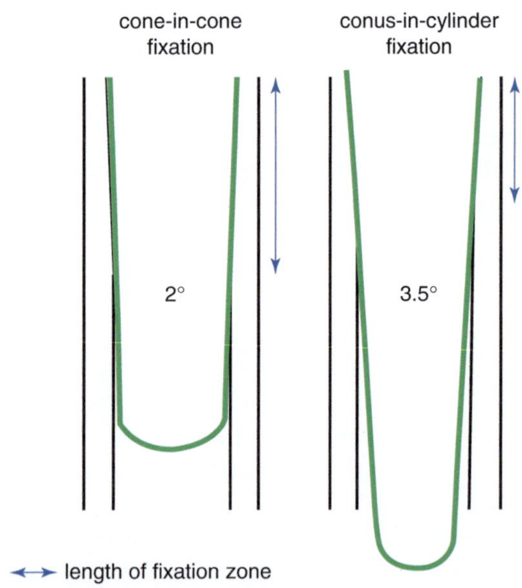

Fig. 7.2 Principle of cone-in-cylinder fixation for a 2-degree tapered revision stem on the left and a 3.5-degree tapered revision stem on the right

modular version of the Wagner stem, the Revitan Straight (Zimmer Biomet, Winterthur, Switzerland), is round in the cross section of the longitudinal ribs, but the core of the stem is flattened in the frontal plane to ensure better elasticity (Fig. 7.3). Bircher et al. [7] used pathological and histological preparations to show that there is adequate bone growth onto the star-shaped profile of the stem.

Cone-in-cone is a well-known method of firm fixation from the world of engineering. In femoral revision arthroplasty, it functions reliably over a fixation distance of 3–5 cm [8, 9]. It is not possible to prepare a longer conical fixation bed in the cortex of the femur without significantly reducing the thickness of the cortex and, thus, weakening it. In biomechanical studies, Kirk et al. [10] and Russell et al. [11] demonstrated that a tapered stem with splines (Link MP, Waldemar Link, Hamburg, Germany, for Kirk et al. [10], and Wagner SL Stem, Zimmer Biomet, Warsaw, IN, USA, for Russell et al. [11]) and a cone-in-cone fixation in the isthmus produces greater stability than a cylindrical fully coated, roughly structured stem with a scratch-fit fixation (Solution, DePuy Synthes, Warsaw, IN, USA, for Kirk et al. [10] and Versys, Zimmer Biomet, Warsaw, IN, USA, for Russell et al. [11]).

Many revision stems have been developed on the basis of the original Wagner revision stem, some of which use the same taper of 2° (Revitan, Zimmer Biomet Winterthur, Switzerland; MRP stem, Peter Brehm Germany; MP Stem, Waldemar Link, Hamburg, Germany) and other angles (2.5° for the Reclaim Stem, DePuy Synthes, Warsaw, IN; 3° for the Arcos Stem, Zimmer Biomet, Warsaw, IN, USA; 3.5° for the ZMR Stem, Zimmer Biomet, Warsaw, IN, USA)

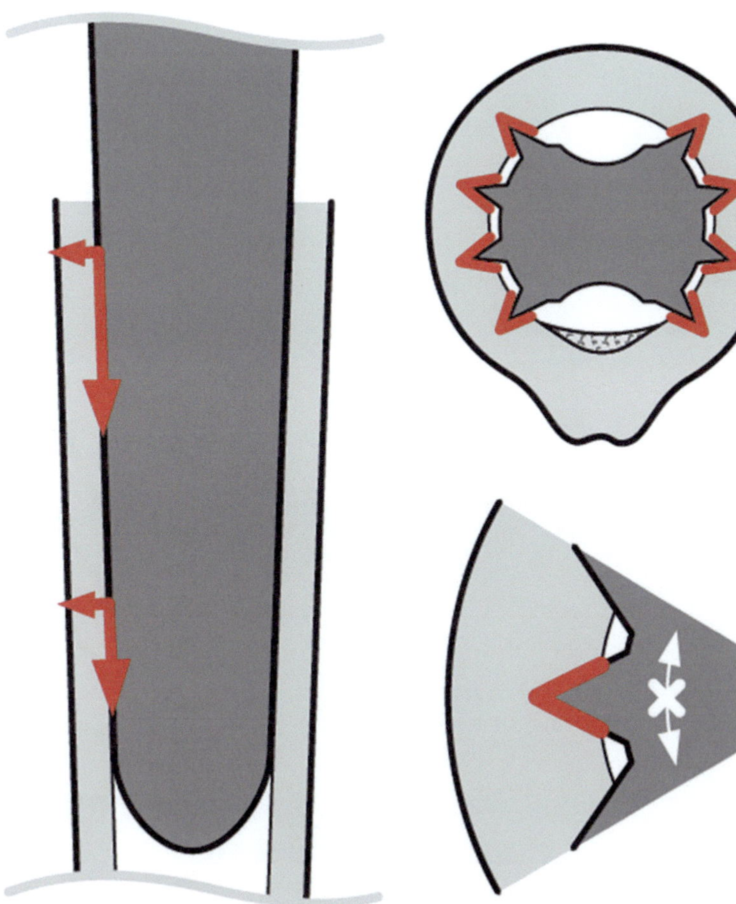

Fig. 7.3 Cone-in-cone fixation with the Wagner SL Stem or the modular variant Revitan Straight (Zimmer Biomet, Winterthur, Switzerland)

(Fig. 7.2). The details of the differences are discussed in the next chapter (Chap. 8).

There are also tapered, curved modular stems, where the fixation bed is first prepared cylindrically with flexible medullary reamers and then conically with conical rasps increasing in size. One of these is the Revitan Curved stem (Zimmer Biomet, Winterthur, Switzerland). Here, the curved distal component is octagonal in cross section and also has a 2-degree taper. Its rotational stability is created by the ribs (longitudinal flutes) of the octagonal cross section.

There are two approaches that can be applied to the implantation of revision stems: endofemoral and transfemoral approaches. Longer straight stems, usually more than 225 mm long, have to be implanted via a transfemoral approach in order to avoid ventral perforation of the femur [5–7]. Curved stems, on the other hand, can be implanted endofemorally with greater lengths provided there is no deformity of the femur.

Transfemoral and endofemoral implantation results in different cone-in-cone fixations, as shown in our own cadaver studies involving contact radiographs [8]. The transfemoral implantation of the Revitan Straight revision stem (Zimmer Biomet, Winterthur, Switzerland) revealed a circular cone-in-cone fixation of all splines in the cortex of the isthmus and resulted in a firm press-fit fixation (Fig. 7.4). A similar distal press-fit fixation was observed with the Revitan Curved stem (Zimmer Biomet Winterthur, Switzerland) after transfemoral implantation, with the preparation of the fixation bed in the isthmus of the femur by rasping. There was similar circular penetration of all splines of the octagonal stem into the cortical bone of the isthmus (Fig. 7.5). Endofemoral implantation of

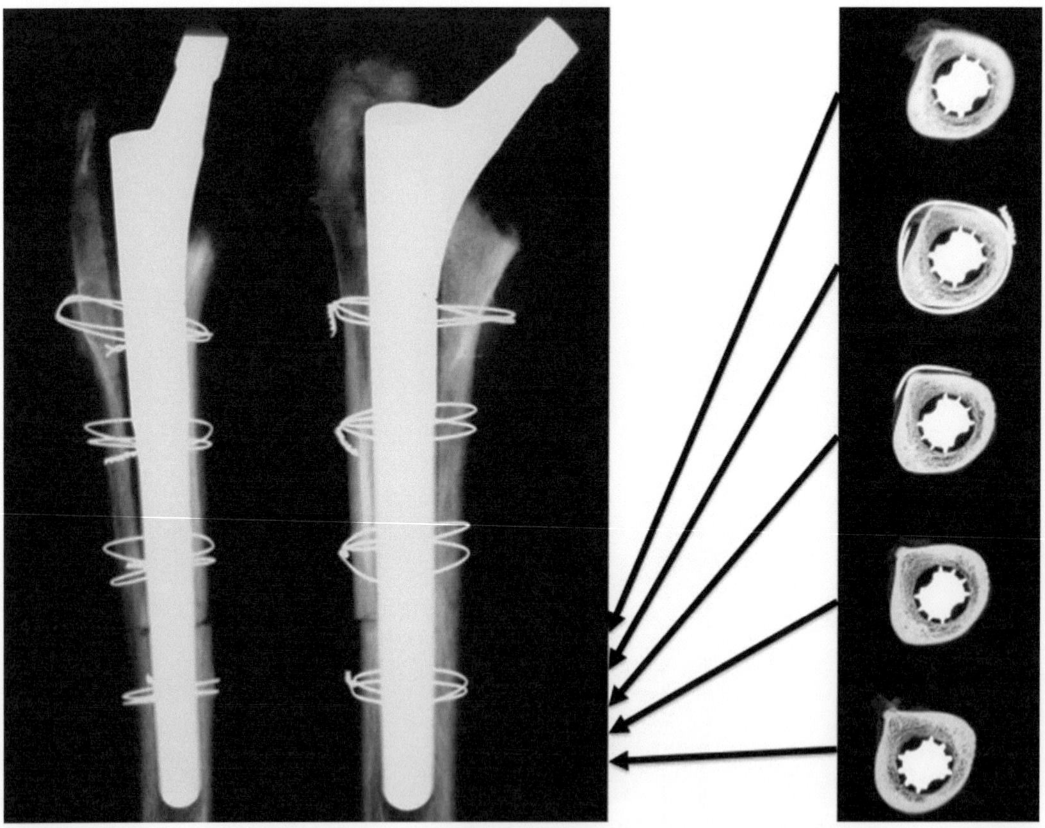

Fig. 7.4 Contact radiography of the distal cone-in-cone fixation with the Revitan Straight stem

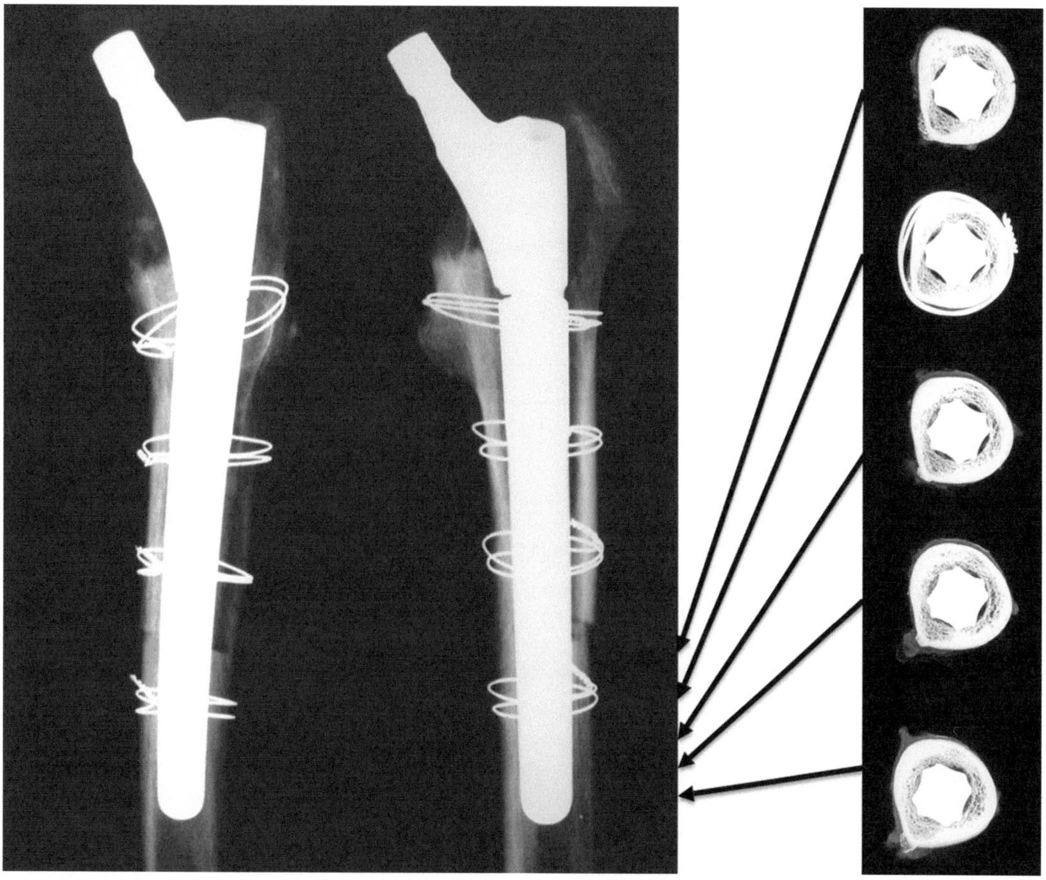

Fig. 7.5 Contact radiography of the distal cone-in-cone fixation with the Revitan Curved stem

the Revitan Curved stem on the opposite side of the cadaver (as with the transfemoral implantation of the Revitan Curved) showed a different cone-in-cone fixation, which we have called three-surface fixation [8]. Here, three splines of the octagonal structure of the stem cut distally into the bone for several centimeters (3–4 cm), while, further proximally in the diaphysis and/or meta-diaphyseal transition, three other splines also cut into the bone for several centimeters (3–4 cm) (Fig. 7.6). Even further proximal, in the metaphysis, only 2 ribs of the octagonal structure were in contact with the bone, and no longer participated in the rotational stability of the stem or in the primary fixation of the stem. They only served for secondary osteointegration and thus for secondary stability of the stem (Fig. 7.6). Thus, instead of a circular cone-in-cone fixation of 3–5 cm (Fig. 7.7) as in transfemoral implantation, a cone-in-cone fixation of two times 3/4 of the circumference of 3–4 cm is produced (Fig. 7.8). This results in an overall cone-in-cone fixation of 6–8 cm and for a 3/4 circumference, which gives the stem its axial fixation and rotational stability. Circular incision of all 4 splines of the octagonal Revitan Curved stem during endofemoral implantation would only be possible if the radius of the antecurvature of the femur was exactly equal to that of the revision stem (1.2 m for the Revitan Curved). However, this can never be assumed, or only extremely rarely. The different lengths of the fixation zones of the three-surface fixation and the differences in the implant diameter to that of the transfemoral implanted stem on the opposite side of the cadaver were the result of the different antecurvatures and cross sections of the femurs involved [8].

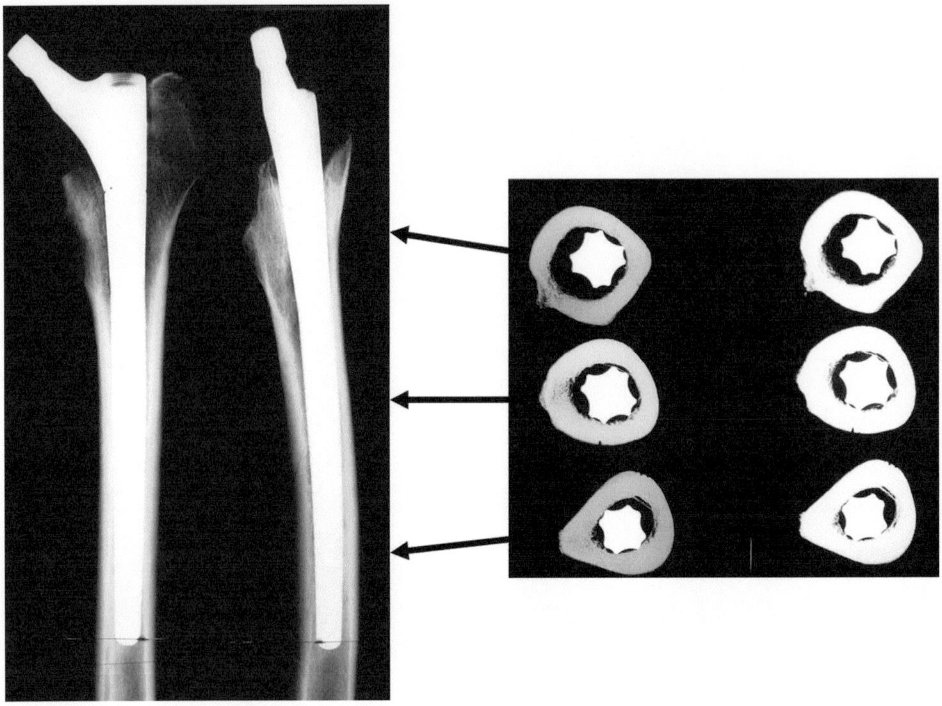

Fig. 7.6 Contact radiograph of the fixation zones of the three-surface fixation of the endofemorally implanted Revitan Curved stems

Fig. 7.7 Distal fixation zone in a transfemorally implanted Revitan Curved stem (left) with follow-up radiograph 3 years after surgery (right)

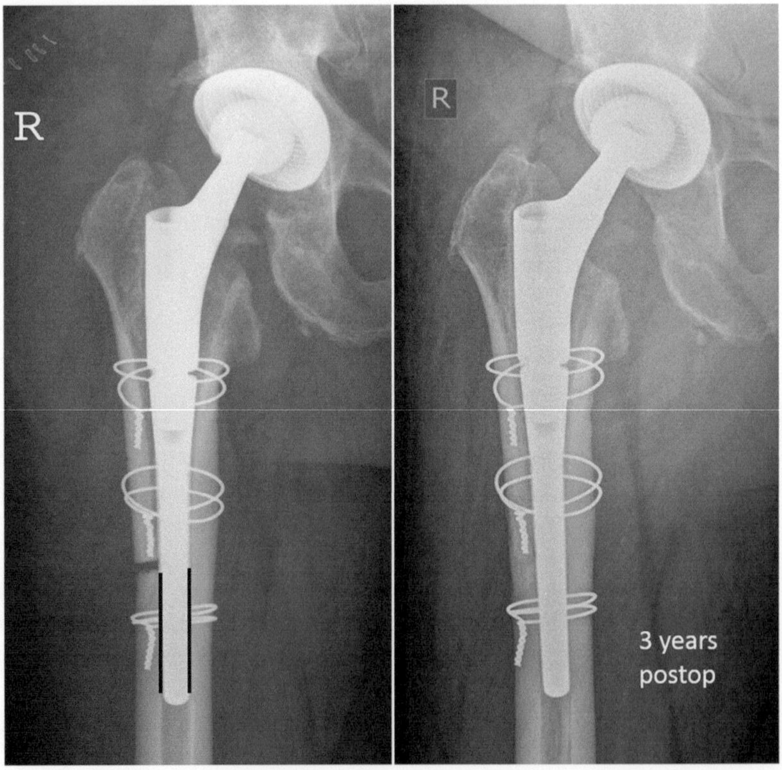

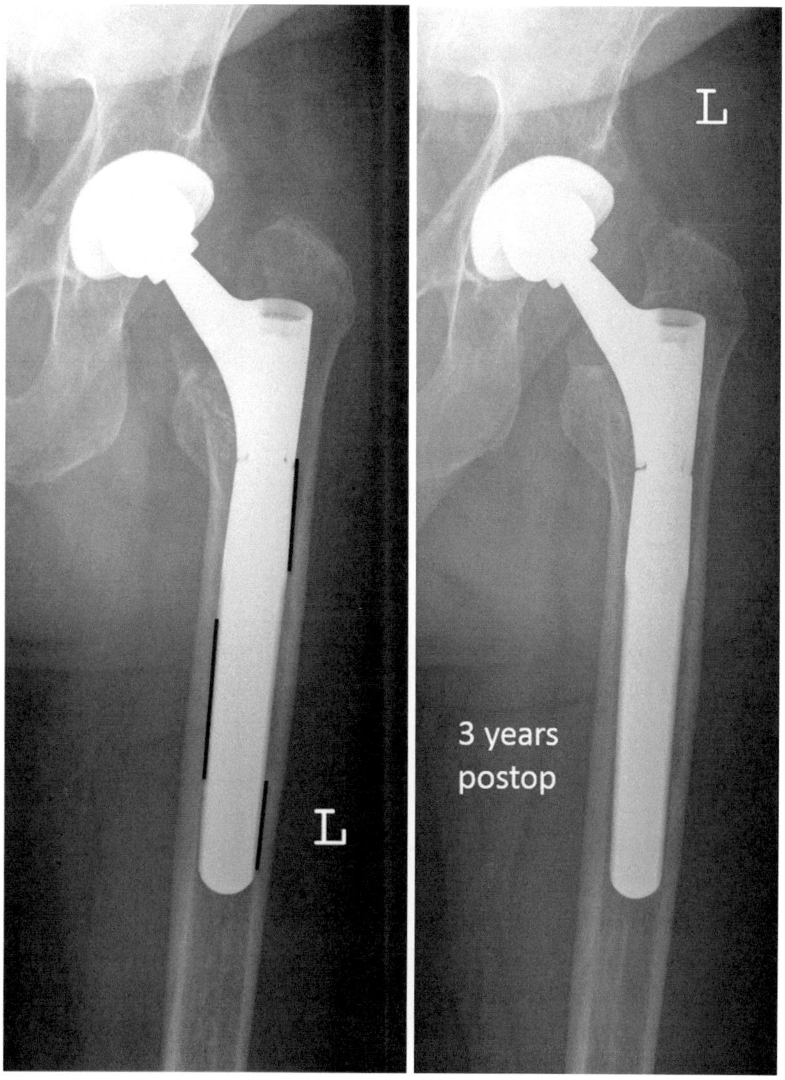

Fig. 7.8 Three-surface fixation of an endofemorally implanted Revitan Curved stem (left) with follow-up radiograph 3 years after surgery (right)

Comparing these two categories of cone-in-cone fixation (circular for transfemoral and three surfaces for endofemoral implantation) shows that different prosthesis component combinations will need to be selected for the same femur. Endofemoral implantation results in thinner and slightly longer component combinations than transfemoral implantation, as shown for the Revitan Curved stem in our cadaver study [8] (Figs. 7.7 and 7.8). This is also apparent during the intraoperative implantation of the Revitan Curved stem. In a transfemoral approach, after cylindrical reaming of the isthmus with a flexible medullary reamer, the conical fixation bed is gradually prepared with conical rasps. In this process, the final rasp, which creates a conical fixation at the tip of the stem, has a nominal diameter that is 4 mm greater than the thickness of the final medullary reamer. However, this in no way implies a press fit of 4 mm. The 4-mm difference results from the fact that the nominal thickness of the Revitan stem is measured 11 cm above the tip of the stem. With a taper of 2°, this results in the appropriate dimension at the tip of the stem for cone-in-cone fixation. However, the endofemoral approach never results in a difference of 4 mm but rather, depending on the radius of the curvature, a difference of 2 or 3 mm between the medullary reamer on the one hand and rasp and/or distal component diameter on the other.

As our cadaver studies were able to show, the endofemoral implantation of the Revitan Curved stem also results in a distal fixation in the femoral diaphysis, whereby this cone-in-cone fixation is a function of the two distal surfaces of the three-surface fixation. This knowledge can be used in the endofemoral implantation of these types of stem, so that in situ assembly of the modular components can be performed after secure fixation of the distal component and trial positioning with the proximal trial component. This will be discussed in more detail in the corresponding Chaps. 11 and 16.

The three-surface fixation described here, which involves cone-in-cone fixation of the stem by two distal surfaces, must not be confused with the three-point fixation of a straight stem. The latter implies only short-range bone contact of a to thin, and usually to long, straight stem in the curved femur, which results in insufficient fixation of the stem and leads to subsidence of the stem.

7.3.1 Length of Fixation Zone

As shown in our own clinical studies and radiographic evaluations of 120 revision operations with the Revitan Curved system, transfemoral implantation to give a 3 cm long, circular cone-in-cone fixation in the isthmus of the femur is sufficient for adequate fixation without subsidence of the 2-degree tapered stem [9]. The 5 of the 78 transfemoral implanted stems that exhibited subsidence all had fixation zones less than 3 cm because of defects or fractures in the isthmus of the femur. None of the transfemorally implanted stems with a fixation zone of 3 cm or more showed any subsidence [9]. Thus, for distal cone-in-cone fixation of a 2-degree tapered revision stem, a fixation zone of 3 cm in the isthmus of the shaft is sufficient. In contrast, a scratch fit (cylinder-in-cylinder fixation) requires at least 4 cm [2]. The length of the fixation zone required for distal cone-in-cone fixation depends, in part, on the thickness of the cortex of the isthmus. A thick cortex allows deeper incision of the ribs or splines of the stem and therefore necessitates only a short fixation zone. A thinner cortex does not allow as much penetration because of the risk of fracture, so fixation needs to be accomplished over a longer region of contact in the isthmus (Figs. 7.7 and 7.9a, b). This can be achieved with the transfemoral implantation of the 2-degree tapered stem, when the difference between the final intramedullary reamer diameter and that of the implanted stem is 3 mm instead of 4 mm (as mentioned above).

Secondly, the length of the required fixation zone depends on the degree of taper of the distal stem. Pierson et al. [12] demonstrated in a biomechanical study that the axial stability of the tapered stem increases with increasing taper, because there is more spline penetration over a shorter distance of cortical bone. In line with this, Tangsataporn et al. [13] found that for the ZMR stem (Zimmer Biomet, Warsaw, IN, USA) with a taper of 3.5°, the risk of subsidence was related to a fixation zone of less than 2 cm. Thus, increasing taper results in a shorter minimum fixation zone (Fig. 7.2). However, a sufficiently thick cortex is also necessary.

According to our own studies, the fixation zone for a 2-degree tapered stem must be at least 3 cm, as already mentioned [9]. For the 2-degree tapered stems with distal cone-in-cone fixation, this can be in the isthmus of the femur at the tip of the stem. The fixation zone in the isthmus of the femur is prepared and predetermined with conical reamers (for a straight stem) or rasps (for the Revitan Curved stem). The tapered stem of a defined length is now fixed in this predetermined fixation zone. This can be at the tip of the stem (with a taper of 2°). A longer stem or distal component does not result in a longer fixation zone; instead, the same length of fixation is achieved, but the zone is located above the tip of the stem or of the distal component (Fig. 7.10). Longer stems thus do not result in a longer fixation zone, but in some cases may even lead to a worse fixation, namely when the circular press-fit fixation is replaced by a three-point fixation in the isthmus of the femur [14]. De Menezes et al. [14] evaluated 100 transfemorally implanted Revitan Straight stems and showed that short stems with

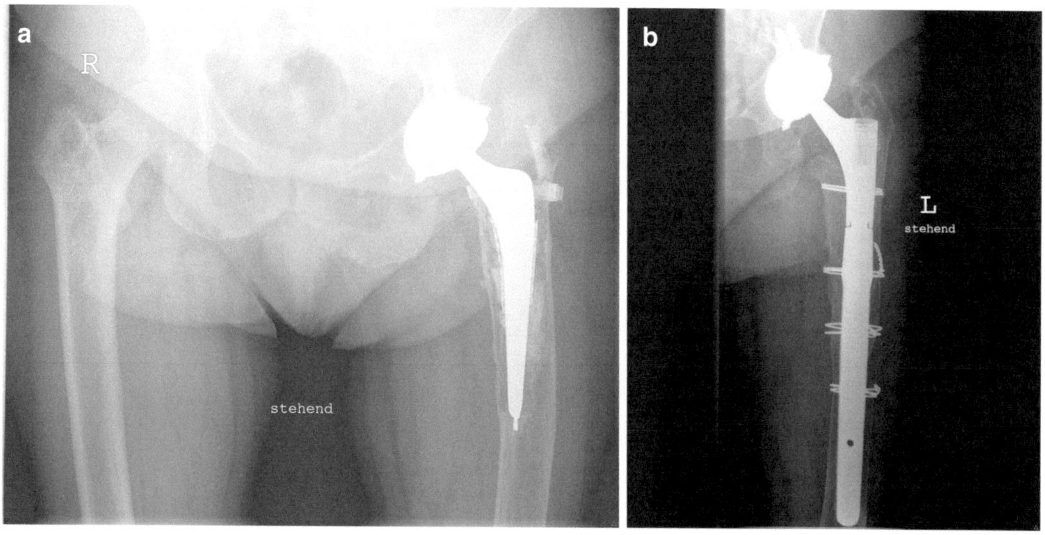

Fig. 7.9 (**a**) Stem loosening on the left with variation of the femur and thin cortical bone in the isthmus of the femur. (**b**) Radiograph 2 years postoperatively after transfemoral stem revision to Revitan Curved stem. The contact area in the distal femur is longer than in the example of Fig. 7.7 because of the thin cortical bone. Here, a difference of 3 mm between the last medullary reamer and nominal stem thickness was chosen because of the thin cortical bone

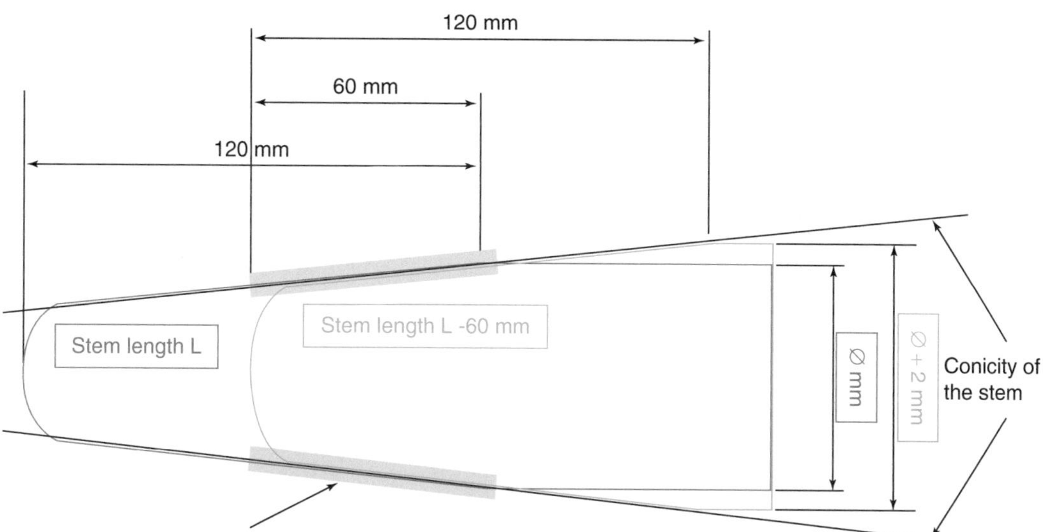

Fig. 7.10 Schematic representation of the localization of the fixation zone with a thicker (green) and thinner longer (red) tapered stem

fixation at the tip of the stem in the isthmus had a lower rate of subsidence than longer stems.

The height of the fixation zone on the stem, that is, the regions on the stem that penetrate the distal cortex, depends on the degree of taper of the stem. Two-degree tapered stems, as mentioned, can produce fixation at the tip, i.e., the distal end. In stems with higher degrees of taper, this zone is more proximal, and the greater the angle of taper, the higher the location on the stem

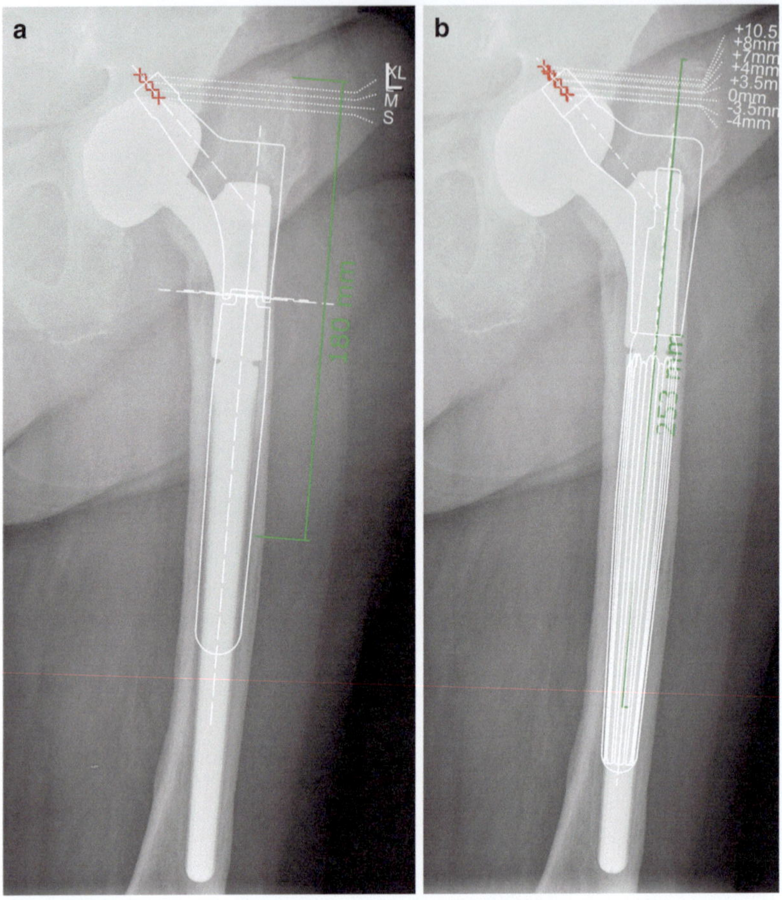

Fig. 7.11 (**a**) Planning of a transfemoral stem revision using the 2-degree tapered Revitan Curved modular revision stem. (**b**) Component planning when using the 3.5-degree tapered modular revision stem ZMR (Zimmer Biomet, Warsaw, IN, USA), which would also be implanted transfemorally. Because of the greater taper, the fixation zone here is more proximal on the distal component, resulting in a longer stem combination than in Fig. 4.50a

that cuts into the distal cortex (the isthmus in the transfemoral approach) (Fig. 7.11a, b).

7.3.2 Distal Interlocking

If the fixation zone in the isthmus of the femur is less than 3 cm because of a defect or fracture associated with a Vancouver B3 type periprosthetic fracture, then according to the above, the isthmus is not suitable for either scratch-fit fixation (at least 4 cm) or for cone-in-cone fixation of a 2-degree tapered stem alone. According to our earlier discussion, a distally fixed stem with greater taper (3.5°) would still work in these cases up to a minimum fixation zone of 2 cm provided there is good cortical thickness over this shorter distance [13]. Alternatively, if a 2-degree tapered stem is used, additional fixation support in the form of distal locking screws is required (Fig. 7.12a–c). In biomechanical studies, Mohamed et al. [15] demonstrated that distal locking screws could significantly increase the axial and rotational stability of distally fixed stems.

However, anchorage of the stem is still based on, and requires, cone-in-cone fixation, in this case in a zone less than 3 cm, which is created via a transfemoral approach according to the same principles (cylindrical reaming with medullary reamer, followed by preparation of the fixation bed using conical shaping rasps). After careful positioning of the stem with a cone-in-cone fixation of less than 3 cm in the deficient isthmus, adjunctive fixation is then created below the isthmus with locking screws (Fig. 7.12b, c). These provide additional stability until callus formation resulting from the transfemoral approach has enabled bone to grow onto the proximal portions of the newly implanted stem. This type of locking

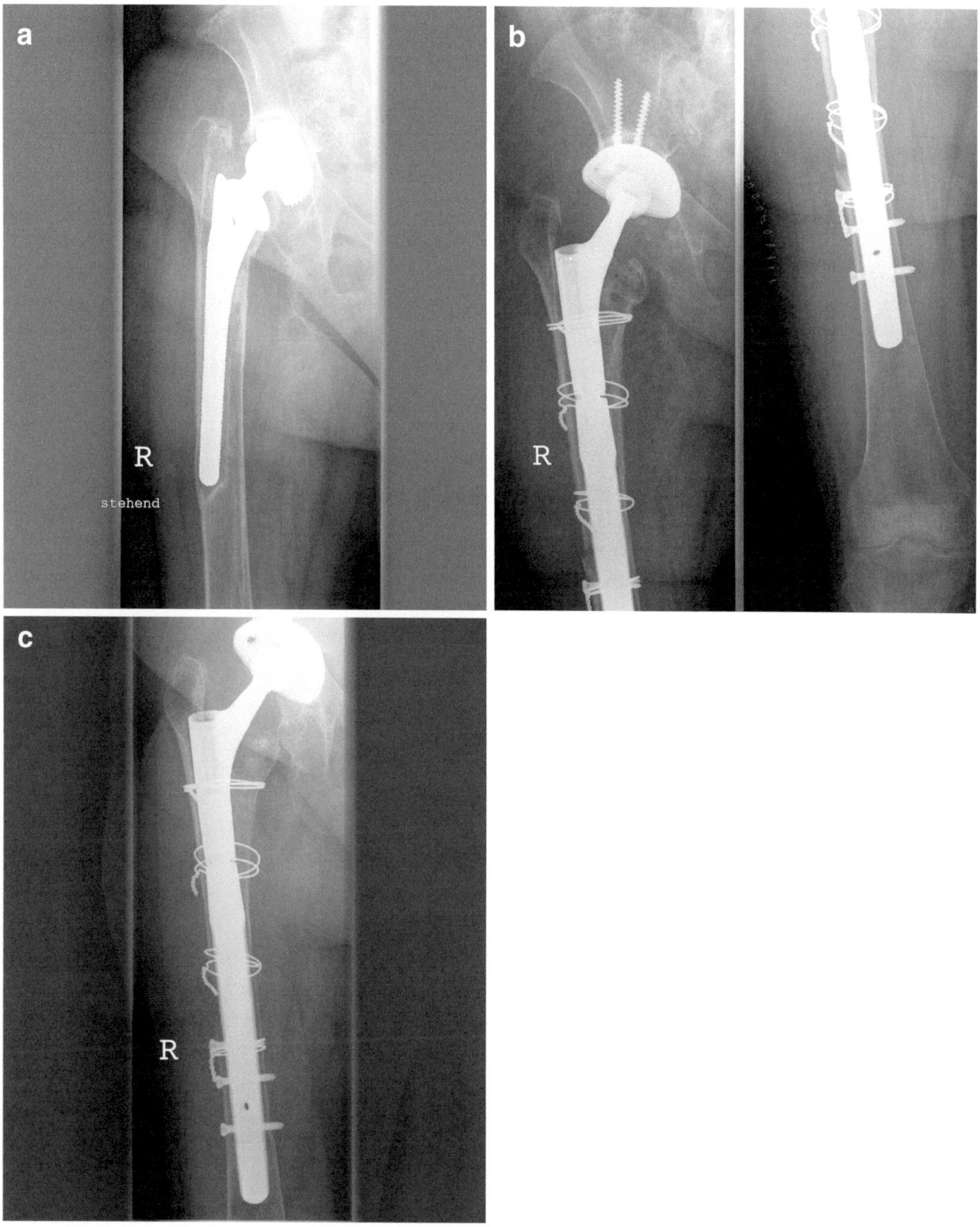

Fig. 7.12 (**a**) Prosthesis loosening on the right with femoral bone defect of the Paprosky IV type with missing isthmus. (**b**) Transfemoral prosthesis revision to Revitan Curved modular revision stem and Allofit-S press-fit cup (Zimmer Biomet, Winterthur, Switzerland). Short cone-in-cone fixation of the stem can be seen above the adjunctive distal locking. (**c**) Radiograph 8 years after surgery showing unchanged position of the implants

system constitutes a method for supporting the short cone-in-cone fixation in the deficient isthmus. It should not be confused with multiple locking over a long section of a cylindrical revision stem (e.g., Huckstep stem, Downs Surgical, Chapeltown, UK, or a variant of the Acros stem,

Zimmer Biomet, Warsaw, IN, USA). I do not recommend the latter because of the significantly greater trauma to the soft tissues and the impaired ability to retract or revise, for example, in the event of a periprosthetic infection.

In a follow-up study of 15 cases in which locking was necessary because of defects or fractures in the isthmus, 14 cases showed stable fixation without subsidence of the stem, radiolucency around the locking screws, or even breakage of the same [16] (Fig. 7.12a–c). Only in one case, where fixation was based on the locking screws alone and a short cone-in-cone fixation could not be achieved, did the fixation fail with fracture of the locking screws [16]. Fixation by locking screws alone is not sufficient to achieve reproducibly good outcomes. This was confirmed by the findings of Eingärnter et al. [17], who saw system failure in more than 12% (5 cases) of 41 periprosthetic fractures (2 Vancouver type A, 14 B1, 8 B2, and 13 Vancouver B3 fractures) with the low-taper Bicontact Revision stem (Aesculap, Tuttlingen, Germany) (0.6° of taper) and additional locking. Because of this stem's low taper of 0.6°, fixation relied heavily on the locking screws. In addition, poorer outcomes for multiple locking have also been reported for the cylindrical Huckstep stem. Aspinall et al. [18] reported short-term results of the Huckstep stem in 57 patients who had difficult primary implantations and revisions with femoral defects. Revisions were required in 19.3%, 7% suffered screw fractures as a sign of stem instability, 3.5% periprosthetic fractures, and 8.8% periprosthetic infections.

Some modular revision stem systems (e.g., Restoration (Stryker, Kalamazoo, MI, USA), Arcos (Zimmer Biomet, Warsaw, IN, USA)) offer a number of distal components with different fixation principles (scratch fit, cone-in-cone) that can be combined with several proximal components of different designs and principles (cylindrical, conical, calcar). However, the company's efforts to offer the surgeon all possible options do not make it any easier for him/her to choose the right one. Instead, it requires a high level of understanding on the part of the surgeon of the various fixation principles. In such cases, I recommend the surgeon chooses either one of the distal fixation principles, so that the learning curve with the handling of this system is as short and steep as possible, or he/she establishes a clear, defect-oriented concept for the selection of stems or fixation principles. In my opinion, it makes no sense here to mix different principles. If, for example, because of the type of defect, a decision has been made in favor of a distal fixation modular revision system and, for example, the conically fixed distal component is firmly fixed in situ, the proximal component is used purely for correct adjustment of the leg length and antetorsion as well as reconstruction of the center of rotation and offsets. Therefore, there is no need for a voluminous proximal component with the aim of achieving additional proximal fixation. Distal fixation and proximal fixation do not work together, either distally or proximally, never both. A voluminous proximal component risks unnecessary pressure on the greater trochanter with the consequent risk of fracture, especially in the case of a tapered form.

Some distal components of some multifaceted modular revision systems attempt to improve fixation in the femur by combining different principles. For example, the Arcos modular revision system (Zimmer Biomet, Warsaw, IN) features a cylindrical, coarse-textured, curved component that can be locked along its entire length in three additional locations (Fig. 6.24). In my opinion, it is very difficult for the surgeon to plan preoperatively and gauge intraoperatively when he or she will need additional locking screws with this approach. This is different with the Revitan Curved tapered revision stem, where it is possible to measure preoperatively whether there is a fixation zone in the isthmus of 3 cm (no locking) or not (locking). In the case of a deficient isthmus, a scratch fit is no longer an option, and the fixation of an insufficiently fixed stem using only locking screws does not promise reproducibly achievable good outcomes. Moreover, additional locking along the entire length of the stem is associated with further traumatization of the musculature that is important for the blood supply to the femur.

References

1. Paprosky WG, Greidanus NV, Antoniou J. Minimum 10-year-results of extensively porous-coated stems in revision hip arthroplasty. Clin Orthop. 1999;369:230–42.
2. Weeden SH, Paprosky WG. Minimal 11-year follow-up of extensively porous-coated stems in femoral revision total hip arthroplasty. J Arthroplasty. 2002;17 Suppl:134–7.
3. Mumme T, Müller-Rath AS, Wirtz DC. Zementfreier Femurschaftwechsel in der Moularen Revisions Prothese MRP-Titan-Revisionsschaft. Oper Orthop Traumatol. 2007;19:56–77.
4. Wimmer MD, Randau TM, Deml MC, Ascherl R, Nöth U, Forst R, Gravius N, Wirtz D, Gravius S. Impaction grafting in femur in cementless modular revision total hip arthroplasty: a descriptive outcome analysis of 243 cases with the MRP-Titan revision implant. BMC Musculoskelet Disord. 2013;14:19.
5. Wagner H. Revisionsprothese für das Hüftgelenk. Orthopäde. 1989;18:438–53.
6. Wagner H, Wagner M. Femur-Revisionsprothese. Z Orthop. 1993;131:574–7.
7. Bircher HP, Riede U, Lüem M, Ochsner PE. Der Wert der SL-Revisionsprothese nach Wagner zur Überbrückung großer Femurdefekte. Technik und Resultate. Orthopäde. 2001;30:294–303.
8. Fink B, Hahn M, Fuerst M, Thybaut L, Delling G. Principle of fixation of the cementless modular revision stem Revitan. Unfallchirurg. 2005;108:1029–37.
9. Fink B, Grossman A, Schubring S, Schulz MS, Fuerst M. Short-term results of hip revisions with a curved cementless modular stem in association with the surgical approach. Arch Orthop Trauma Surg. 2009;129:65–73.
10. Kirk KL, Potter BK, Lehman R, Xenos JS. Effect of distal stem geometry on interface motion in uncemented revision total hip prostheses. Am J Orthop. 2007;36:545–9.
11. Russell RD, Pierce W, Huo MH. Tapered vs cylindrical stem fixation in a model of femoral bone deficiency in revision total hip arthroplasty. J Arthroplasty. 2016;31:1352–5.
12. Pierson JL, Small SR, Rodriguez JA, et al. The effect of taper angle and spline geometry on the initial stability of tapered, splined modular titanium stems. J Arthroplasty. 2015;30:1254–9.
13. Tangsataporn S, Safir OA, Vincent AD, Abdelbary H, Gross AE, Kuzyk PRT. Risk factors for subsidence of a modular tapered femoral stem used for revision total hip arthroplasty. J Arthroplasty. 2015;30:1030–134.
14. De Menezes DFA, Le Béguec P, Sieber HP, Goldschild M. Stem and osteotomy length are critical for the transfemoral approach and cementless stem revision. Clin Orthop Relat Res. 2012;470:883–8.
15. Mohamed N, Schatzker J, Hearn T. Biomechanical analysis of a distally interlocked press-fit femoral total hip prosthesis. J Arthroplasty. 1993;8:129–32.
16. Fink B, Grossmann A, Fuerst M. Distal interlocking screws with a modular revision stem for revision total hip arthroplasty in severe bone defects. J Arthroplasty. 2010;25:759–65.
17. Eingärtner C, Ochs U, Egetemeyer D, Volkmann R. Treatment of periprosthetic femoral fractures with the Bicontact revision stem. Z Orthop Unfall. 2007;145(Suppl 1):S29–33.
18. Aspinall GR, Nicholls A, Kerry RM, Hamer AJ, Stockley I. The short term outcome of the Huckstep hip prosthesis. Orthop Proc. 2004;86-A(Suppl I):72.

Differences in Distal Fixated Revision Stems

8

Content

References 97

The various stem systems with distal fixation have different characteristics that the surgeon should be aware of. For example, the length of the tapered portion of the distal components of the different stem systems varies. In addition, the length of the tapered portion of the distal components of one and the same system can vary. For example, in the Revitan system (Zimmer Biomet, Winterthur, Switzerland), the tapered section is 10 cm long for the shorter distal component and 12 cm for the longer distal components (Fig. 8.1). Similarly, long tapered sections exist for the ZMR stem (Zimmer Biomet, Warsaw, IN, USA), the Redapt (Smith & Nephew, Memphis, TN, USA), the Profemur R (Microport Orthopedics, Arlington, TN, USA), and the Prevision stem (Aesculap, Tuttlingen, Germany) (Table 8.1). The Link MP stem (Waldemar Link, Hamburg, Germany) has a tapered section of 83 mm for the three lengths 160 mm, 180 mm, and 210 mm and then increases with increasing length of the distal component (Table 8.1). Other stems, such as the MRP stem (Peter Brehm, Weisendorf, Germany), the Arcos stem (Zimmer Biomet, Warsaw, IN, USA), and the Prevision stem (Stryker, Kalamazoo, MI, USA), have a taper over the entire length of the distal component of all lengths.

Furthermore, the nomenclature for the thickness of the shaft is not uniform. The height that determines the designation of the stem thickness for the monoblock stem or the distal component of the modular system differs from stem to stem. This is not even uniform for different stems within a single manufacturer, because of the company mergers that have taken place. In the case of the Revitan stem system, for example, the thickness of the stem is defined by the diameter of the stem at a height of 11 cm above the tip of the stem. Paradoxically, since the short distal component of the Revitan system, with a length of 140 mm, has a taper of only 10 cm, it does not actually attain the thickness indicated by its name. For the longer distal components, the length of the tapered section is 12 cm. In the Arcos system (Zimmer Biomet, Warsaw, IN, USA), the thickness reference point is 10.3 cm above the tip for the shorter tapered distal component (150 mm) and the ETO variant (250 mm), and 14.3 cm above the tip for the 190 mm distal component. For the Restoration stem (Stryker, Kalamazoo, MI, USA), the thickness is measured 12 cm above the tip, for the Prevision stem (Aesculap, Tuttlingen, Germany) 4 cm, and for the Profemur R (Microport Orthopedics,

B. Fink, *Femoral Revision Arthroplasty*, https://doi.org/10.1007/978-3-030-84821-7_8

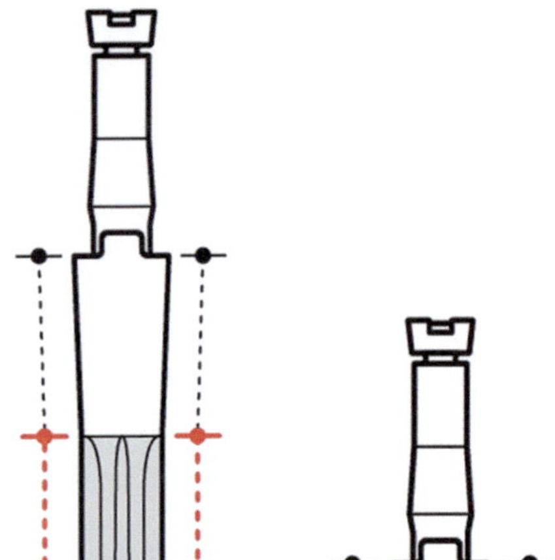

Fig. 8.1 Tapered portion of the distal components of the Revitan system (Zimmer Biomet, Winterthur, Switzerland)

Arlington, TN, USA) 3 cm above the tip. For the Link MP stem (Waldemar Link, Hamburg, Germany), the diameter of the stem is determined at a height of 84.5 mm from distal for the three distal components of length 160 mm, 180 mm, and 210 mm. With increasing length of the subsequent distal components, the thickness is defined more proximally (Table 8.1). For the MRP stem (Peter Brehm, Weisendorf, Germany), the height of the nominal diameter also changes with the length of the distal component, but only for the first three lengths, since the distance from proximal for those thereafter remains constant. The nominal diameter is set at 5.5 cm from the distal tip of the 80 mm long distal component, 9.5 cm for the 140 mm long component, and 13.5 cm for the 200 mm long distal component. For the distal components of 260 mm and 320 mm length, the thickness of the stem is determined directly at the prosthesis distal tip (Table 8.1). The Reclaim stem (DePuy Synthes, Warsaw, IN, USA) and the MUTARS revision stem (implantcast, Buxtehude, Germany) follow a similar principle. Here, too, the distance from the distal prosthesis tip to the height of the nominal diameter marking changes with the length of the distal component. However, the increase in this distance remains constant with the increase in length of the distal component. Thus, different stems cannot necessarily be compared with each other in terms of their thickness specifications (Table 8.1).

From the above, it follows that a difference with respect to the nominal diameter definition for the different lengths is whether the distance to the point of nominal diameter definition is measured from distal or proximal and whether it remains constant for the different lengths. On the one hand, there are stems in which the thickness is measured at a defined point on the stem from the distal tip and this remains constant for all lengths of the distal components. In the case of the Revitan stem (Zimmer Biomet, Winterthur, Switzerland), as already mentioned, the thickness is always 11 cm from the distal tip, whereas in the case of the Profemur R (Microport Orthopedics, Arlington, TN, USA) the thickness is always 3 cm from the tip. On the other hand, there are stems where the thickness is always measured from the proximal end at a defined point for all lengths. For example, the measuring point of the Reclaim stem (DePuy Synthes, Warsaw, IN, USA) is always 3.8 cm distal to the junction, while the measuring point of the ZMR stem (Zimmer Biomet, Warsaw, IN, USA) is always 3.0 cm from the junction (Table 8.1). This means that the thickness of the 140 mm long distal component of the Reclaim stem is fixed at 11.2 cm from the distal side, but for the next size 190 mm at 16.2 cm, etc. The situation is similar for the distal components of the ZMR stem (105 mm, 155 mm, and 205 mm for the lengths of the distal component 135 mm, 185 mm, and

Table 8.1 Details of tapered modular distal components and tapered nonmodular revision stems

Stem	Company	Modularity	Straight/Curved	Taper amount	Length of the tapered region	Distance from the tip to the diameter marking	Difference between the nominal diameter and the diameter at the distal start of the taper
Arcos	Zimmer Biomet	Modular	Straight	3°	Over the whole length of the tapered part of the DC	103 mm for 150 DC and ETO Version; 143 mm for 190 DC	150 DC: 4.17 mm for ND 12 reducing to 3.70 mm for ND 30 190 DC: 6.32 mm for ND 12 reducing to 5.85 mm for ND 30 250 ETO-DC: 4.20 mm for ND 12 reducing to 3.74 mm for ND 30
MRP	Peter Brehm	Modular	Very short and short straight Medium and long curved	2°	Over the whole length of the tapered part of the DC	5.5 cm for 80 DC 9.5 cm for 140 DC 13.5 cm for 200 DC 0 cm for 260 and 300 DC	4 mm for 80, 140, and 200 DC 0 mm for 260 and 320 DC
MP	Waldemar Link	Modular	3° angled	2°	83 mm for 160, 180, 210 DC 123 mm for 250 DC, 163 for 290 DC, 203 for 330 DC	84.5 mm for 160, 180, 210 DC 124.5 mm for 250 DC; 164.5 mm for 290 DC; 204.5 mm for 330 DC	2.5 mm
MUTARS R	implantcast	Modular	Curved	1.5°	150 mm (70 mm with splines) for 150 and 200 DC 190 mm (140 mm with splines) for 250 DC	14 cm for 150 DC 19 cm for 200 DC	4 mm for 150 and 200 DC 6 mm for 250 DC
Prevision	Aesculap	Modular	Straight Curved	2° 0.6°	100 mm for 180 DC, 110 mm for the longer straight DC	4 cm	1 mm

(continued)

Table 8.1 (continued)

Stem	Company	Modularity	Straight/Curved	Taper amount	Length of the tapered region	Distance from the tip to the diameter marking	Difference between the nominal diameter and the diameter at the distal start of the taper
Profemur R	Microport	Modular	135 mm straight 175 and 215 mm curved	2°	105 mm for 135 DC	3 cm	0 mm
Reclaim	DePuy Synthes	Modular	140 mm straight 190 mm straight and 3° angled 240 and 290 mm 3° angled	2.5°	105 mm for 140 DC, 155 mm for 190 DC, 205 mm for 240 DC, 255 mm for 290 DC	112 mm for 140 DC, 162 mm for 190 DC, 212 mm for 240 DC, 262 mm for 290 DC	4 mm for 140 DC, 6 mm for 190 DC, 8 mm for 240 DC, 10 mm for 290 DC
Redapt	Smith & Nephew	Monoblock and with sleeve	Straight	3°	100 mm	12.5 cm	3 mm for 190 stem 5 mm for 240 and 300 stem
Restoration	Stryker	Modular	Straight	3° center 2° splines	Over the whole length of the DC	12 cm	4 mm
Revitan	Zimmer Biomet	Modular	Straight series Curved series	2°	100 mm for 140 DC 120 mm for 200 and 260 DC	11 cm	3.8 mm
Wagner	Zimmer Biomet	Monoblock	Straight	2°	107.7 mm for 190 DC, 143.7 mm for 225 DC, 183.7 mm for 285 DC, 223.7 mm for 305 DC	11.9 cm	3.8 mm
ZMR	Zimmer Biomet	Modular	Straight	3.5°	99.7 mm for ND 17–19 98.2 mm for ND from 20	105 mm for 135 DC, 155 mm for 185 DC, 205 mm for 235 DC	6.1 mm for ND 17–19 6.0 mm for ND from 20

DC distal component, *ND* nominal diameter

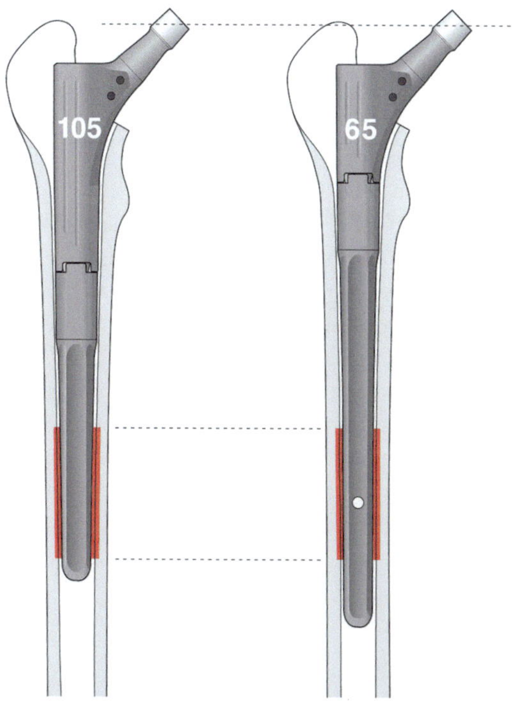

Fig. 8.2 Change from a shorter distal component to a longer distal component. If the diameter of the stem is determined from the distal side, the same thickness is used to move the junction more proximally (with permission of Zimmer Biomet, Winterthur, Switzerland)

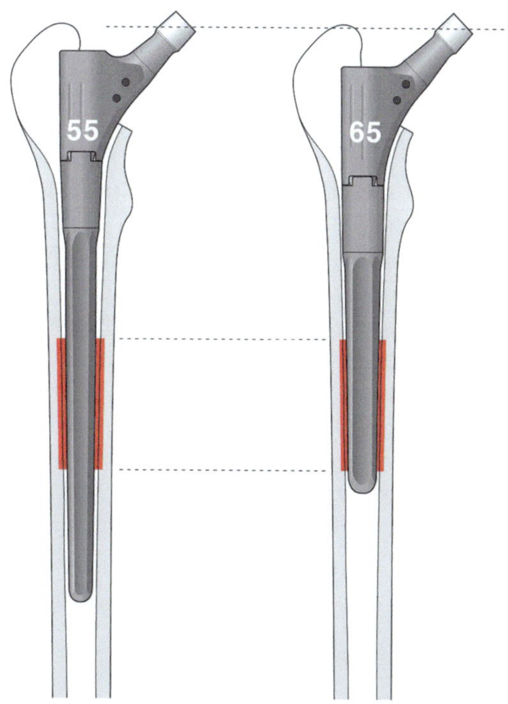

Fig. 8.3 Change from a distally longer to a distally shorter component in a stem system with a thickness determined from the distal side. With the same fixation distance, a thicker distal component is required to bring the junction slightly more distal in this system (with permission of Zimmer Biomet, Winterthur, Switzerland)

235 mm) (Table 8.1). This difference and understanding its relevance are particularly important during intraoperative change from one distal component length to another, for example, to reconstruct the leg length correctly. In the case of a stem where the thickness is measured at the same distance for all lengths from the distal side, the same thickness can be used for this change from a shorter to a longer distal component in order to move the junction further proximally (Fig. 8.2). In the case of a stem such as the Reclaim stem or the MUTARS RS (implantcast, Buxtehude, Germany), in which the distance of the thickness measurement from proximal remains constant for the different distal component lengths, a thicker, longer distal component must be used for this change in order to bring the junction further proximally. Conversely, when revising from a longer to a shorter distal component, a thicker distal component is required for the first types of stem (determination of the thickness from distal) so that the junction is only slightly deeper (Fig. 8.3). In the stems with the thickness nomination set from the proximal side, the junction is reduced distally by the difference in length between the longer and shorter distal components when a change to the shorter one is performed.

Another important difference between the various tapered stems is the degree of taper. Following the 2-degree taper of the original Wagner stem, its successors Wagner SL and Revitan (Straight and Curved) (Zimmer Biomet, Winterthur, Switzerland, formerly Sulzer GmbH) also have a 2-degree taper. The Link MP stem (Waldemar Link, Hamburg, Germany) and the MRP stem (Peter Brehm GmbH, Weisendorf, Germany) have also adopted this 2-degree taper. For the Prevision stem (Aesculap, Tuttlingen, Germany), the taper was changed from 0.6 to 2° in the newer straight version, no doubt to improve the distal fixation in the isthmus of the femur. The older version with a 0.6-degree taper (Bicontact revision) was not capable of producing an adequate press fit in the isthmus and was therefore frequently dependent on additional fixation with locking screws, although this did not result in reproducibly good outcomes either [1]. Eingärnter et al. [1] had to revise stems implanted in over 12% of cases because of early loosening. The curved distal version of the Prevision stem retained the 0.6-degree taper. Other stem systems have different degrees of taper, probably in part due to patent considerations or the desire for greater differentiation and specialization. The Reclaim stem (DePuy, Warsaw, IN) has a taper of 2.5°, the Arcos stem (Zimmer Biomet, Warsaw, IN, formerly Biomet) and Redapt stem (Smith & Nephew, Memphis, TN, USA) have a taper of 3°, and the ZMR stem (Zimmer Biomet, Warsaw, IN, formerly Zimmer) has a taper of 3.5° (Table 8.1). Thus, there is a range of tapers between 0.6 and 3.5° (Table 8.1). These differences in taper result in a different height of the stem or the distal component, where the cone-in-cone fixation in the isthmus of the shaft can be created. The greater the degree of taper, the more proximal to the tip is the fixation zone (Figs. 7.2 and 8.4a–c). While the fixation zone can be created at the tip of the stem with 2° of taper, it is significantly higher, for example, with the ZMR stem (Figs. 7.2 and 8.4a–c).

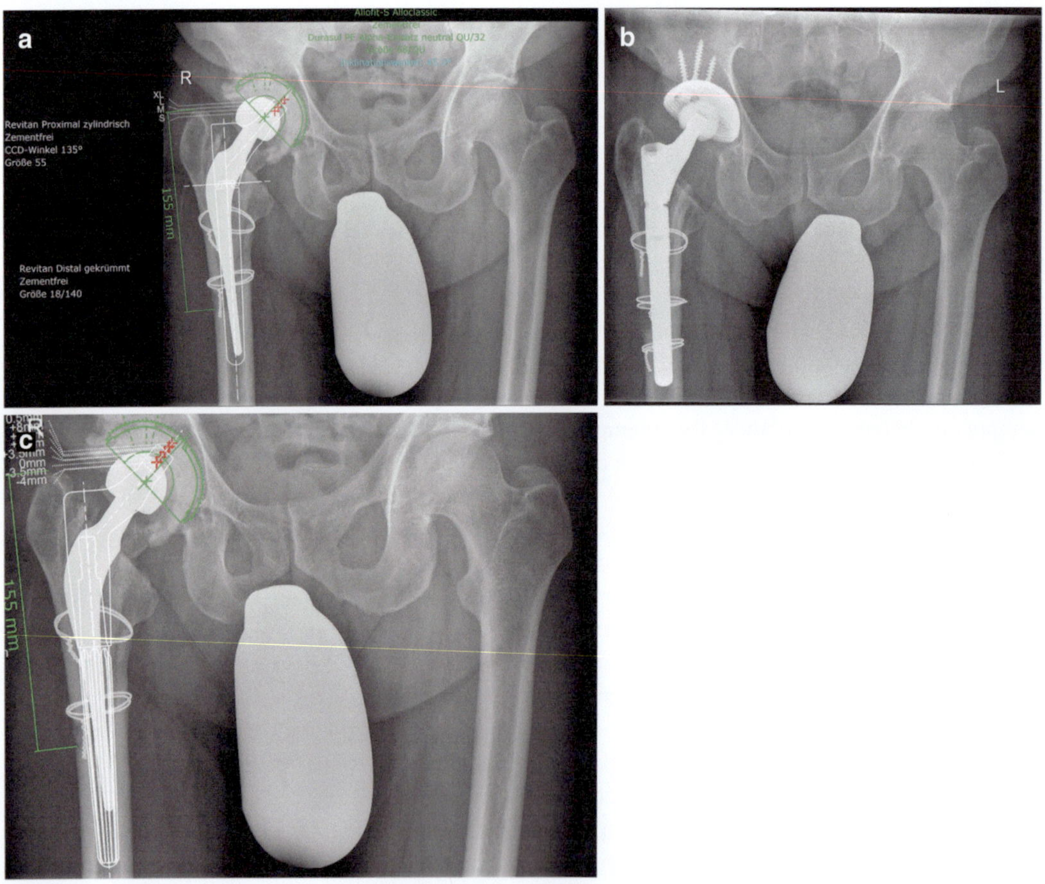

Fig. 8.4 (**a**) Planning a transfemoral stem revision with a 2° tapered Revitan stem with fixation at the tip of the distal component. (**b**) Radiograph 6 months after surgery and implementation of the planned procedure. (**c**) Planning a transfemoral stem revision with a 3.5-degree tapered ZMR stem with fixation proximal to the tip of the distal component

A greater taper of the stem leads to the necessity of implanting longer stems or distal components. With the 2-degree tapered stems, fixation in the isthmus of the femur can be achieved at the tip of the shortest distal components such that the isthmus is not traversed. With stems of greater taper, however, the higher level of the fixation zone means that it passes through the isthmus of the femur. This in turn then leads to a higher risk of ventral perforation of the femur or periprosthetic fracture, especially with straight stems. For example, van Houwelingen et al. [2] observed a periprosthetic fracture in 16% of 48 stem revisions with the ZMR system. In addition, Huddleston et al. [3] in a multicenter study compared modular revision stems (mostly ZMR stems with 3.5° of taper) and nonmodular revision stems (with 2° of taper) for bone defects from Paprosky I to IIIA, and found a greater risk of intraoperative fractures for the modular revision stems (11% versus 7%). However, this is not due to the modularity, but rather to the different taper. Another reason for the increasing fracture rates with increasing stem taper, as observed by Swanson et al. [4], is the higher force applied to shorter bone sections with greater taper, according to the biomechanical study by Pierson et al. [5]. Stems with a greater taper will be fixed over a shorter length of bone. However, axial stability is improved with increasing taper [5]. If the cortical bone in which the stem is to be fixed is thick enough, highly tapered stems can also become fixed in the isthmus of the femur even if the fixation zone is intact for only a short distance. Therefore, these stems are especially indicated for Paprosky IIIB defects with good cortical bone in the still intact isthmus. However, if the short intact isthmus section exhibits only thin cortical bone, the greater forces exerted over such a short distance lead to a higher risk of fracture.

Conversely, the smaller the taper, the longer the required fixation zone in the isthmus. Here, there should also be a minimum taper that is necessary for a sufficient cone-in-cone fixation. There are no precise calculations or experience in this respect, except that an additional distal locking was always necessary for the older version of the Previsions stem (Bicontact Revision) with a taper of 0.6° [1].

The distal fixation stems are available in straight and curved versions. In some cases, both forms are offered in all lengths in one system (e.g., Revitan and Arcos, Zimmer Biomet, Warsaw, IN), so that the surgeon must decide in principle between one of these two systems (Fig. 6.22). In other modular systems, the distal components are straight in the shorter versions and curved in the longer ones (Reclaim, DePuy, Warsaw, IN; MRP stem, Peter Brehm GmbH, Weisendorf) (Fig. 6.23). The radius of the antecurvation of the stem is also different in the various stem systems. For the Revitan Curved and Profemur R, the radius is 1.2 m, for the Prevision curved stem 1.0 m, and for the MRP stem 1.35 m for all distal component lengths (Table 8.1). For the MUTARS RS, it changes with the length of the distal components: For the 120 and 150 mm lengths, it is 1.6 m, and for the 200 and 250 mm lengths of the distal components, it is 1.1 m (Table 8.1).

Some systems feature an additional coating of hydroxyapatite, in some only as a variant of the proximal component (e.g., Restoration, Stryker, Memphis, TN), and in others the complete stem is coated with hydroxyapatite (e.g., Reef stem, DePuy Synthes, Warsaw, IN, USA, or MUTARS R, implantcast, Buxtehude, Germany). In the fully hydroxyapatite-coated stems, where the distal component of the stem system is also coated, the stems are only slightly tapered so that additional distal locking is used to achieve adjunctive fixation and the hydroxyapatite coating accelerates osteointegration of the stem (Fig. 6.28 and Table 8.1).

It is also important to know the specifics of the preparation of the fixation bed for the respective system. In most straight tapered systems, the conical bed is created with conical reamers, resulting in a cone-in-cone fixation. Only the Profemur R (Microport Orthopedics, Arlington, MI) uses a cylindrical reamer, resulting in a cone-in-cylinder fixation with this straight stem system.

The preparation of the fixation bed in the curved versions differs between the different systems. The Revitan Curved (Zimmer Biomet, Winterthur Switzerland) is the only curved stem system that creates a conical fixation bed with a conical rasp (after cylindrical reaming with medullary reamers), thus creating a cone-in-cone fixation with the curved version as well. With other curved stems (MRP), a cylindrical bed is created with an intramedullary reamer so that a cone-in-cylinder fixation is created with the tapered stem. In the Prevision stem (Aesculap, Tuttlingen, Germany), the fixation bed of the tapered curved distal component is prepared with a conical straight reamer, and in the Profemur R stem (Microport Orthopedics, Arlington, MI), a cylindrical straight reamer is used. In these cases, the prepared fixation bed may not exactly match the shape of the stem, making controlled distal fixation of the curved stems, as determined by the surgeon, more difficult to achieve. In a biomechanical study, Heinecke et al. [6] showed that a form-fit preparation of the fixation bed for the Link MP stem with a 3-degree angle using appropriately angled reamers resulted in significantly higher axial strength than the preparation with a non-form-fit straight conical reamer without the appropriate angulation.

In the Arcos system (Zimmer Biomet, Warsaw, IN, USA), the straight distal components are fixed conically by preparing the fixation bed with conical reamers (Fig. 6.24). However, the curved distal components are cylindrical and are fixed with a scratch fit after cylindrical reaming of the femur. This results in different fixation distances for the same diameter of stem and different minimum fixation zones (longer for the stem with cylinder-in-cylinder fixation).

The Link MP stem (Waldemar Link, Hamburg, Germany) and a variant of the Reclaim stem (DePuy Synthes, Warsaw, IN, USA) have distal components angled at 3° and represent one variant of straight stem fixation (Fig. 6.20 and Table 8.1). This is intended to help reduce the occurrence of ventral perforation of the femur or periprosthetic fractures caused by longer distal components. Very good results with low fracture rates have been achieved with this system (Table 6.9). However, Klauser et al. [7] and Wang et al. [8] reported intraoperative fractures in 17% and Amanatullalh et al. [9] in 12% of cases. In the Reclaim revision system (DePuy Synthes, Warsaw, IN), there is a straight version for the shorter 140 mm long and the middle 190 mm long distal component, and also a version with a 3-degree angle for the middle length. The long 240-mm distal components only exist with a 3-degree angle. A similar concept exists for the Arcos stem system (Zimmer Biomet, Warsaw, IN, USA). The two shorter lengths of the tapered distal components (150 mm and 190 mm) are straight, and the so-called ETO version of 250 mm has a kink above the tapered portion and then transitions to a cylindrical, coarse-structured portion (Fig. 6.24, left distal component). In this case, the angle is also used for adaptation to the anatomical curve of the femur and thus for better closure of the osteotomy.

Another special feature of the Link MP system (Waldemar Link, Hamburg, Germany) is represented by components that can be cemented distally, resulting in a modular system of distally cemented components and proximally cementless components (Fig. 8.5).

As a further differentiation between the various distal fixation stem systems with double-conical fixation, there are those that increase in thickness in 1-mm increments (ZMR, Arcos, Reclaim, Wagner, MRP, MUTARS) and those that increase in 2-mm increments (Revitan, Link MP stem). The two thickest distal stem components of the Link MP system (22.5 mm and 25 mm) even show a 2.5 mm step. Since these stems have a cone-in-cone fixation, the 2-mm increment has no disadvantages. However, the 1-mm gradation has the advantage of being somewhat finer. Systems based on scratch-fit fixation, on the other hand, require 1-mm gradation, as otherwise the risk of fracture would be increased.

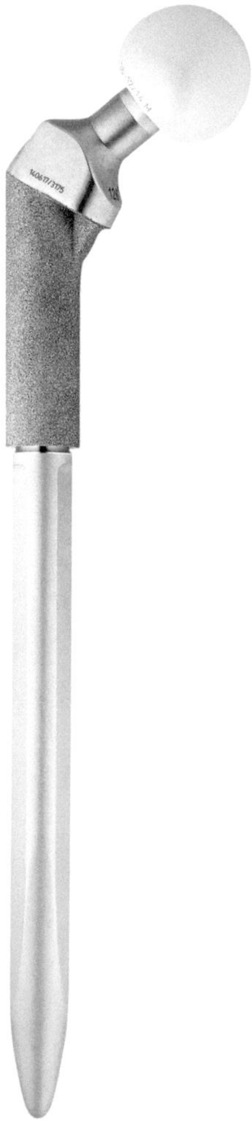

Fig. 8.5 Modular Link MP stem with a distally cementable component (Waldemar Link, Hamburg, Germany)

References

1. Eingärtner C, Ochs U, Egetemeyer D, Volkmann R. Treatment of periprosthetic femoral fractures with the Bicontact revision stem. Z Orthop Unfall. 2007;145(Suppl 1):S29–33.
2. van Houwelingen AP, Duncan CP, Masri BA, Greidanus NV, Garbuz DS. High survival of modular tapered stems for proximal femoral bone defects at 5 to 10 years follow-up. Clin Orthop Relat Res. 2013;471:454–62.
3. Huddleston JI, Testreault MW, Yu M, Bedair H, Hansen VJ, Choi H-R, Goodman SB, Sporer MD, Della Valle CJ. Is there a benefit to modularity in "simpler" femoral revisions? Clin Orthop Relat Res. 2016;474:415–20.
4. Swanson TV. Tapered, fluted femoral fixation. In: Brown TF, Cui Q, Mihalko WM, et al., editors. Arthritis and arthroplasty. Philadelphia: Elsevier; 2009. p. 354–62.
5. Pierson JL, Small SR, Rodriguez JA, et al. The effect of taper angle and spline geometry on the initial stability of tapered, splined modular titanium stems. J Arthroplasty. 2015;30:1254–9.
6. Heinecke M, Layer F, Matziolis G. Anchoring of a kinked uncemented femoral stem after preparation with a straight or a kinked reamer. Orthop Surg. 2019;11:705–11.
7. Klauser W, Bangert Y, Lubinus P, Kendoff D. Medium-term follow-up of a modular tapered titanium stem in revision total hip arthroplasty: a single-surgeon experience. J Arthroplasty. 2013;28:84–9.
8. Wang L, Dai Z, Wen T, Li M, Hu Y. Three to seven year follow-up of a tapered modular femoral prosthesis in revision total hip arthroplasty. Arch Orthop Trauma Surg. 2013;133:275–81.
9. Ammanatullah DF, Howard JL, Siman H, Trousdale RT, Mabry TM, Berry DJ. Revision total hip arthroplasty in patients with extensive proximal femoral bone loss using a fluted tapered modular femoral component. Bone Joint J. 2015;97-B:312–7.

Allograft Prosthesis Composite (APC) and Megaprostheses

9

Contents

9.1 **Allograft Prosthesis Composite (APC)** 99
9.1.1 Surgical Technique 99
9.1.2 Outcomes 101

9.2 **Proximal Femoral Replacement (Megaprostheses)** 101
9.2.1 Surgical Technique 103
9.2.2 Outcomes 105

9.3 **Total Femoral Replacement** 105
9.3.1 Surgical Technique 105
9.3.2 Outcomes 110

References 110

9.1 Allograft Prosthesis Composite (APC)

In an allograft prosthesis composite (APC), the proximal femur is replaced with an allograft and a prosthesis is cemented into it with its tip anchored in the host bone. The APC is indicated in cases of extensive destruction of the proximal femur, such as a Vancouver B3 type periprosthetic fracture and concomitant extensive segmental bone defects extending at least 8 cm into the diaphysis [1]. This technique is recommended only in younger patients (<75 years), as there must be sufficient capacity for osteoneogenesis to facilitate osteointegration or healing of the allograft into the host bone [2]. The advantages of the APC include the potential for the biological reconstruction of the deficiency, facilitating the attachment of soft tissue to the construct, union of the host greater trochanter, and the advantageous mechanical properties of the allograft that are similar to those of the host bone [3]. The disadvantages of APC continue to be the possibility of disease transmission, resorption of the allograft, the potential for the patient to mount an immune response against it, and the difficulty in obtaining such allografts.

9.1.1 Surgical Technique

For this surgical technique, the head of an irradiated, fresh frozen (−70 °C) allograft of the proximal femur, which, after thawing, is smaller in diameter than the patient's, is first resected approximately 1 cm proximal to the lesser trochanter. In order to increase the rotational stability of the subsequent construct, a step osteotomy is performed at the distal end of the allograft at a level determined during planning (Fig. 9.1a). If

B. Fink, *Femoral Revision Arthroplasty*, https://doi.org/10.1007/978-3-030-84821-7_9

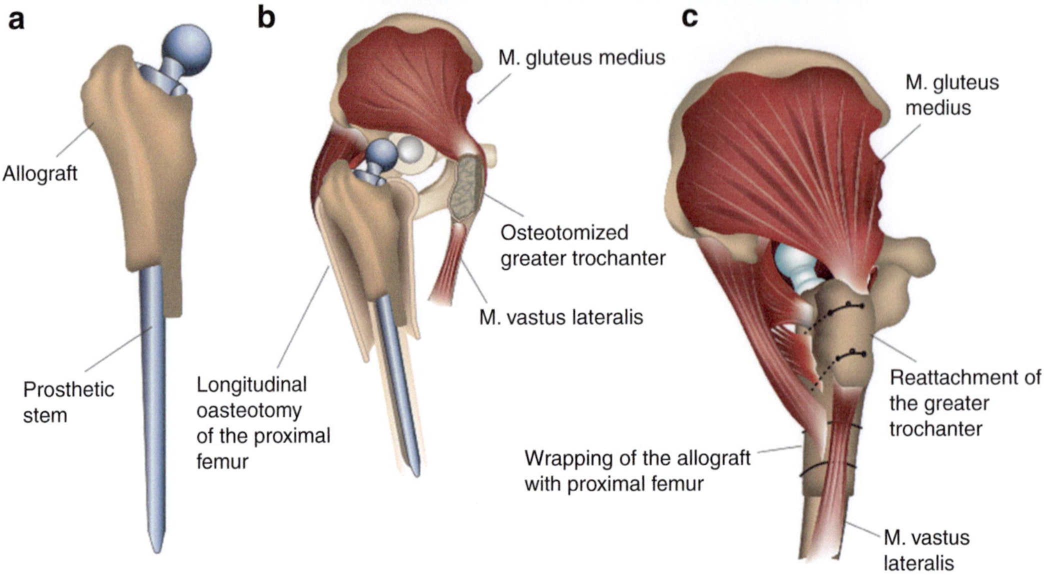

Fig. 9.1 (**a**) Implantation of the revision stem into the proximal allograft. (**b**) Implantation of the allograft prosthesis composite into the distal femur. Proximally, the femur is divided lengthwise and the greater trochanter with the attached vasto-gluteal sling is folded away ventrally by means of a so-called trochanteric slide. (**c**) Proximal femur is bound around the allograft prosthesis composite, and the greater trochanter is folded back into place and secured with cerclages

the greater trochanter with inserted muscles is available from the patient, it should be osteotomized and retained. The patient's distal femur is exposed via a transfemoral approach or so-called trochanteric slide. Both approaches have the advantage of preserving and sparing both the vasto-gluteal muscle sling and the insertion of the gluteal muscles in the greater trochanter. As a result, both of these approaches yield higher rates of bony trochanteric union than the transgluteal approach [4]. The proximal femur is exposed via the intermuscular lateral septum, and from there, the vastus lateralis muscle is undercut slightly to anterior. The deficient proximal femoral bone portion is divided above the osteotomy and/or bisected as in the transfemoral approach, leaving the musculature on the bony flaps as undamaged as possible (Fig. 9.1b). This preserves the vascularity of the bony flaps and later promotes osteointegration of the allograft. The patient's femur should be prepared according to the length of the allograft with a step cut in the healthy bone that corresponds to the allograft. Alternatively, an oblique osteotomy can be carried out. Purely transverse osteotomies are not recommended because of the low rotational stability and the lack of contact area required for effective union of the bone. Before the osteotomy, it makes sense to place a Steinmann nail in the os ilium as a reference point from which the distance to the osteotomy can be measured. After the osteotomy, the patient's femur is prepared with appropriate broaches or cylindrical medullary reamers (depending on the type of prosthetic stem) for cementless distal fixation. A trial prosthesis may be used to verify the correct leg length and determine the necessary allograft length. The allograft is then processed with increasing diameter rasps, and a prosthetic stem, which has been selected according to the distal dimensions, is cemented into the allograft with the correct antetorsion (Fig. 9.1b). The cement mantle should ideally be 2 mm [5–7]. The APC should be inserted approximately 1–2 cm into the patient's femur and trimmed appropriately. Implantation of the prosthetic stem into the femur can be with cement or cementless [6, 8]. Cementless implantation requires a sufficient length of the prosthetic stem in the distal femur for effective fixation. Maury et al. [6] recommend 4 stem diameters. The remaining proximal host bone is secured around the implanted construct with cerclages or cables (Fig. 9.1c). It is primarily at the junction between the allograft and the host bone that the residual bone surrounding the construct acts as a sort of vascularized autograft, thereby promoting bony union with the allograft. The greater trochanter is now attached to the proximal region of the allograft using a tension strap or cerclages (Fig. 9.1c).

Postoperative follow-up depends on the type of fixation of the allograft in the host bone:

- In the case of cementless implantation, partial weight bearing of approximately 20 kg should be applied until the first signs of incorporation of the allograft are radiologically visible. Some authors recommend a low partial weight bearing of 3 months [6].
- Full weight bearing may be permissible with a cemented implantation.
- Active abduction and aggressive physiotherapy with weight training should be avoided for the first 3 months.

9.1.2 Outcomes

APCs are associated with a high incidence of complications (Table 9.1). Babis et al. [18] reported a complication rate of 26.5% (allograft nonunion, allograft fracture, allograft resorption, aseptic loosening, stem fracture, infection) and a rate of revision of 33.4%. Two studies by Head et al. [10], for example, reported complications in 67% and 53% of cases, respectively. Wang and Wang [15] studied 15 patients with APC and found an allograft nonunion rate of 13%, allograft fracture in 6.7%, trochanteric dislocation in 26.7%, infection in 20%, and cup loosening in 6.7% of cases. In addition, mild-to-moderate resorption of the allograft was reported in 25% of cases by Blackley et al. [14], and in 11.4% by Vastel et al. [7].

9.2 Proximal Femoral Replacement (Megaprostheses)

Proximal femoral replacement with prosthetic components is technically much simpler than the APC technique and has the advantage (with cemented fixation) of tolerating immediate weight bearing (Fig. 9.2a, b). Therefore, in differentiating between APC and megaprostheses in the setting of pronounced femoral defects, the latter is especially indicated in older patients.

In proximal femoral replacement, a distal component is fixed distal to the deficient proximal femur bone (either cementless or cemented, depending on age and bone structure), and modular proximal prosthetic components are added to replace the proximal femur and restore leg length. The greater trochanter with attached gluteal muscles should be preserved and fixed to the prosthetic construct. A proximal femoral replacement cannot be used if infection is present and the distal femoral bone is not suitable for adequate fixation. The proximal femoral replacement has the disadvantage that the risk and rate of infection are significantly higher compared to revision prostheses because of the larger metal surface area (see outcomes). To reduce the risk of infection, some companies offer special anti-infective surface finishes, such as silver coatings (MUTARS, implantcast, Buxtehude, Germany). Furthermore, the fixation of these megaprostheses in the distal bone is no better than that of revision prostheses. On the contrary, the more rigid and heavier construct of the proximal femoral replacement requires a longer fixation zone in the distal bone than the more flexible revision stems. Thus, higher rates of radiolucency are seen after cemented proximal femoral replacements than with proximally coated or extensively coated revision stems [21]. In cases of distally insufficient bone (Paprosky type IV defects), the only option often left in revision arthroplasty is a long zone of cemented fixation where the megaprosthesis offers no particular advantage over and above the distal cemented fixation of a revision stem (e.g., Link MP stem, Waldemar Link GmbH, Hamburg, Germany) and still shows the same

Table 9.1 Allograft prosthesis composites for implant revision in cases of prosthesis loosening, infection, or periprosthetic fracture

Author	Cases, *n*	Age (years)	Follow-up (years)	Revision (%)	Nonunion (%)	Loosening (%)	Dislocation (%)	Infection (%)	Fracture (%)	Survival, *a* = years
Head [9]	22	51	2.3	40.9	18.2		27.3	6	4.5	73%, 2a
Head [10]	70	58	2.5		20		16	4	6	
Zmolek [11]	15	59	4	26.7	18	13.3*	55	6.7		73%, 2a
Chandler [12]	30	62	2	10	13.6/10T	13.3*	16.7	3.3		90%, 2a
Gross [13]	130		4.8							85%; 4.8a
Haddad [8]	40		8.8	10	8/46T	10	10	5		85%; 8.8a
Blackley [14]	48	62.5	11	21	6.3/22T	6.3	8.3	10.4		77%, 11a
Graham [5]	25	64	4.5	8	20/36T	8*	0	4		92%, 4.5a
Wang [15]	15	58.7	7.6	33.4	13.3	6.7	6.7	20	6.7	67%; 5a
Maury [6]	25	70.2	5.1	16	16/24T	12	8	0		84%; 5.1a
Vastel [7]	44	60.2	7.1	9.1	56.8T	4.5	13.6	2.3	4.5	91%, 7a
Safir [16]	50	63	16.2	6	24	12	8	4		82.2%, 15a
Lee [17]	15	60.9	4.2	20	6.7	13.3	6.7	6.7		87%, 4.2a
Babis [18]	72	59.9	12	26.4	2.7	5.5	11.1	6.9	5.5	66%, 12a
Sternheim [19]	30	58.1	15	20						75.5%, 15a
Sternheim [20]	21	64	8		9.5	4.8				83.5%, 10a

T trochanteric nonunion

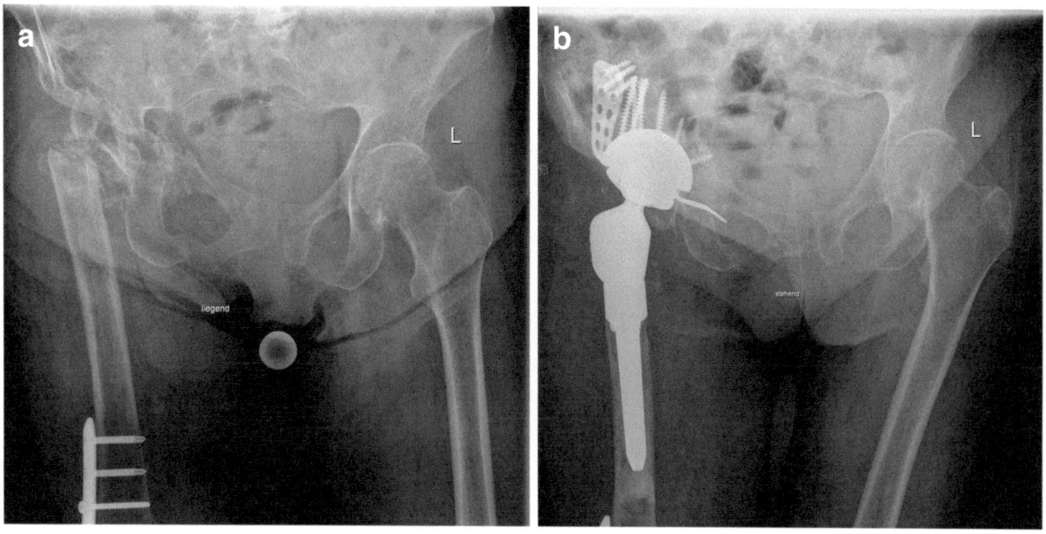

Fig. 9.2 (**a**) Girdlestone situation with significant leg shortening and pelvic discontinuity after extramural removal of an infected firmly fixed hip total endoprosthesis. (**b**) Postoperative radiograph after implantation of a proximal femoral replacement (Waldemar Link, Hamburg, Germany) and a cup-and-cage system with Duo-Mobility Cup (Zimmer Biomet, Warsaw, IN, USA)

disadvantages. This equivalence in fixation quality is countered by the higher complication rates so I try to avoid the use of proximal femoral replacements in favor of revision prostheses (Fig. 9.3a–c).

9.2.1 Surgical Technique

The femur is exposed via an extended approach (vastus slide, trochanteric slide, or extended trochanteric osteotomy = transfemoral). If the proximal part of the femur is intact, a longitudinal osteotomy should be performed (preferably as a transfemoral approach) to remove the existing prosthesis. This is followed by a transverse osteotomy of the distal femur. The goal should be to preserve as much as possible of the distal femoral segment because the outcomes of proximal femoral replacement depend on the length of this particular section of the femur [21]. The distal component is then fixed into the remaining portion of the distal femur. Depending on the bone quality, this is cemented in place or implanted with a cementless fixation. In revision arthroplasty and cases that are candidates for proximal femoral replacement, cemented implantation is usually recommended because, in most cases, bone quality is very poor. The length of the fixation zone for the megaprosthesis in the distal femur should be at least 6 cm [6]. Subsequently, the proximal trial components of the modular system are placed in position and a trial reduction is performed. Special attention must be paid to establishing the correct rotation and leg length in order to avoid instabilities on the one hand and overstretching of the sciatic nerve on the other. For correct adjustment of leg length, before the transverse distal osteotomy is carried out, it is helpful to place a Steinmann nail in the os ilium as a reference point and to measure out the distance from this nail to the planned transverse osteotomy. This distance represents the length of the proximal part of the megaprosthesis. After a successful trial, the final implants are fitted to the distal component. Alternatively, only trial prosthesis components are first positioned in the distal femur, and the successfully tested combination of modular components is assembled on the operating table and then implanted as a complete unit. However, I consider the first procedure to be somewhat easier, especially if cementless distal

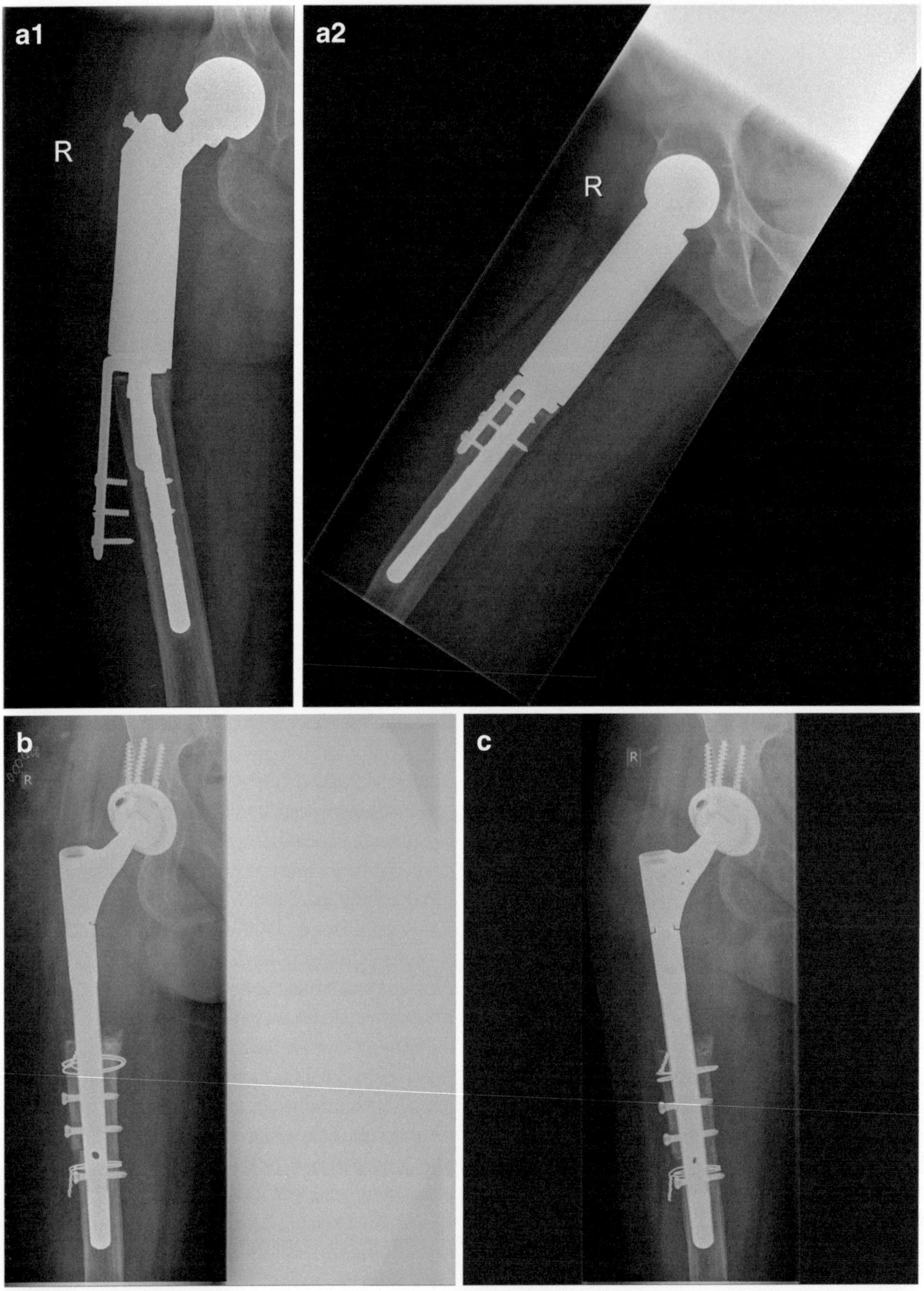

Fig. 9.3 (**a**) Fractured Kotz tumor prosthesis (Howmedica) 18 years after implantation because of chondrosarcoma. (**a1**) Radiograph a.p., (**a2**) Lateral radiograph. (**b**) Postoperative radiograph after "transfemoral" procedure with distal flap and implantation of a modular revision system (Revitan Curved, Zimmer Biomet, Winterthur, Switzerland) with distal locking and use of the same for closure of the flap. The proximal prosthesis is exposed. (**c**) Radiograph 12 months after surgery. The flap shows bony consolidation

fixation is chosen. In this way, the advantages of the modular system with separation of the distal fixation and correct adjustment of leg length, offset, and antetorsion can also be exploited in such cases.

One problem with megaprostheses is the high risk of dislocation, partly because of alteration to the abductor muscles by previous surgery. Therefore, the proximal femoral portion with its integrated musculature (especially the greater trochanter with the gluteal muscles) should be preserved as much as possible (no matter how deficient) and attached to the proximal femoral replacement with cerclages. Dual-mobility cup systems may also be used to further improve stability.

9.2.2 Outcomes

Satisfactory clinical outcomes can be achieved with proximal femoral replacement prostheses, although Al-Taki et al. [22] and Muhyeddine et al. [23] found significantly better WOMAC functional scores and Oxford hip scores for revision prostheses in a comparative study. Instabilities and infections constitute the main problems. Dislocation rates of between 18% and 50% were reported in a review by Rasouli et al. [2], which is also reflected in the lists in Table 9.2. A contributing factor is the weakening of the abductor muscles due to the difficulty of reattachment of the greater trochanter and/or the muscles to the prosthesis. Thus, most authors have reported positive Trendelenburg signs [2, 26].

9.3 Total Femoral Replacement

If the defect of the femur is so pronounced that, in the case of a Paprosky type IV defect, there is no bone stock left into which the distal stem of a prosthesis can be fixed, with or without cement, and the only remaining option is to replace the entire femur with a intramedullary femoral replacement (push-through endoprosthesis) or total femoral replacement (extramedullary femoral replacement) (Fig. 9.4). These complex and expensive endoprosthesis constructions serve to avoid amputation and thus to preserve the limb. Indications may include significant bone loss due to osteolysis or debridement required in cases of periprosthetic infections and interprosthetic fractures between two long prostheses (Figs. 9.5a–c and 9.6a, b). The difference between the intramedullary and extramedullary femoral replacement is that in the former one the bony femoral diaphysis into which the femoral endoprosthesis is inserted is preserved as far as possible with its attaching muscles. Both forms of total femoral replacement are attached to the tibia by means of an axis-guided knee prosthesis. The difference in indication is based on the amount of bone that is still present and worth preserving. If the greater trochanter, diaphyseal bone, and sufficient distal femur are available for fixation of a femoral component and a rotating-hinge prosthesis (with augmentations if necessary), I believe that an intramedullary total femoral replacement (push-through endoprosthesis) is indicated. If the diaphyseal bone with attached musculature is less than 12 cm and the distal femur is no longer suitable for fixation of a femoral rotating-hinge component, extramedullary total femoral replacement is preferable. If the greater trochanter is still present, it should also be preserved during extramedullary total femoral replacement.

9.3.1 Surgical Technique

Implantation of both forms of total femoral replacement requires obtaining access to the proximal femur and to the distal femur and the knee joint. With the intramedullary femoral replacement (push-through prosthesis), this can be done via two separate approaches (one being the extended femoral approach in combination with a medial Payr approach) to the knee joint. In this case, the patient can be operated on in the reclined or lateral position (depending on the selected extended femoral access). Alternatively, implantation is performed via an extended transfemoral approach that leads distally into a lateral Payr approach to the knee joint. After removal of the old prostheses, either proximal from endofemoral or transfemoral, the tibial component is

Table 9.2 Proximal femoral replacements in prosthesis revision in cases of non-neoplastic indications (prosthesis loosening, infection, or periprosthetic fracture)

Author	Cases, *n*	Age (years)	Follow-up (years)	Revision (%)	Loosening (%)	Dislocation (%)	Infection (%)	Periprosthetic fracture (%)	Survival
Sim [24]	21	59.3	2–7	19	5	14	5	5	90%, 6a
Malkani [25]	50	60.6	11.1	32	8	22	6.3	0	64%, 12a
Haentjens [26]	19	78	5	47.4	5	37	16	0	
Klein [27]	21	78.3	3.2	14.3	0	9.5	9.5	4.8	
Parvizi [28]	48	73.8	3	20.8	4.2	16.7	2.1	0	73%, 5a
Shih [29]	12	59	5.7	41.7	8.3	41.7	33.3	0	
Schoenfeld [30]	19	76	3.7	15.8	0	16	5	5	
Bertani [31]	10	65	5.4	40	0	30	10	10	
Gebert [32]	45	62	3.2	17.8	4	2	11	0	
Sewell [33]	15	67	5	13.3	0	13	13	0	
Al-Taki [22]	63	73	3.2	9.5	0	6	2	0	
Muhyeddine [23]	36	73	3.2		3	8.3	3		
Dean [34]	8	67.5	1.5	0	0	0	0	0	
McLean [35]	20	72	4	30	0	15	5	10	
Colman [36]	21	75	1.3	38	0	19	19	0	
Lundh [37]	5	56	4	40	0	40	20	0	
Korim [38]	356	69.6	3.8	24	2.5	16	7.6	1	83%
Artiaco [39]	5 inf					33	20		
Grammato-pulos [40]	80	69	5	11.3		3.8	11.3		87%, 5a
Curtin [41]	16	75	1.6			12.5			
Viste [42]	44	79	6	4.5	2.3	13.6	2.3	9.1	66%, 10a

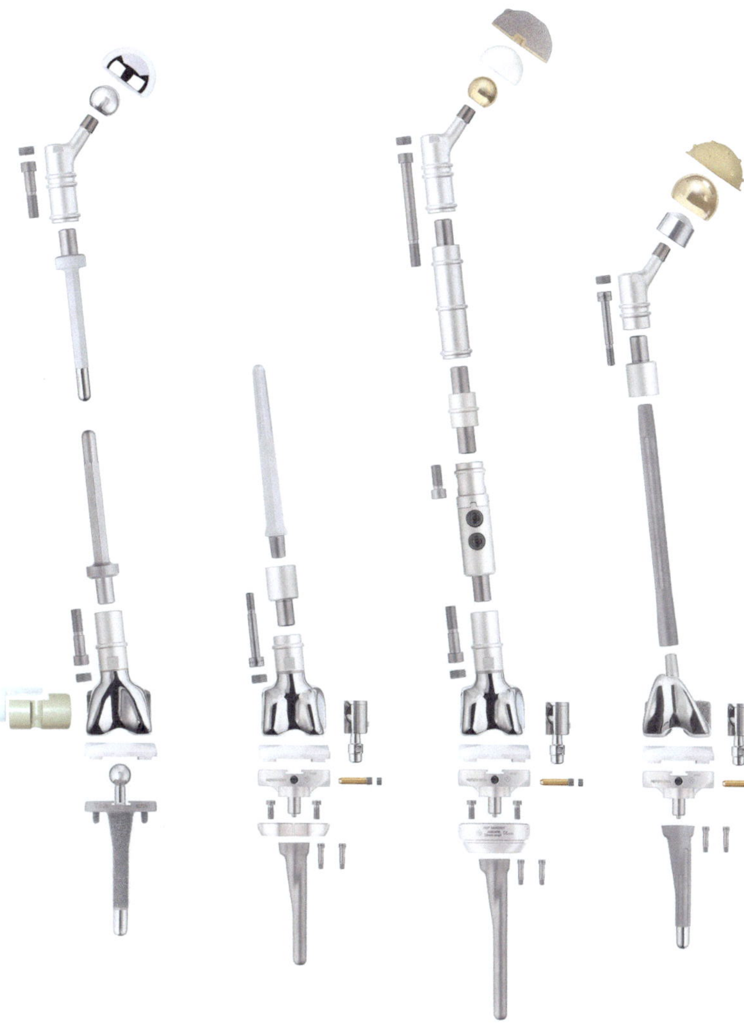

Fig. 9.4 MUTARS total femoral replacement system as extramedullary and intramedullary system (push-through) (implantcast, Buxtehude, Germany)

prepared accordingly and a trial tibial prosthesis is inserted. Following on from this, the trial femoral prosthesis with any femoral condylar augmentations is then passed through the distal femoral diaphysis with a trial stem and paired proximally with the modular proximal components. This complete construct is then used to perform a trial reduction and, most importantly, to check leg length and stability of the joint. Depending on the soft tissue situation in the area of the knee joint, it may be useful to insert the femoral components first and then the tibial components, and then connect them for the trial run. If this trial is satisfactory, the final components are assembled in the same order. The final distal femoral component is cemented in place with its stem attached, followed by proximal connection in situ of the proximal component with reduction in the hip joint. The tibial component is assembled on the operating table and cemented into position before the knee joint is assembled with the corresponding axis-guided knee prosthesis. If a transfemoral approach has been performed, then the proximal part of the prosthesis can be encased in cement and the flap closed by tightening previously applied cerclages (Fig. 9.5b, left).

In extramedullary total femoral replacement, the diaphyseal bone is not preserved and is released from its soft tissue union. Various extended approaches are possible for this purpose. The greater trochanter with the attaching gluteal musculature should be preserved

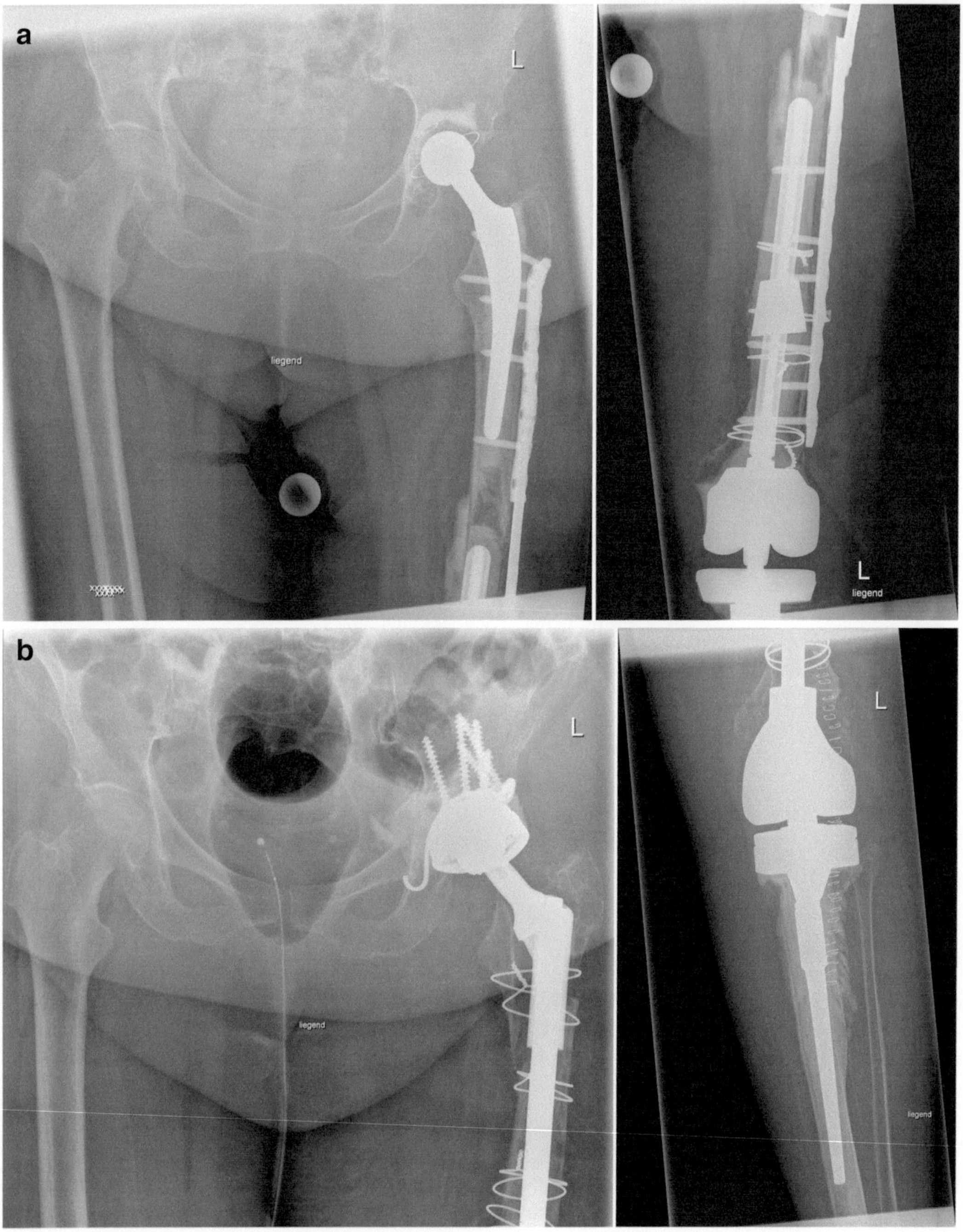

Fig. 9.5 (**a**-left and right) Interprosthetic fracture with fracture of an osteosynthesis plate. (**b**-left and right) Postoperative radiographs after revision to a push-through prosthesis

whenever possible, for example, by a trochanteric slide approach and later attached to the proximal component of the extramedullary total femoral replacement using, for example, clamping devices. Implantation of the trial and final components is similar to the procedure used for the intramedullary femoral replacement (push-through prosthesis), but without passing the

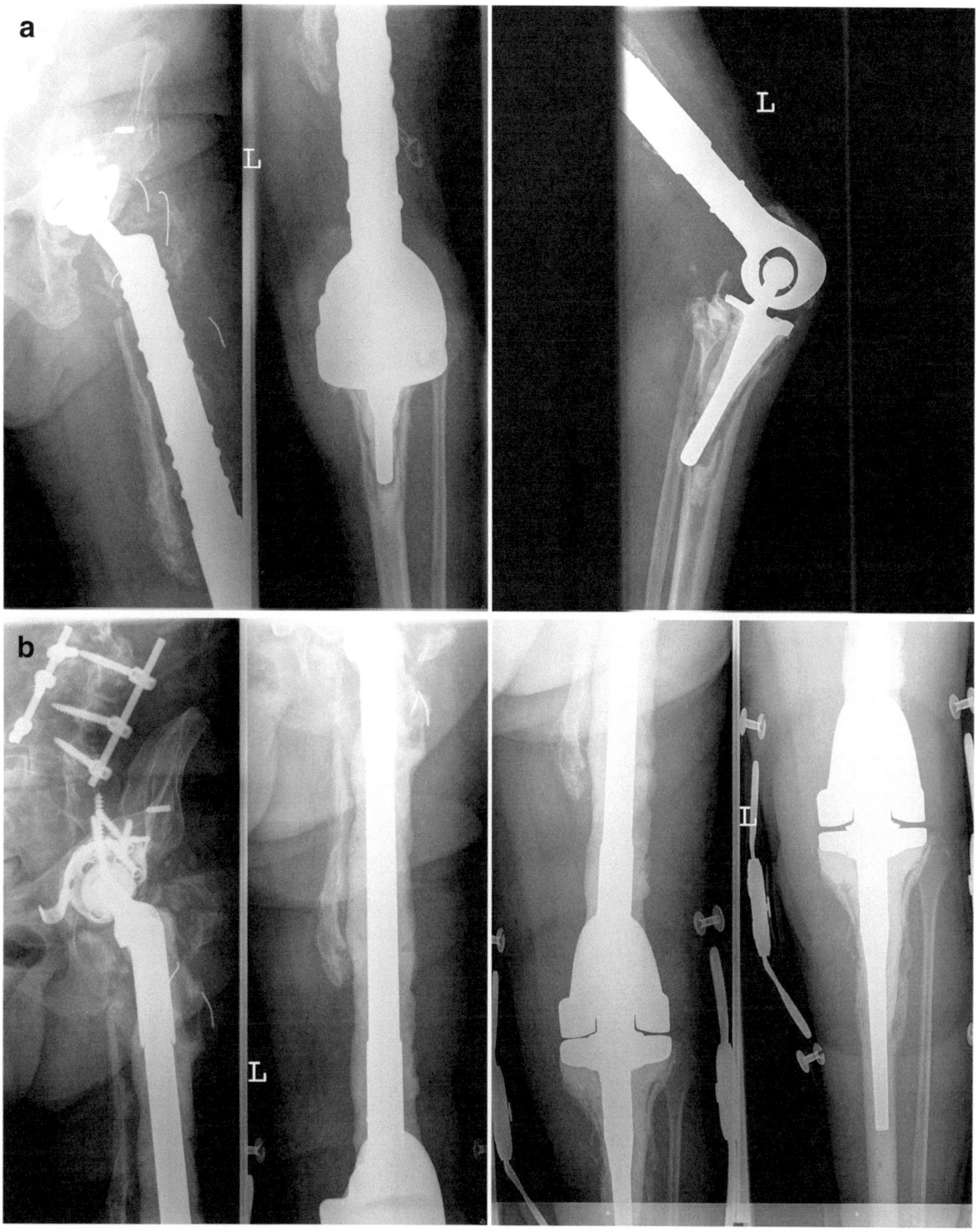

Fig. 9.6 (**a**-left and right) Total femoral replacement infected with Candida albicans after 2 previous extramural septic revision surgeries and one aseptic revision surgery. (**b**-left and right) Postoperative radiographs after one-stage septic revision of a total femoral replacement (Waldemar Link, Hamburg, Germany)

prosthesis through the diaphyseal bone. Since the distal femur is no longer present, it is more difficult to set the correct rotation of the distal femoral component within the total femoral replacement. Rotational errors must also be avoided with this prosthesis. To improve function and protect the prosthesis, the detached musculature should be sutured as securely as possible to

Table 9.3 Total femoral replacement for prosthesis revision in cases of prosthesis loosening, infection, or periprosthetic fracture

Author	Cases, *n*	Age (years)	Follow-up (years)	Revision (%)	Loosening (%)	Dislocation (%)	Infection (%)	Survival, *a* = years
Amanatullah [44]	20	65	6.1	30		25	35	70%, 5a
Berend [45]	58	74	4.8	30.5	3.4	12.1	13.8	65%, 5a
Fontain [46]	14	63	7.5	35		41.6	25	
Friesecke [47]	100	68	4.9	21		9.8	14.8	
Lombardi [48]	50	73	3.5	30.7	4	14	22	
Töpfer [49]	18	78	6.6	72		11.1	44.4	56%, 5a

the implant. Special tubing systems (e.g., Dacron or Trevira tubing), which are placed around the prosthesis and connected to it with purse string sutures, are helpful here. Nowadays, dual-mobility cup systems are preferred for improving the overall stability of the hip joint (Figs. 9.2b and 9.5b1).

9.3.2 Outcomes

In general, both forms of total femoral replacement exhibit high levels of complications. Implantation of a intramedullary femoral replacement (push-through prosthesis) is certainly technically more complex, and problems related to surgical technique are more frequent here. This probably explains the higher complication rate of 33% in 15 cases of push-through prostheses compared to 4% in 12 extramedullary total femoral replacements reported by Hoell et al. [43]. However, this report is in stark contrast to all other published data on the outcomes of total femoral replacements (Table 9.3). The major disadvantage of extramedullary total femoral replacement is the large metal surface area that is not protected by bone and muscle, and so carries a high risk of infection. Infection rates of 14–44% have been reported. In the relatively few publications, lower infection rates are reported for the intramedullary femoral replacement (push-through prosthesis) (because of better coverage of the prosthesis with bone and soft tissue). Peters et al. [50] observed infection and dislocation (9.1%) in 2 cases each in their study of 22 push-through prostheses. Because of the high complication rate, either type of total femoral replacement is indicated in revision arthroplasty only as the last resort for preservation of the limb.

References

1. Kellett CF, Boscainos PJ, Maury AC, et al. Proximal femoral allograft treatment of Vancouver type-B3 periprosthetic femoral fractures after total hip arthroplasty. Surgical technique. J Bone Joint Surg Am. 2007;89-A(Suppl 2):S68–79.
2. Rasouli MR, Porat MD, Hozack WJ, Parvizi J. Proximal femoral replacement and allograft prosthesis composite in the treatment of periprosthetic fractures with significant bone loss. Orthop Surg. 2012;4:203–10.
3. Sakellariou VI, Babis GC. Management bone loss of the proximal femur in revision hip arthroplasty: update on reconstructive options. World J Orthop. 2014;5:614–22.
4. Lakstein D, Kosashvili Y, Backstein D, et al. Modified trochanteric slide for complex hip arthroplasty: clinical outcomes and complication rates. J Arthroplast. 2010;25:363.
5. Graham NM, Stockley I. The use of structural proximal femoral allografts in complex revision hip arthroplasty. J Bone Joint Surg. 2004;86:337–43.
6. Maury AC, Pressman A, Cayen B, et al. Proximal femoral allograft treatment of Vancouver type-B3 periprosthetic femoral fractures after total hip arthroplasty. J Bone Joint Surg Am. 2006;88:953–8.
7. Vastel L, Lemoine CT, Kerboull M, Courpied JP. Structural allograft and cemented long-stem prosthesis for complex revision hip arthroplasty: use of a trochanteric claw plate improves final hip function. Int Orthop. 2007;31:851–7.
8. Haddad FS, Spangehl MJ, Masri BA, et al. Circumferential allograft replacement of the proximal femur. A critical analysis. Clin Orthop Relat Res. 2000;371:98–107.
9. Head WC, Berklacich FM, Malinin TI, Emerson HC Jr. Proximal femoral allografts in revision total hip arthroplasty. Clin Orthop Relat Res. 1987;225:22–36.

10. Head WC, Hillyard JM, Emerson RH, Peters PC Jr. Proximal femoral allografts in revision total hip arthroplasty. Semin Arthroplasty. 1993;4:92–8.
11. Zmolek JC, Dorr LD. Revision total hip arthroplasty: the use of solid allograft. J Arthroplasty. 1993;8:361–70.
12. Chandler H, Clark J, Murphy S, et al. Reconstruction of major segmental loss of the proximal femur in revision total hip arthroplasty. Clin Orthop Relat Res. 1994;298:67–74.
13. Gross AE, Hutchison CR, Alexeeff M, et al. Proximal femoral allografts for reconstruction of bone stock in revision arthroplasty of the hip. Clin Orthop Relat Res. 1995;319:151–8.
14. Blackley HR, Davis AM, Htichson CR, et al. Proximal femoral allografts for reconstruction of bone stock in revision arthroplasty of the hip. A nine to fifteen-year follow-up. J Bone Joint Surg Am. 2001;83-A:346–54.
15. Wang JW, Wang CJ. Proximal femoral allografts for bone deficiencies in revision hip arthroplasty: a medium-term follow-up study. J Arthroplasty. 2004;19:845–52.
16. Safir O, Kellett CF, Flint M, Backstein D, Gross AE. Revision of the deficient proximal femur with a proximal femoral allograft. Clin Orthop Relat Res. 2009;467:206–12.
17. Lee SH, Ahn YJ, Chung SJ, Kim BK, Hwang JH. The use of allograft prosthesis composite for extensive proximal bone deficiencies: a 2- to 9.8-year follow-up study. J Arthroplasty. 2009;24:1241–8.
18. Babis GC, Sakellariou VI, O'Connor MI, et al. Proximal femoral allograft prosthesis composites in revision hip replacement: a 12 year follow-up study. J Bone Joint Surg Br. 2010;92-B:349–55.
19. Sternheim A, Rogers BA, Kuzyk PR, Safir OA, Backstein D, Gross AE. Segmental proximal femoral bone loss and revision total hip replacement in patients with developmental dysplasia of the hip. J Bone Joint Surg Br. 2012;94:762–7.
20. Sternheim A, Drexler M, Kuzyk PR, Safir OA, Backstein DJ, Gross AE. Treatment of failed allograft prosthesis composites used for hip arthroplasty in the setting of severe proximal femoral bone defects. J Arthroplasty. 2014;29:1058–62.
21. Parvizi J, Sim FH. Proximal femoral replacements with megaprostheses. Clin Orthop Relat Res. 2004;420:169–75.
22. Al-Taki MM, Masri BA, Duncan CP, et al. Quality of life following proximal femoral replacement using a modular system in revision THA. Clin Orthop Relat Res. 2011;469:470–5.
23. Muhyeddine M, Al-Taki MD, Masri BA, Duncan CP, Garbuz DS. Quality of life following proximal femoral replacement using a modular system in revision THA. Clin Orthop Relat Res. 2011;469:470–5.
24. Sim FH, Chao EY. Hip salvage by proximal femoral replacement. J Bone Joint Surg Am. 1998;63-A:1228–32.
25. Malkani AL, Settecem JJ, Sim FH, et al. Long-term results of proximal femoral replacement for non-neoplastic disorders. J Bone Joint Surg Br. 1995;77-B:351–6.
26. Haentjens P, De Boeck H, Opdecam P. Proximal femoral replacement prosthesis for salvage of failed hip arthroplasty: complications in a 2–11 year follow-up study in 19 elderly patients. Acta Orthop Scand. 1996;67:37–42.
27. Klein GR, Parvizi J, Rapuri V, Wolf CF, Hozack WJ, Sharkey PF, Purtill JJ. Proximal femoral replacement for the treatment of periprosthetic fractures. J Bone Joint Surg Am. 2005;87-A:1777–81.
28. Parvizi J, Tarity TD, Slenker N, et al. Proximal femoral replacement in patients with non-neoplastic conditions. J Bone Joint Surg Am. 2007;89-A:1036–43.
29. Shih ST, Wang JW, Hsu CC. Proximal femoral megaprosthesis for failed total hip arthroplasty. Chang Gung Med J. 2007;30:73–80.
30. Schoenfeld AJ, Leeson MC, Vrabec GA, Scaglione J, Stonestreet MJ. Outcomes of modular proximal femoral replacement in treatment of complex proximal femoral fractures: a case series. Int J Surg. 2008;6:140–6.
31. Bertani A, Helix M, Louis ML, et al. Total hip arthroplasty in severe segmental femoral bone loss situations: use of a reconstruction modular stem design (JVC IX). Retrospective study of 23 cases. Orthop Traumatol Surg Res. 2009;95:491.
32. Gebert C, Wessling M, Götze C, et al. The modular universal tumour and revision system (MUTARS) in endoprosthetic revision surgery. Int Orthop. 2010;34:1261–5.
33. Sewell MD, Hanna SA, Carrington RW, et al. Modular proximal femoral replacement in salvage hip surgery for non-neoplastic conditions. Acta Orthop Belg. 2010;76:493.
34. Dean BJF, Matthews JJ, Pric A, et al. Modular endoprosthetic replacement for failed internal fixation of proximal femur following trauma. Int Orthop. 2012;36:731.
35. McLean AI, Patton JT, Moran M. Femoral replacement for salvage of periprosthetic fracture around a total hip replacement. Injury. 2012;43:1166–9.
36. Colman M, Choi I, Chen A, et al. Proximal femoral replacement in the management of acute periprosthetic fractures of the hip: a competing risks survival analysis. J Arthroplasty. 2014;29:422.
37. Lundh F, Sayed-Noor AS, Brosjö O, et al. Megaprosthetic reconstruction for periprosthetic of highly comminuted fractures of the hip and knee. Eur J Orthop Surg Traumatol. 2014;24:553.
38. Korim MT, Esler CN, Ashford RU. Systematic review of proximal femoral arthroplasty for non-neoplastic conditions. J Arthroplasty. 2014;29:2117–21.
39. Artiaco S, Boggop F, Colzani G, Titolo P, Zoccola K, Bainchi P, Bellomo F. Megaprostheses in the revision of infected total hip arthroplasty. Clinical series and literature review. Bul Hosp J Dis. 2015;73: 229–32.
40. Grammatopulos G, Alvand A, Martin H, Whitwell D, Taylor A, Gibbons CL. Five-year outcome of proximal

femoral endoprosthetic arthroplasty for non-tumour indications. Bone Joint J. 2016;98-B:1463–70.
41. Curtin M, Bryan C, Murphy E, Murphy CG, Curtin W. Early results of the LPS limb preservation system in the management of periprosthetic femoral fractures. J Orthop. 2016;14:34–7.
42. Viste A, Perry KL, Taunton MJ, Hanssen AD, Abdel MP. Proximal femoral replacement in contemporary revision total hip arthroplasty for severe femoral bone loss: a review of outcomes. Bone Joint J. 2017;99-B:325–9.
43. Hoell S, Butschek S, Gosheger G, Dedy N, Dieckmann R, Henrichs M, Daniilidis K, Hardes J. Intramedullary and total femur replacement in revision arthroplasty as a last limb-saving option: is there any benefit from the less invasive intramedullary replacement? J Bone Joint Surg Br. 2011;93-B:1545–9.
44. Amanatullah DF, Trousdale RT, Hanssen AD, Lewallen DG, Taunton MJ. Non-oncologic total femoral arthroplasty: retrospective review. J Arthroplasty. 2014;29:2013–5.
45. Berend KR, Lombardi AV Jr, Mallory TH, Adams JB, Dodds KL. Total femoral arthroplasty for salvage of end-stage prosthesis disease. Clin Orthop Relat Res. 2004;2:162–70.
46. Fontain JR, Dalby-Bell J, Caroll FA, Stockley I. The use of total femoral arthroplasty as a limb salvage procedure: the Sheffield experience. J Arthroplasty. 2007;22:663–9.
47. Friesecke C, Plutat J, Block A. Revision arthroplasty with use of a total femur prosthesis. J Bone Joint Surg Am. 2005;87-A:2693–701.
48. Lombardi AV Jr, Berend KR. The shattered femur: radical solution options. J Arthroplasty. 2006;21:107–11.
49. Töpfer A, Harrasser N, Petzschner I, Pohlig F, Lenze U, Gerdesmeyer L, Pförringer D, Töpfer M, Beier M, Crönlein M, von Eisenhart-Rothe R, Mühlhofer H. Short- to long-term follow-up of total femoral replacement in non-oncologic patients. BMC Musculoskelet Disord. 2016;17:498.
50. Peters CJ, Hickman JM, Erickson J, Lombardi AV, Berend KR, Mallory TH. Intramedullary total femoral replacement for salvage of the compromised femur associated with hip and knee arthroplasty. J Arthroplasty. 2006;21:53–8.

Choice of the Implant Depending on the Type of Defect

10

Contents

10.1 **Paprosky Type I Defects** ... 113
10.2 **Paprosky Type IIA Defects** ... 114
10.3 **Paprosky Type IIB Defects** ... 115
10.4 **Paprosky Type IIC Defects** ... 115
10.5 **Paprosky Type IIIA Defects** ... 116
10.6 **Paprosky Type IIIB Defects** ... 117
10.7 **Paprosky Type IV Defects** ... 120
References ... 122

Before selecting the implant, the bone must be evaluated with respect to the extent of the defect, its expected quality or stability (especially in the proposed fixation bed of the selected stem), and its conformation (axial deviations that require a corrective osteotomy). The final choice of implant will depend on this analysis and the location (proximal or distal) of the fixation zone to be selected. This analysis is essential because not all stem systems are equally suitable for all defects. The defect analysis therefore determines the choice of the appropriate stem systems, with the exact fixation zone and size to be determined during preoperative planning (see also Chap. 11). Although Wayne Paprosky [1, 2] removed the type II subcategories from his classification, they will be retained here in order to help clarify implant selection.

10.1 Paprosky Type I Defects

The metaphyseal defect is minor, and proximal rotational stability is not significantly reduced compared to primary implantation of a prosthetic stem. Cemented prosthetic stems may be used in elderly patients with only minor osseous defects [3]. Otherwise, cementless metaphyseal or metaphyseal–diaphyseal anchored primary stems are the implants of choice (Fig. 10.1a–c). Rectangular prostheses or prosthesis geometries adapted to the defect are often used to achieve rotational stability. In a systematic literature search, Cavagnoro et al. [4] evaluated eight publications with 454 stem revisions with Paprosky type I and II defects and found a stem-related survival rate of 95.6% for cementless primary stems after an average follow-up of 4.7 years. Iorio

B. Fink, *Femoral Revision Arthroplasty*, https://doi.org/10.1007/978-3-030-84821-7_10

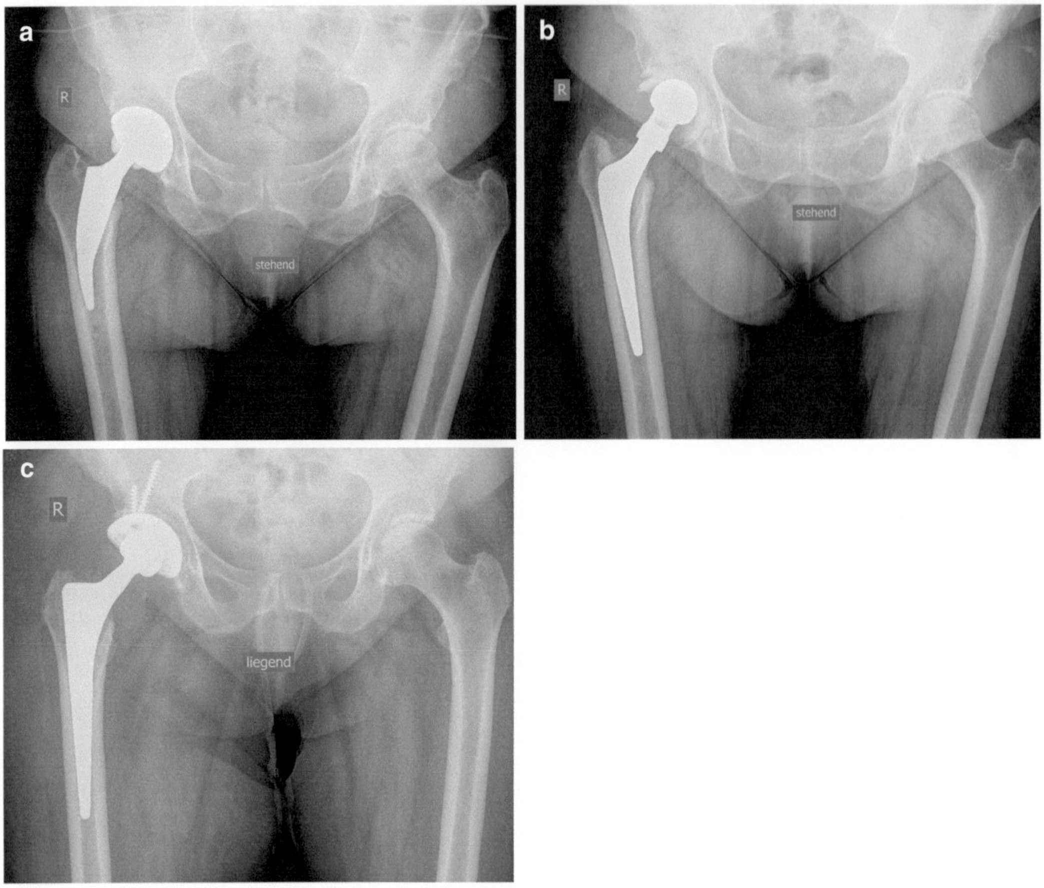

Fig. 10.1 (**a**) Periprosthetic infection of a total hip replacement on the right side. (**b**) Interim prosthesis (spacer) after removal of the infected hip prosthesis with a femoral defect Paprosky type I. (**c**) Reimplantation of a cementless standard prosthesis (CLS stem and Allofit-S cup, Zimmer Biomet, Winterthur, Switzerland)

et al. [5] compared cemented stems with modular metaphyseal fixed, cementless revision stems (S-ROM, DePuy Synthes, Warsaw, IN, USA) in Paprosky I and II defects and found no differences in clinical outcome and 5-year survival (94% cementless versus 92% cemented).

10.2 Paprosky Type IIA Defects

Proximal rotational stability of the remaining metaphyseal bone is present, but reduced compared to Paprosky type I defects. Primary stems with proximal fixation and usually coarsely structured surface and/or hydroxyapatite coating can still be used if sufficient rotational stability can be achieved (Fig. 10.2a, b). This depends on the mechanical quality of the remaining metaphyseal bone and must be carefully checked intraoperatively with the trial prosthesis or rasp. Longer primary prostheses that serve as revision prostheses can also be used here (e.g., Zweymüller Alloclassic SLL, Zimmer Biomet, Winterthur, Switzerland, or CoreHip Extended, Aesculap, Tuttlingen, Germany). Artiaco et al. [6] found a 100% stem survival rate after 12.25 years with 32 stem revisions using a Zweymüller SLL stem (extended primary stem). The revision stems to be considered are proximal fixation stems, which are usually coarsely structured in the proximal portion and/or hydroxyapatite-coated. They may also have a direct contact in the area of the calcar, which must be sawn to the correct shape during the operation. Alternatively, impaction grafting is

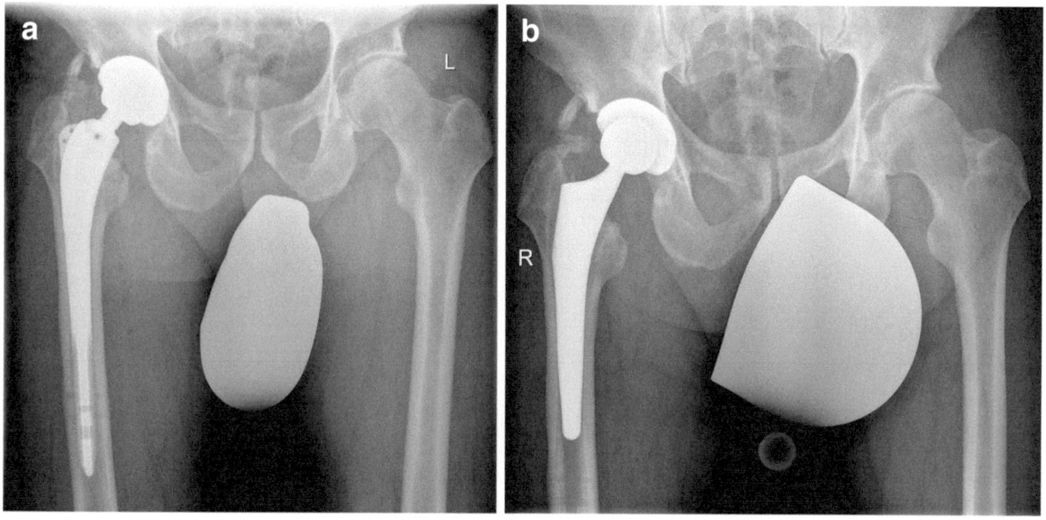

Fig. 10.2 (**a**) Stem loosening with subsidence of a distally locked revision stem with a Paprosky IIA type bone defect. (**b**) Revision to a hydroxyapatite-coated standard stem (Exception, Zimmer Biomet, Winterthur, Switzerland)

possible in such cases where the medial bone is thin, but still sufficiently stable to ensure that the inserted bone chips remain firmly in place during impaction. In such cases, supporters of impaction grafting often reinforce the stability of the medial bone area in the calcar with a medial metal mesh fixed around the femur with cerclages.

10.3 Paprosky Type IIB Defects

This is an anterolateral defect of the subtrochanteric region of the metaphysis. The lateral femur is defective below the greater trochanter. Rotational stability is only partially ensured by this proximal metaphyseal bone and is no longer suitable for proximally anchoring primary stems. In such cases, proximally anchoring longer stems (Zweymüller Alloclassic SLL, Zimmer Biomet, Winterthur, Switzerland) or proximally anchoring revision prostheses are suitable in the form of monoblock prostheses (e.g., CORAIL (DePuy Synthes, Warsaw, IN, USA) or Mallory-Head (Biomet, Warsaw, IN, USA)) with coarse structuring proximally, hydroxyapatite coating, and/or the calcar replacement variant. Alternatively, modular proximal fixation revision stems (S-ROM (DePuy Synthes, Warsaw, IN, USA), Arcos proximal fixation stem (Zimmer Biomet, Warsaw, IN, USA)) can be used. Li et al. [7] found no differences in Paprosky I and II defects with respect to clinical outcomes and 5-year survival when comparing the modular S-ROM stem and a cementless longer monoblock stem (SLR-Plus, Smith & Nephew) of the Zweymüller type (92.3% for S-ROM and 85.7% for SLR-Plus). However, distally fixed nonmodular and modular revision prostheses can also be used (Fig. 10.3a, b). The metaphyseal bone no longer provides sufficient cancellous bone for good interdigitation of the cement during standard cementation, so that cemented standard stems are no longer indicated. This also limits the implant survival of cemented long stem prostheses. Therefore, standard cementation should only be considered in older patients with reduced life expectancy. Impaction grafting is possible if the remaining bone is sufficiently stable to withstand the forces applied during impaction. Minor lateral segmental defects can be repaired with a metal mesh or a strut graft, which is fixed using cerclage around the femur.

10.4 Paprosky Type IIC Defects

In this case, metaphyseal fixation is no longer stable enough for load bearing and fixation due to the defect of the entire metaphyseal region.

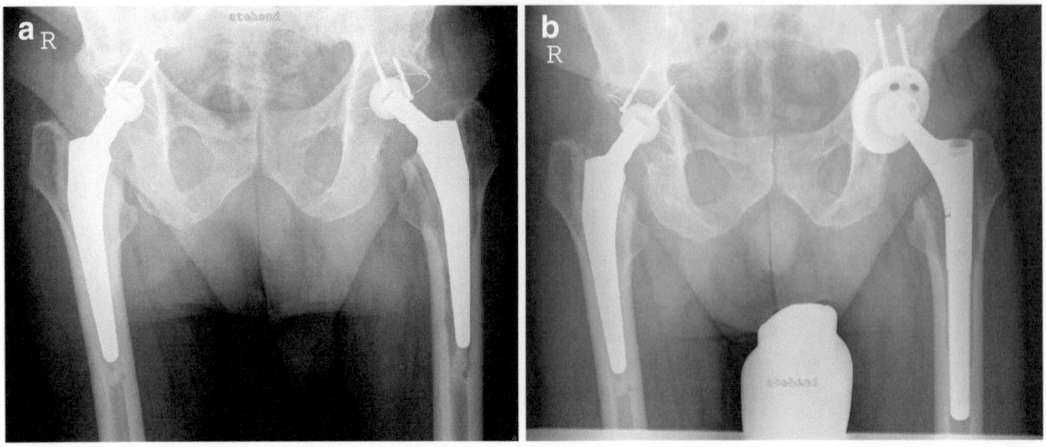

Fig. 10.3 (**a**) Loosening of a hybrid endoprosthesis on the left with a femoral bone defect of the Paprosky IIB type. (**b**) Revision to a modular distal fixation revision stem Revitan Curved with proximal medial bone grafting in the calcar region and an Allofit-S cementless press-fit cup (Zimmer Biomet, Winterthur, Switzerland)

Longer stem prostheses must be used and, if necessary, the medial bone defect must be repaired with a medial strut graft if the stem is still to be anchored in the metaphyseal region. In this case, we recommend bridging the defective zone with a nonmodular or modular distal fixation revision stem (Revitan, Arcos, MRP, MP, etc.) (Fig. 10.4a, b). In my opinion, neither standard cementation nor impaction grafting is an option. Impaction grafting would require extensive support of the medial femoral region with larger metal meshes and would require extensive preparation of the proximal femur with denudation of the bone through dissection of the musculature. Although this technique has been described in the literature by advocates of impaction grafting, I do not recommend it because there are better cementless alternatives with less traumatization of the soft tissues and reproducibly good outcomes reported in many publications.

10.5 Paprosky Type IIIA Defects

This type of defect represents the classic indication for distally fixed prostheses with any of the fixation principles (scratch fit, cone-in-cylinder, or cone-in-cone anchorage). The defective zone is no longer able to support the prosthesis and the fixation is sought in the distal femur, which must be sufficiently intact. In Paprosky type IIIA defects, the isthmus has an intact zone of at least 4 cm. The modular distal revision stems make the operation technically easier for these types of defects, since the distal component is used to achieve distal fixation under the control of the surgeon(s) before the proximal component is used to set the correct leg length, antetorsion, and offset (Fig. 10.5a, b). Monoblock revision stems are also indicated, but make the surgery technically more difficult, since all goals (distal fixation, correct leg length, antetorsion, and offset) must be achieved with just one step of insertion of the nonmodular revision stem. In the case of extensively porous-coated stems, the stability of the stem can be improved by the additional application of strut grafts, which in some cases are reported to be effective even in more severe defects (Paprosky IIIB and IV) [8]. Ding et al. [8] achieved a 10-year survival rate of 96.2% in 44 revisions (19 IIIA defects, 9 IIIB defects, and 4 IV defects) and complete integration of the strut grafts in 31 patients. Strut grafts are indicated for supportive use during surgery if the trial prosthesis indicates that sufficient rotational stability of the implant cannot be achieved. Two to three strut allografts with a mean length of approximately 16 cm are placed around the deficient proximal

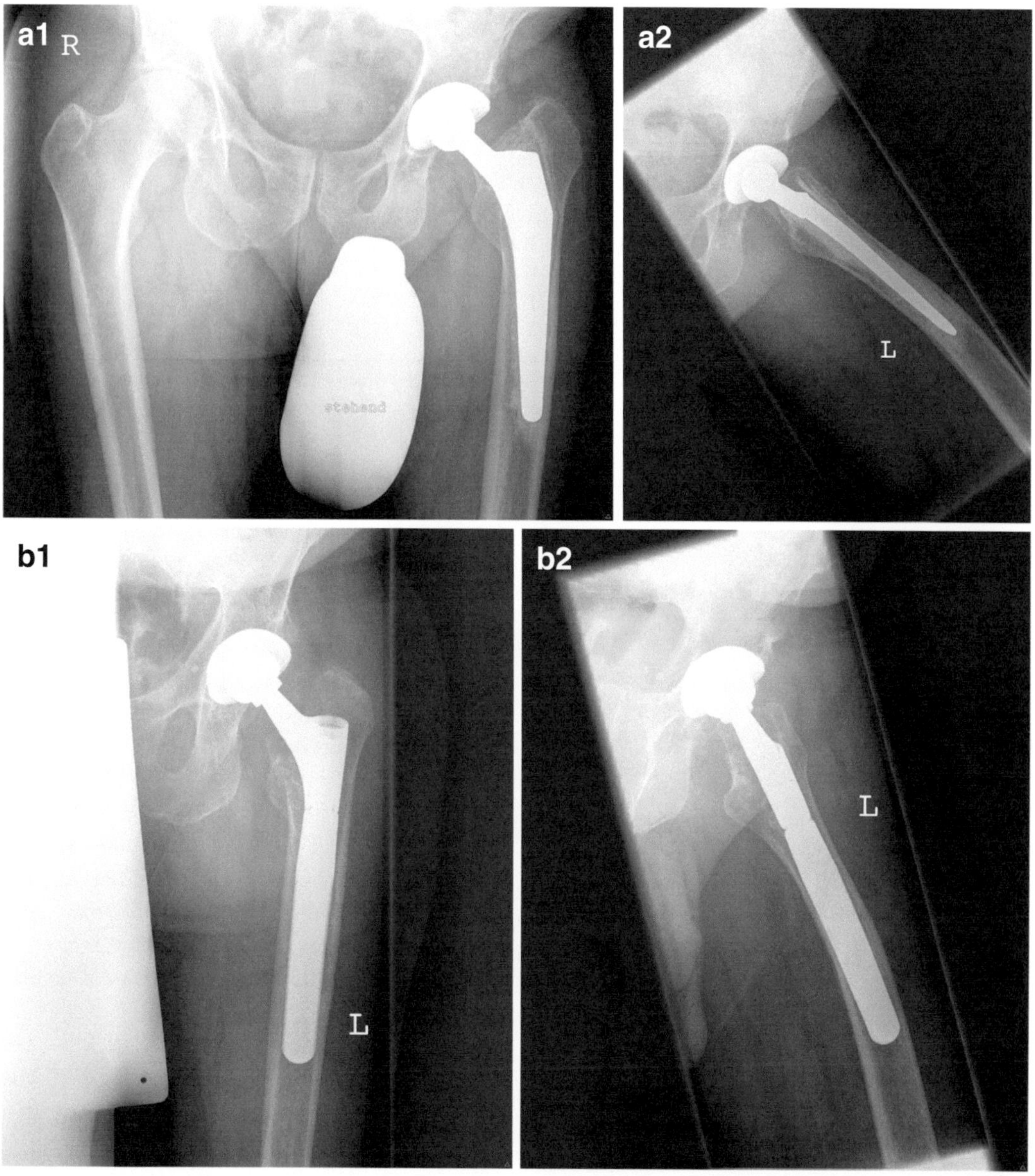

Fig. 10.4 (**a**) Loosening of a cemented stem with variation and a femoral bone defect of the Paprosky IIC type extending to the lesser trochanter. (**a1**) Pelvic overview. (**a2**) Lateral radiograph, showing the greater antecurvature of the femur. (**b**) Revision to the modular distal fixation revision stem Revitan Curved (Zimmer Biomet, Winterthur, Switzerland). (**b1**) A.p. radiograph. (**b2**) Lateral radiograph

femur with double cerclages, and then, the actual stem is implanted [8]. In general, strut grafts are suitable for bridging and constructing non-circumferential segmental bone defects [9]. However, calcar allografts have not proven successful due to their high resorption rates [9].

10.6 Paprosky Type IIIB Defects

By definition, the isthmus of the femur with this defect has a fixation distance of less than 4 cm [1, 2]. Therefore, distal scratch-fit fixation (cylinder-in-cylinder fixation) in the isthmus of the femur

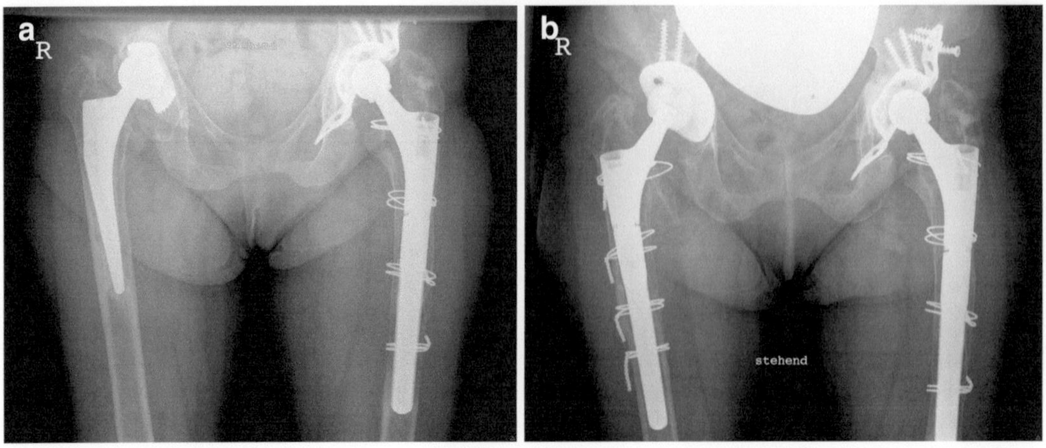

Fig. 10.5 (**a**) Prosthesis loosening on the right with a Paprosky IIIA type femoral defect and, on the left, a transfemoral stem revision to the modular revision stem Revitan Curved (Zimmer Biomet, Winterthur, Switzerland) carried out 3 months earlier for a type IIIA defect. (**b**) Radiograph 6 weeks postoperatively after transfemoral prosthesis revision on the right with a modular revision stem Revitan Curved and a press-fit cup Allofit-S (Zimmer Biomet, Winterthur, Switzerland)

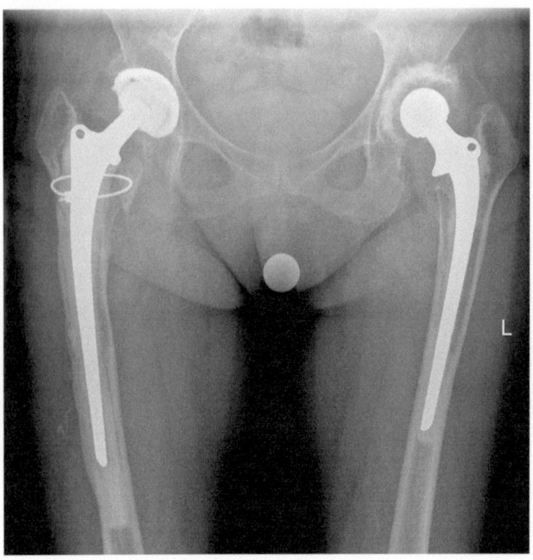

Fig. 10.6 Stem loosening of a cemented revision prosthesis on the right 1.5 years after endofemoral revision of a Paprosky IIIB type femoral defect

is no longer an option (personal communication from Paprosky [10]). The cementing of long cemented revision stems does not result in sufficient interdigitation of the cement or adequate fixation of the stem, so that early loosening must be expected (Fig. 10.6). Therefore, in my opinion, this method should not be performed at all, even in older patients.

According to our own studies of a distally fixing, 2-degree tapered titanium revision stem, a minimum fixation distance of 3 cm is sufficient for adequate distal fixation [11]. Thus, distal tapered revision stems would still be possible in the isthmus of the femur if the fixation zone is between 3 and 4 cm long. However, not only the length of the still intact isthmus is important here, but also the thickness of the undamaged cortex of the isthmus. The thicker the cortex, the shorter the fixation distance can be. Tangsataporn et al. [12] identified a fixation distance of less than 2 cm as a risk factor for subsidence for the ZMR stem (Zimmer Biomet, Warsaw, IN, USA) with a taper of 3.5°. A higher degree of conicity during preparation automatically leads to a shorter fixation distance (Fig. 7.2).

If a minimum fixation distance of 3 cm is not reached with 2° conical revision stems, an additional supplementary fixation technique or another fixation method is required. Our own studies have shown that an additional distal locking device, placed below the isthmus, is effective for a cone-in-cone fixation zone of less than 3 cm [13] (Fig. 10.7a–c). These studies involved the curved modular revision stem Revitan Curved (Zimmer Biomet GmbH, Winterthur, Switzerland), implanted in these cases via a

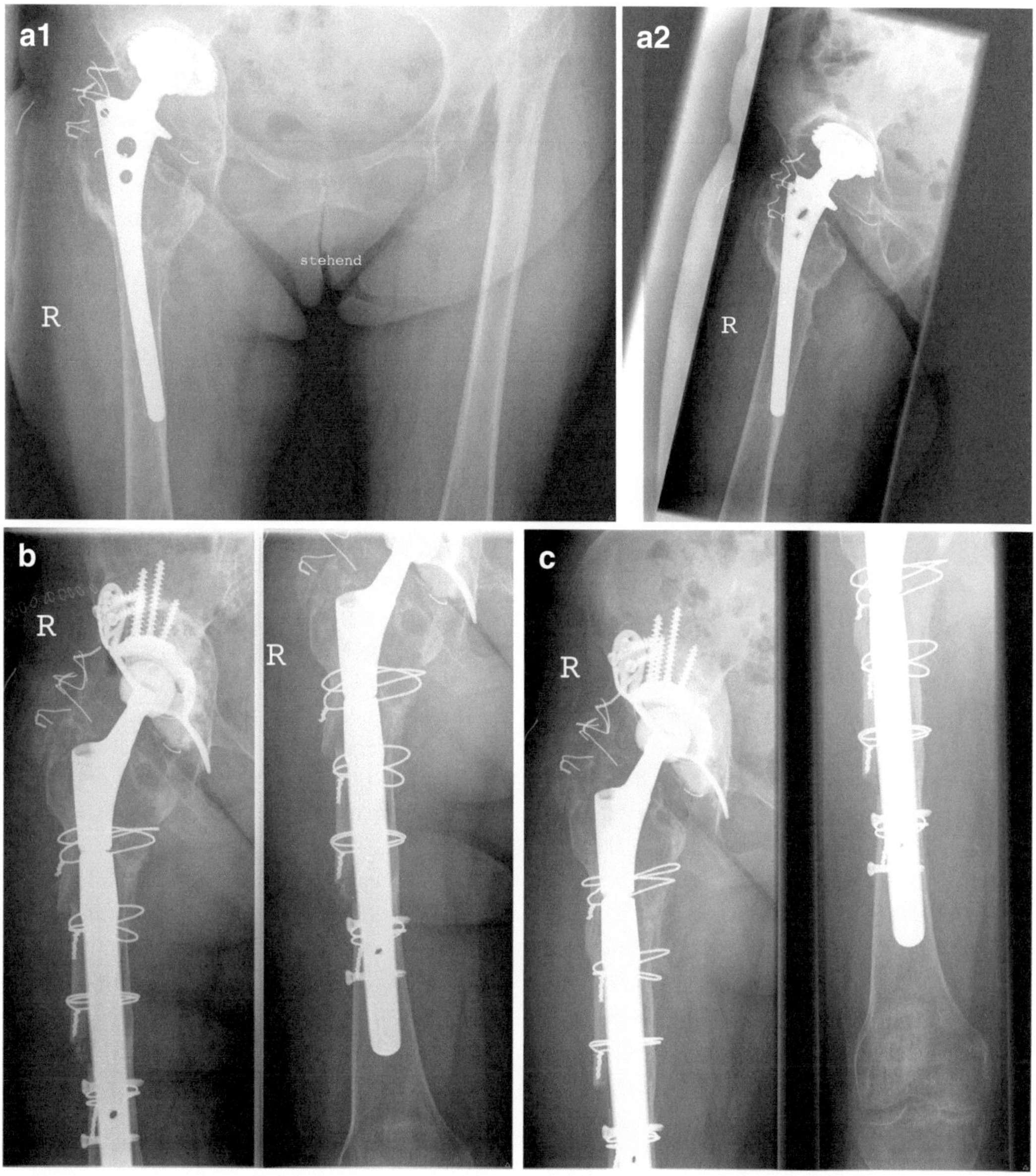

Fig. 10.7 (**a**) Right prosthesis loosening with femoral and acetabular defects of type Paprosky IIIB. (**a1**) Pelvic overview image. (**a2**) Lateral radiograph. (**b**) Transfemoral prosthesis revision to the modular revision stem Revitan Curved with distal locking and a Burch–Schneider reinforcement ring (Zimmer Biomet, Winterthur, Switzerland) with homologous acetabular floor grafting. Intraoperative fracture of the bony flap occurred because of the thin cortical bone. (**c**) Radiograph 1 year after surgery. Bony consolidation of the proximal flap fracture and bone regeneration in the region of the proximal femur and the acetabular floor

transfemoral approach (extended trochanteric osteotomy). The additional fixation by the distal locking device is subsequently superseded postoperatively by callus-induced bone formation and osteointegration of the proximal prosthetic part in the region of the extended trochanteric osteotomy [13]. It is not clear whether this also applies to other straight and curved modular revision stems with distal locking capabilities (MRP stem, Peter Brehm, Weisendorf, Germany;

Prevision Revision Stem, Aesculap, Tuttlingen, Germany; Reef Stem, DePuy Synthes, Warsaw, IN, USA), as different fixation principles (e.g., MRP stem, Peter Brehm, Weisendorf, Germany; Prevision Revision Stem, Aesculap, Tuttlingen, Germany; Reef Stem, DePuy Synthes, Warsaw, IN, USA) are used, e.g., cone-in-cylinder fixation with the MRP stem, cylinder-in-cylinder fixation with the Reef Stem, and different taper angles (e.g., Reef Stem with a cylindrical distal part without taper). However, to date, there have not been any studies published of these stems in the treatment of Paprosky type IIIB and IV defects.

If a short fixation zone with a stable cortex is available, distally fixing conical stems with a higher degree of taper can also be used without locking (e.g., ZMR stem with 3.5° of taper) [14]. Also, Dzaja et al. [15] and Desai et al. [16] found only minor subsidence and loosening for the 3-degree tapered modular revision stem Restoration (Stryker, Kalamazoo, MI, USA) in Paprosky IIIB and IV defects. Biomechanical studies by Pierson et al. [17] showed that as the angle of taper increases, the fixation distance in the isthmus decreases and axial stability increases. Stems with a greater taper become wedged over a shorter distance and axial stability improves with increasing taper [17]. If the cortical bone layer in which the stem is wedged is thick, more highly tapered stems can be anchored in the isthmus of the femur with short, stable fixation distances. Thus, these stems are suitable for revision of Paprosky IIIB defects. However, if the intact isthmus only has a thin cortical segment, the greater force applied over such a short distance leads to a high risk of fracture. These more severe defect types (Paprosky type IIIB and IV) generally require thicker stems for distally fixing revision prostheses, which in turn leads to an increase in the rigidity of the stem system and promotes stress shielding [18].

10.7 Paprosky Type IV Defects

The isthmus of the femur is nonexistent in these extensive metaphyseal and diaphyseal defects, and the femur cannot be used for normal distal fixation of a revision stem. There is no really good solution for this type of defect. All solutions are compromises that have a variety of disadvantages. On the one hand, long cementless modular revision stems with distal locking below the former isthmus area are again a possibility. It is important to understand that the fixation of the system cannot be solely based on the locking screws (Fig. 10.8a–c). Bone contact is required, and either a short-distance conical fixation or a longer-distance bone contact is required to allow osteointegration of the stem. The Reef revision stem (DePuy Synthes, Warsaw, IN, USA) is coated with hydroxyapatite to promote osteointegration of the stem. We have shown that the principle of additional distal interlocking for the 2-degree tapered Revitan Curved stem also works in Paprosky type IV defects [13]. Similar studies are still pending for the other types of stem with distal locking in cases of type IV defects.

Other options for these difficult situations have also been reported in the literature. For example, distal tapered stems with higher taper angles are reported as possible solutions. However, in such cases, there is only a small amount of contact between the stem and the thin remainder of the isthmus corticalis and/or the distal femur, which is likely to increase the risk of fracture. For example, van Houwelingen et al. [14] found fractures in 16% of cases with the ZMR stem with 3.5-degree taper when used for Paprosky III and IV type defects, and Desai et al. [16] in 15%. The significantly increased risk of fracture in these cases is probably also true for the impaction grafting technique, since considerable forces are applied to the thin bone during impaction. The cementing of a long cemented revision prosthesis also has several disadvantages. It is very difficult to produce an adequate cement plug. The insertion of several cement plugs until a somewhat compression-resistant conglomerate is created is one of the suboptimal solutions. In addition, interdigitation of the cement into the remaining thin, smooth-walled bone is not possible. The same problem exists with the use of tumor prostheses, or megaprostheses, with a proximal femoral replacement as

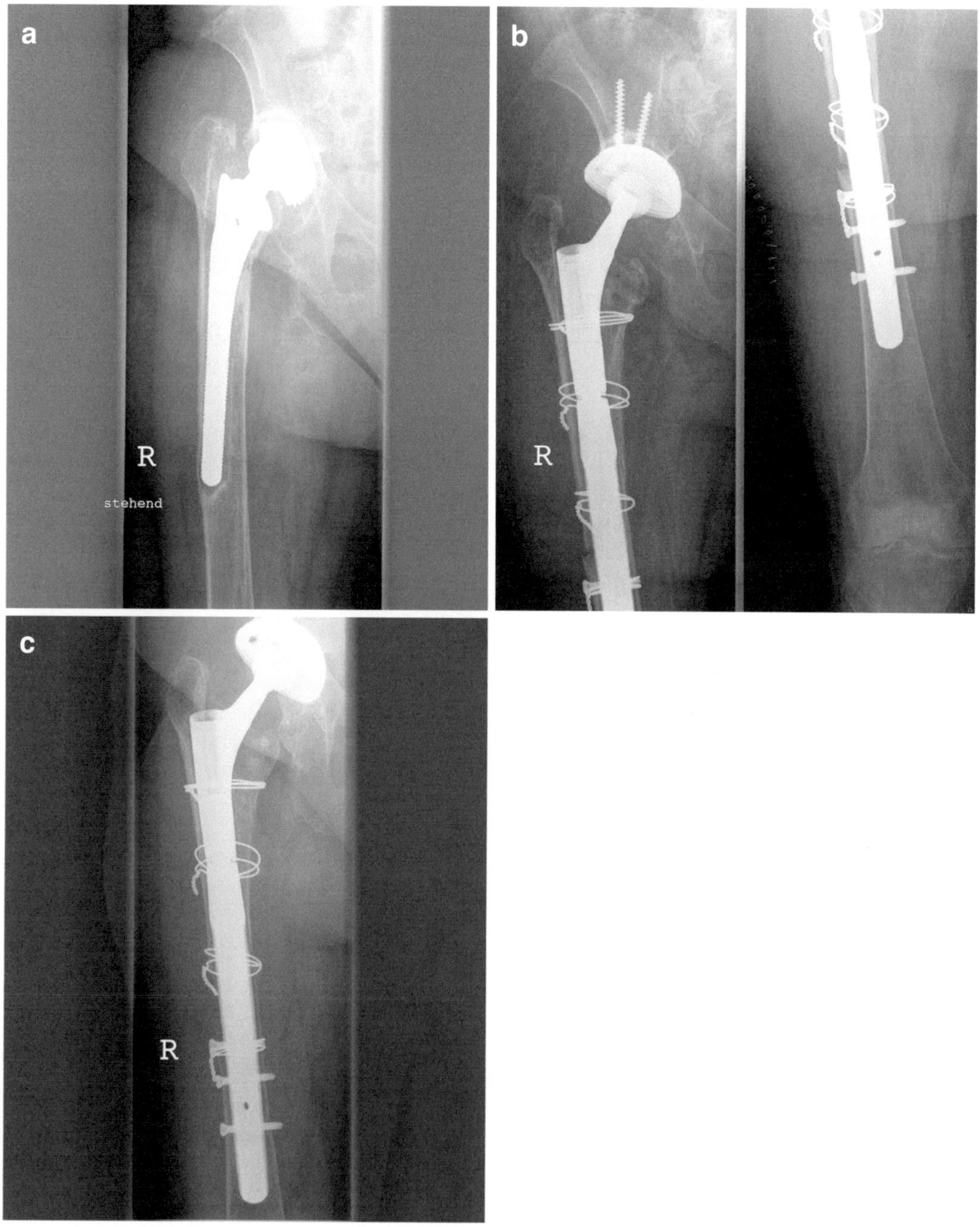

Fig. 10.8 (**a**) Right prosthesis loosening with femoral bone defect of type Paprosky IV with missing isthmus. (**b**) Transfemoral prosthesis revision to the modular revision stem Revitan Curved and a press-fit cup Allofit-S. A short cone-in-cone fixation of the stem can be seen above the additional distal locking system. (**c**) Radiograph 8 years after surgery with unchanged position of the implants. Slight stress shielding in the proximal region has occurred with an overall reduction in the Barnett and Nordin score (Barnett and Nordin 1960, see Chap. 22)

recommended in the literature. These megaprostheses do not provide better distal fixation per se. Thus, 12-year survival rates of tumor prostheses used in revision arthroplasty have been reported to be only 64% [19]. In addition, megaprostheses have the disadvantage that their use results in the alteration of the pelvitrochanteric musculature with ensuing negative effects on muscular function, stability of the hip joint, and an increased risk of periprosthetic infections. Therefore, I consider the cementing of a modular revision system with a cemented distal component (e.g., Link MP revision stem system) to be the better solution. In this case, a transfemoral approach (extended trochanteric osteotomy) is used to wrap the muscles together with the proximal femur around the cementless proximal part of the prosthesis.

In case of extreme proximal bone defects (including periprosthetic fractures type B3), allograft prosthesis composites (APCs) can be performed in younger patients with a proximal femoral allograft [20]. The potential advantage of this method over proximal megaprostheses is the possibility of biological reconstruction of the muscle attachments and bone [9]. The difficulty of obtaining larger allografts, the technical requirements, the risk of nonhealing, and the possible transmission of diseases limit the broad application of this method [21].

As an alternative, the use of megaprostheses in the form of proximal femoral replacements has been recommended for older patients. The disadvantages of this procedure include a higher risk of dislocation, a higher risk of infection, higher aseptic loosening rates, and the risk of further bone loss [22].

References

1. Paprosky WG, Greidanus NV, Antoniou J. Minimum 10-year-results of extensively porous-coated stems in revision hip arthroplasty. Clin Orthop. 1999;369:230–42.
2. Paprosky WG, Aribindi R. Hip replacement: treatment of femoral bone loss using distal bypass fixation. Instr Course Lect. 2000;49:119–30.
3. Wirtz DC, Heller KD, Holzwarth U, et al. A modular femoral implant for uncemented stem revision in THR. Int Orthop. 2000;24:134–8.
4. Cavagnaro L, Formica M, Basso M, Zanirato A, Divano S, Felli L. Femoral revision with primary cementless stems: a systematic review of the literature. Musculoskelet Surg. 2018;102:1–9.
5. Iorio R, Healy WL, Presutti AH. A prospective outcomes analysis of femoral component fixation in revision total hip arthroplasty. J Arthroplasty. 2008;23:662–9.
6. Artiaco S, Fusini F, Colzani G, Aprato A, Zoccola K, Masse A. Long-term results of Zweymüller SLL femoral stem in revision hip arthroplasty for stage II and stage IIIA femoral bone defect: a 9–15-year follow-up study. Musculoskelet Surg. 2020;104(3):273–8. https://doi.org/10.1007/s12306-019-00617-y.
7. Li H, Chen F, Wang Z, Chen Q. Comparison of clinical efficacy between modular cementless stem prostheses and coated cementless long-stem prostheses on bone defect in hip revision arthroplasty. Med Sci Monit. 2016;22:670–7.
8. Ding ZH, Ling TX, Yuan MC, Qin YZ, Mou P, Wang HY, Zhou ZK. Minimum 8-year follow-up of revision THA with severe femoral bone defects using extensively porous-coated stems and cortical strut grafts. BMC Musculoskelet Disord. 2020;21:218.
9. Maurer SG, Baitner AC, Di Cesare PE. Reconstruction of the failed femoral component and proximal femoral bone loss in revision hip surgery. J Am Acad Orthop Surg. 2000;8:354–63.
10. Weeden SH, Paprosky WG. Minimal 11-year follow-up of extensively porous-coated stems in femoral revision total hip arthroplasty. J Arthroplasty. 2002;17 Suppl:134–7.
11. Fink B, Grossmann A, Schubring S, Schulz MS, Fuerst M. Short-term results of hip revisions with a curved cementless modular stem in association with the surgical approach. Arch Orthop Trauma Surg. 2009;129:65–73.
12. Tangsataporn S, Safir OA, Vincent AD, Abdelbary H, Gross AE, Kuzyk PRT. Risk factors for subsidence of a modular tapered femoral stem used for revision total hip arthroplasty. J Arthroplasty. 2015;30:1030–134.
13. Fink B, Grossmann A, Fuerst M. Distal interlocking screws with a modular revision stem for revision total hip arthroplasty in severe bone defects. J Arthroplasty. 2010;25:759–65.
14. van Houwelingen AP, Duncan CP, Masri BA, Greidanus NV, Garbuz DS. High survival of modular tapered stems for proximal femoral bone defects at 5 to 10 years follow-up. Clin Orthop Relat Res. 2013;471:454–62.
15. Dzaja I, Lyons MC, McCalden RW, Naudie DDD, Howard JL. Revision hip arthroplasty using a modular revision system in cases of severe bone loss. J Arthroplasty. 2014;29:1594–7.
16. Desai RR, Malkani AI, Hitt KD, et al. Revision total hip arthroplasty using a modular femoral implant in Paprosky III and IV femoral bone loss. J Arthroplasty. 2012;27:1492–1498.e1.
17. Pierson JL, Small SR, Rodriguez JA, et al. The effect of taper angle and spline geometry on the initial stability of tapered, splined modular titanium stems. J Arthroplasty. 2015;30:1254–9.
18. Fink B, Grossmann A, Schulz MS. Bone regeneration in the proximal femur following implantation of modular revision stems with distal fixation. Arch Orthop Trauma Surg. 2011;131:465–70.

19. Malkani AL, Paiso JM, Sim FH. Proximal femoral replacement with megaprosthesis. Instr Course Lect. 2000;49:141–6.
20. Raousli MR, Porat MD, Hozack WJ, Parvizi J. Proximal femoral replacement and allograft prosthesis composite in the treatment of periprosthetic fractures with significant proximal bone loss. Orthop Surg. 2012;4:203–10.
21. Tomford WW. Transmission of disease through transplantation of musculoskeletal allografts. J Bone Joint Surg Am. 1995;77-A:1742–54.
22. Viste A, Perry KL, Taunton MJ, Hanssen AD, Abdel MP. Proximal femoral replacement in contemporary revision total hip arthroplasty for severe femoral bone loss.: a review of outcomes. Bone Joint J. 2017;99-B:325–9.

Preoperative Planning 11

Contents

11.1 **Exclusion of a Periprosthetic Infection** 126
11.2 **Prosthesis Planning** 127
11.3 **Re 1: Analysis of the Shape of the Femur** 129
11.4 **Re 2: Analysis of the Mechanical Stability of the Femur** 130
11.5 **Re 3: Necessity for Osteotomies** 130
11.6 **Re 4: Selection of Prosthesis Shape (Curved or Straight)** 130
11.7 **Re 5: Selection of the Method of Fixation (Proximal or Distal)** 133
11.8 **Re 6: Selection of Component Sizes** 137
11.9 **Preparation of the Preoperative Planning Sketch** 141
11.9.1 Step 1: Mapping the Axes and, Where Necessary, the Osteotomies 141
11.9.2 Step 2A: Mapping the Distal Components for Distally Fixed Stems 141
11.9.3 Step 2B: Mapping the Distal Components for Proximally Fixed Stems 145
11.9.4 Step 3A: Mapping the Proximal Component for Distally Fixed Stems 146
11.9.5 Step 3B: Mapping the Proximal Component for Proximally Fixed Stems 147
11.9.6 Step 4: Mapping Reference Points and Distances 148
11.9.7 Step 5: Further Steps in Digital Planning 148
References 149

Preoperative planning should be carried out before every prosthesis revision. This not only aids in the selection of prosthetic components, but also allows potential problems, such as the risk of fractures, to be identified and dealt with in a structured manner. The reason for revision surgery should be identified before the operation. Hip prostheses in which the cause of problems cannot be identified should not be surgically explored and certainly not exchanged, as the chances of success in these cases are low [1].

The information relating to the existing implant must be obtained prior to revision surgery. For stand-alone stem revisions, the corresponding inlay of the existing cup must be on hand or at least a strategy devised for the situation when it is no longer available. Several key questions must be answered during the planning of

B. Fink, *Femoral Revision Arthroplasty*, https://doi.org/10.1007/978-3-030-84821-7_11

such revision surgery: Which approach should be taken? How can the existing implant be removed without complications? Which fixation principle and which implant type should be used for the reimplantation? How can the new implant be firmly fixed? How should existing bone defects be dealt with? Possible complications with the selected procedure must be considered and the appropriate solutions planned. This may result in the need to order additional instruments or special implants as a precaution.

Periprosthetic infection must be excluded before every revision. Due to its significance and its necessitating a totally different therapeutic procedure, every prosthesis to be revised or exchanged should be considered to be infected until proven otherwise [2].

11.1 Exclusion of a Periprosthetic Infection

A periprosthetic infection can be the cause of prosthesis loosening or of problems with the prosthesis. The presence of such an infection requires a fundamentally different procedure to that used for aseptic prosthesis revision. Depending on the underlying situation, different time frames are available for reaching a final decision. As a rule, sufficient time is available for the diagnosis. A periprosthetic fracture with a loosened stem and osteolysis, however, may also be associated with a rare but nevertheless possible periprosthetic infection. This is where rapid diagnostic tests (e.g., the alpha-defensin lateral flow test Synovasure, Zimmer Biomet, Warsaw, IN, USA) can help. Due to the considerable significance of this procedure, the diagnostic methodology will be briefly discussed in this section.

Since no test exists with 100% accuracy, a number of different testing strategies are used and different classifications of periprosthetic infection coexist. Not all test procedures and definitions can be discussed in detail in this book, so reference is made to further reading. In the following, I will present, and try to justify, an approach that we use in our clinic that is as pragmatic as possible.

The diagnosis of a periprosthetic infection should always be started preoperatively, since—as I mentioned before—the therapeutic concept changes significantly when such an infection is detected. In doing so, an attempt should always be made to identify the pathogens causing the infection with the corresponding antibiogram. This is the only way to choose a specific local and systemic antibiotic therapy. Not all broad-spectrum antibiotics, which would otherwise be administered on a regular basis, are effective against all pathogens that cause periprosthetic infections, and the development of resistance can be minimized by targeted antibiotic therapy [3–5]. Therefore, in addition to the determination of the C-reactive protein and, if applicable, the D-dimers in serum, the aspiration of the hip joint also plays an important role in diagnostics. In the USA, the erythrocyte sedimentation rate (ESR) is also determined. The number of diagnostic tests that can be performed depends on the amount of fluid obtained. In my opinion, based on the arguments listed above, the culture of the joint aspirate should always be performed as a direct test (with the possibility of detecting bacteria) (Table 2.2) [2]. The following can be considered as suitable indirect tests (without bacterial detection): cell count with determination of the percentage of polymorphonuclear leukocytes, the alpha-defensin test (as ELISA laboratory test or lateral flow rapid test Synovasure, Zimmer Biomet, Warsaw, IN, USA), and the leukocyte esterase test in the form of test strips. The resulting data can now be checked against one of the definitions of periprosthetic infection. We prefer the ICM (International Consensus Meeting) definition from 2018 (Table 11.1) [6]. If one of the so-called major criteria is present (sinus tract from the prosthesis or identical pathogens are detected in 2 tissue samples or aspirates) or if the sum of the tests performed on serum and aspirate yields a total score of at least 6 points, a periprosthetic infection is present. If the score is between 2 and 5, further studies are required and one can either repeat the aspiration or rely on findings from intraoperative diagnostics (Table 11.2) [6]. In view of the above-mentioned arguments, in this situation, we opt for a diagnostic procedure prior to the actual prosthe-

Table 11.1 Weighting of the preoperative diagnostic tests for the diagnosis of a periprosthetic infection according to the ICM definition 2018 [6]

			Score
Major	Sinus tract from prosthesis		
	2 tissue samples/aspirates yielding identical organisms		
Minor	CRP (>10 mg/mL)	Serum	2
	D-dimer (>860 ng/mL)	Serum	2
	ESR (>30 mm/h)	Serum	1
	Cell count in aspirate (>3000/μL)	Synovium	3
	Proportion of PMN in aspirate (>80%)	Synovium	2
	Alpha-defensin (>1)	Synovium	3
	Leukocyte esterase test strip (++)	Synovium	3
	Synovial CRP (>6.9 mg/mL)	Synovium	1

Score ≥ 6 = infection
Score 2 – 5 necessitates intraoperative evaluation

Table 11.2 Weighting of the intraoperative diagnostic tests for the diagnosis of a periprosthetic infection according to the ICM definition 2018 [6]

	Score
Histology: ≥ 5 PMN in ≥ 5 high-power fields (×400)	3
Purulent fluid	3
Single positive culture	2

pre-operative & intraoperative

Score ≥ 6 = infection
Score 4, 5 = equivocal result
Score ≤ 3 = no infection

sis revision and performing biopsies of the periprosthetic tissue together with a further joint aspiration. In a study of 100 hip prosthesis replacement procedures, we were able to achieve a sensitivity of 86.7%, a specificity of 98.2%, a positive predictive value of 97.5%, a negative predictive value of 90%, and an accuracy of 93% in a combination of culture of the aspirate and 5 samples of the periprosthetic tissue and histological examination of 5 samples of the periprosthetic tissue [5]. In a later study of 231 hip prosthesis revisions, the values for the same methodology were 93.8% sensitivity, 94.1% specificity, 93.8% positive predictive value, 94.1% negative predictive value, and 93.9% accuracy [7]. If the results of the preoperative aspiration and biopsy are combined, the 2018 ICM definition (biopsy instead of intraoperative) allows a reliable assessment of whether or not a periprosthetic infection is present. A cumulative score above 6 clearly indicates an infection, and a score of 3 and less clearly indicates no infection [6]. With 4 or 5 points, the situation remains unclear. In such cases, we perform antibiotic shielding with broad-spectrum antibiotics after the revision until the microbiological results for the intraoperative samples have been received. Here, a 14-day culture period, as in the preoperative assessment, is essential because the bacteria often grow very slowly [8]. In addition, in these cases we also carry out a sonification of the implant removed during revision surgery, which further improves results of the diagnostic tests [9].

11.2 Prosthesis Planning

The actual prosthesis planning and planning of the flap length for transfemoral access are carried out on radiographs of the femur in two planes with a film focus distance of 115 cm and a graduated spherical calibration marker for digital planning. These images are used to analyze the shape of the femur with possible axial deviations, to identify defects, osteolyses, and thinning of the femoral cortex with the resulting defect classification, to plan osteotomies with determination of the flap length and/or windows and the choice of component sizes. Depending on the length of the loosened implant, preoperative planning requires radiographs of between 20 and 40 cm length of the corresponding femur in both planes. These should show the entire prosthesis and cement mantle up to its end and at least the whole isthmus of the femur (Fig. 11.1a, b).

It is important in this analysis to determine whether the revision can be performed endofemorally or by using a transfemoral approach (extended trochanteric osteotomy). In particular, it should be determined whether there is a significant risk of an unintentional fracture, due to a femoral axial deviation, cortical thinning, or a coarsely structured cementless stem, or whether there is a risk of perforation due to the presence of a long cement mantle. These can be avoided by means of a transfemoral approach. For this purpose, a line is drawn in the middle of the femoral canal to serve as the centromedullary axis of the femur (Fig. 11.2). If this line runs proximally into the greater trochanter, the endofemoral approach carries an increased risk of an unintentional fracture of the trochanter or more distally of the femur (Fig. 11.2). Therefore, in these cases, correction of the femur should be effected by osteotomy during a transfemoral approach (extended trochanteric osteotomy). The final decision in favor of a transfemoral approach can then be made with an appropriate prosthesis, which, in the example shown here, extends proximally into the lateral cortex and/or the greater trochanter or even beyond it (Fig. 11.3).

In addition to checking the necessity for a transfemoral approach, the length of the associated bony flap is also defined on the radiographs. It is measured from the tip of the greater trochanter, with the aim of preserving the longest possible section of the isthmus, and the apex of the deformity of the femur, which will be subse-

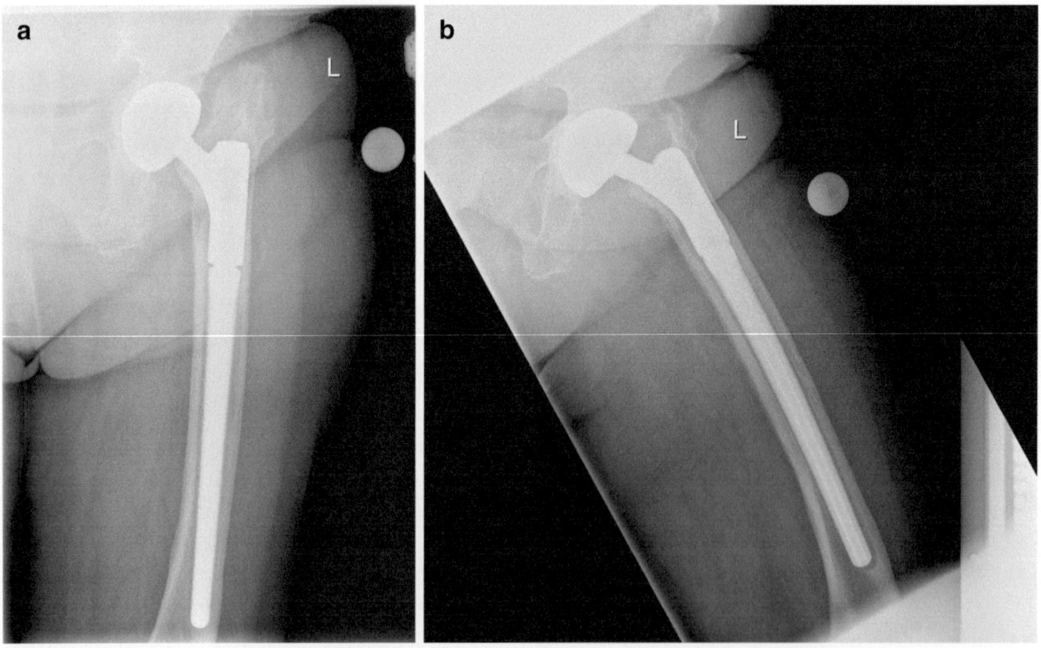

Fig. 11.1 Full-length radiograph of the left hip joint and thigh for planning a stem revision of a loosened, subsided, cementless revision stem. (**a**) Radiograph a.p. with calibration sphere. (**b**) Lateral radiograph with calibration sphere

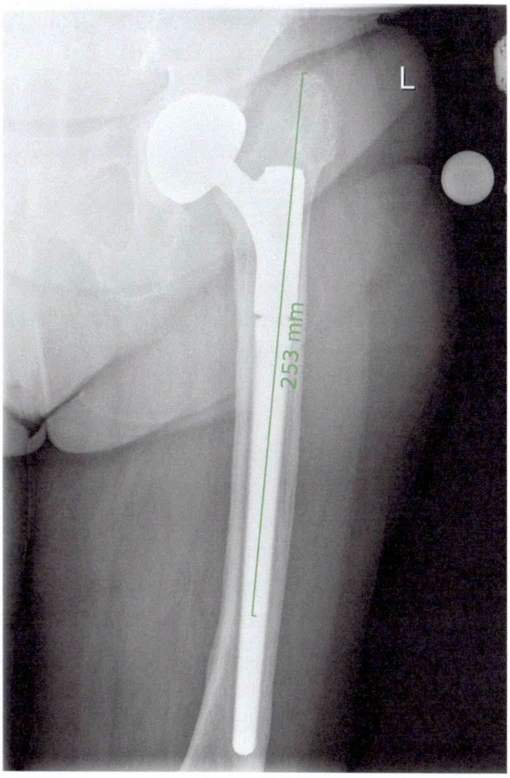

Fig. 11.2 Mapping the centromedullary axis in the center of the femoral canal. The axis here runs through the greater trochanter, and due to the additional thinning of the subtrochanteric cortical bone, there is an increased risk of an unintentional trochanteric fracture in the case of an endofemoral implantation

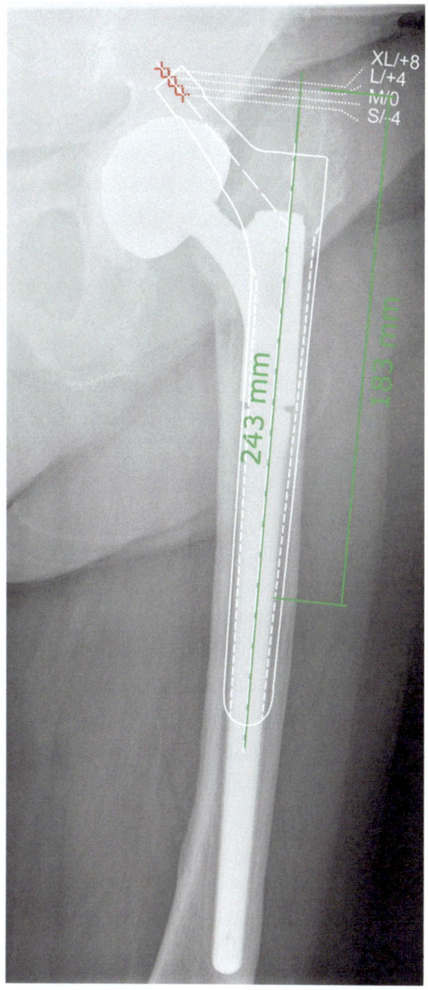

Fig. 11.3 Planning a nonmodular revision stem with distal fixation in the isthmus along the centromedullary axis. The proximal part of the prosthesis penetrates the trochanter. This indicates the risk of unintentional trochanteric fracture if an endofemoral implantation would be carried out. The length of the bony flap for the required transfemoral approach is shown on the side

quently corrected via the transfemoral approach (extended trochanteric osteotomy) (Fig. 11.3).

Therefore, the following points must be analyzed or defined on the radiographs during preoperative planning:

1. shape of the femur with possible axial deviations
2. mechanical stability of the bone and defect analysis
3. necessity of osteotomies (transfemoral approach, double osteotomy of the femur) and planning the length of the flap or flaps (for double osteotomies)
4. choice of prosthesis shape (curved or straight)
5. choice of fixation type (proximal or distal)
6. choice of component sizes and lengths.

11.3 Re 1: Analysis of the Shape of the Femur

The loss of bone substance during implant loosening can cause curvature of the femur in the frontal plane, the sagittal plane, and in both planes in combination (Fig. 11.2). Curvature in the frontal plane occurs as a varus of the metaphyseal bone and as a varus of the metaphyseal and diaphyseal femur. During the loosening process, the force applied to the prosthetic head results in a varus of the prosthetic stem. The bone will be remodeled and aligned with the prosthesis in part according to Wolff's law [10]. Varus of the femur usually requires a correction osteotomy. In the case of slight varus deformities, transfemoral access is usually sufficient for secure stem implantation; in the case of more severe varus deformities, a double osteotomy will be necessary (Fig. 11.4a, b). Curvatures in the sagittal plane occur as antecurvature of the diaphysis with a double curvature of the femur due to an opposing proximal and diaphyseal concavity, and also as an accentuated antecurvature of the femur with dorsal concave curvature of the proximal and diaphyseal femur running in the same direction. The use of a curved stem may reduce the need for femoral osteotomy, but nevertheless it is still necessary to analyze this need during preoperative planning by comparing the femoral curvature with that of the curved stem. Axial deviations in the frontal and sagittal plane can occur in principle in all combinations (Fig. 11.4a–d).

11.4 Re 2: Analysis of the Mechanical Stability of the Femur

The mechanical stability of the femur requires analysis of the bone quality of the metaphyseal and diaphyseal bone. The primary goal is to determine whether the remaining metaphyseal bone is still capable of bearing loads and is therefore suitable for a metaphyseal anchored stem (Fig. 11.5, b). If it is weakened by the loosening process, a proximally anchored prosthesis would carry the risk of an intra- or postoperative periprosthetic fracture (in particular detachment of the greater trochanter) (Fig. 11.6, b). In this case, a distally fixed revision stem should be favored. Furthermore, distal fixation is indicated for periprosthetic fractures requiring prosthesis revision. A periprosthetic fracture should be bridged with the distally fixed implant, and the fixation of the stem should be distal to the fracture.

11.5 Re 3: Necessity for Osteotomies

The transfemoral approach (extended trochanteric osteotomy) is suitable for facilitating the easy removal of stem endoprostheses:

- that are fractured,
- that have an extensive, robust cement mantle,
- that as a cementless stem are only partially loosened (especially in case of a coarsely porous surface structure),
- that are firmly fixed, but infected,
- that sit in a fracture-prone, weakened bone,
- that are loosened in a fractured femur, and/or.
- in a femur with a more pronounced curvature in the frontal and/or sagittal plane.

In the case of more severe deviations, especially in the frontal plane, double osteotomies of the femur may be necessary for complete correction. Preoperative planning is used to determine the position of the osteotomy and of the distal fixation zones (Fig. 11.4a–d).

11.6 Re 4: Selection of Prosthesis Shape (Curved or Straight)

In principle, both types of prosthesis are suitable for endofemoral and for transfemoral access. The only difference is that the curved version approximates the anatomy of the femur, and therefore, a femoral osteotomy, i.e., a transfemoral approach or double osteotomy, is required less frequently than with the straight stem version. Without femoral osteotomy, i.e., without transfemoral access, short stems up to a total length of approx. 220 mm can be implanted in both curved and straight versions if the femur is straight in the frontal plane

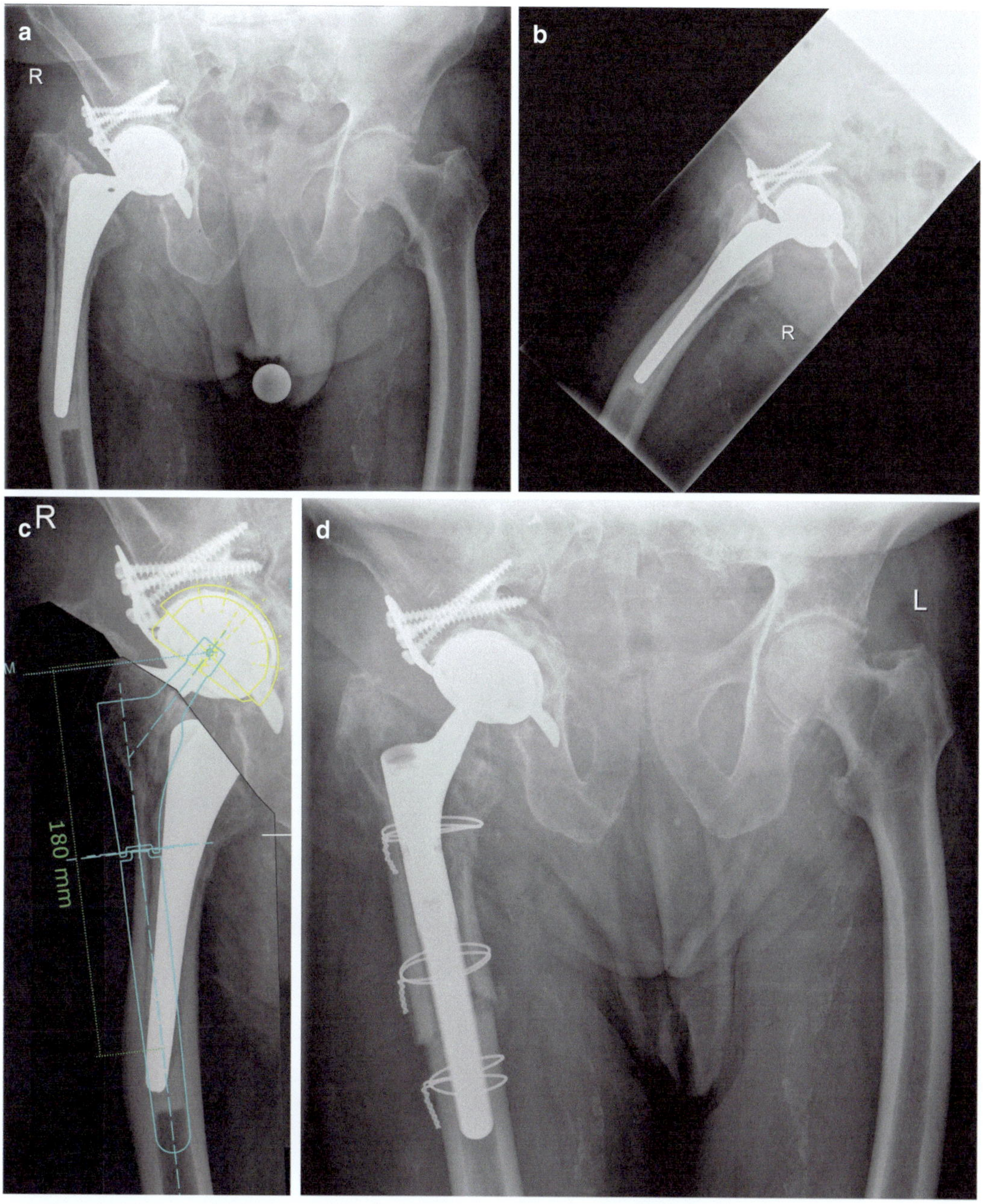

Fig. 11.4 Stem loosening of a cemented stem with axial deviation of the femur in both planes, which requires correction by double osteotomy. (**a**) A.p. radiograph shows the increased varus of the femur. (**b**) Lateral radiograph showing the increased antecurvature of the femur. (**c**) Preoperative planning showing the necessity for the double osteotomy. (**d**) Radiograph 6 weeks postoperatively after stem revision using the modular revision stem Revitan Curved (Zimmer Biomet, Winterthur, Switzerland) implanted via a transfemoral approach with a double osteotomy. The osteotomies show signs of callus formation

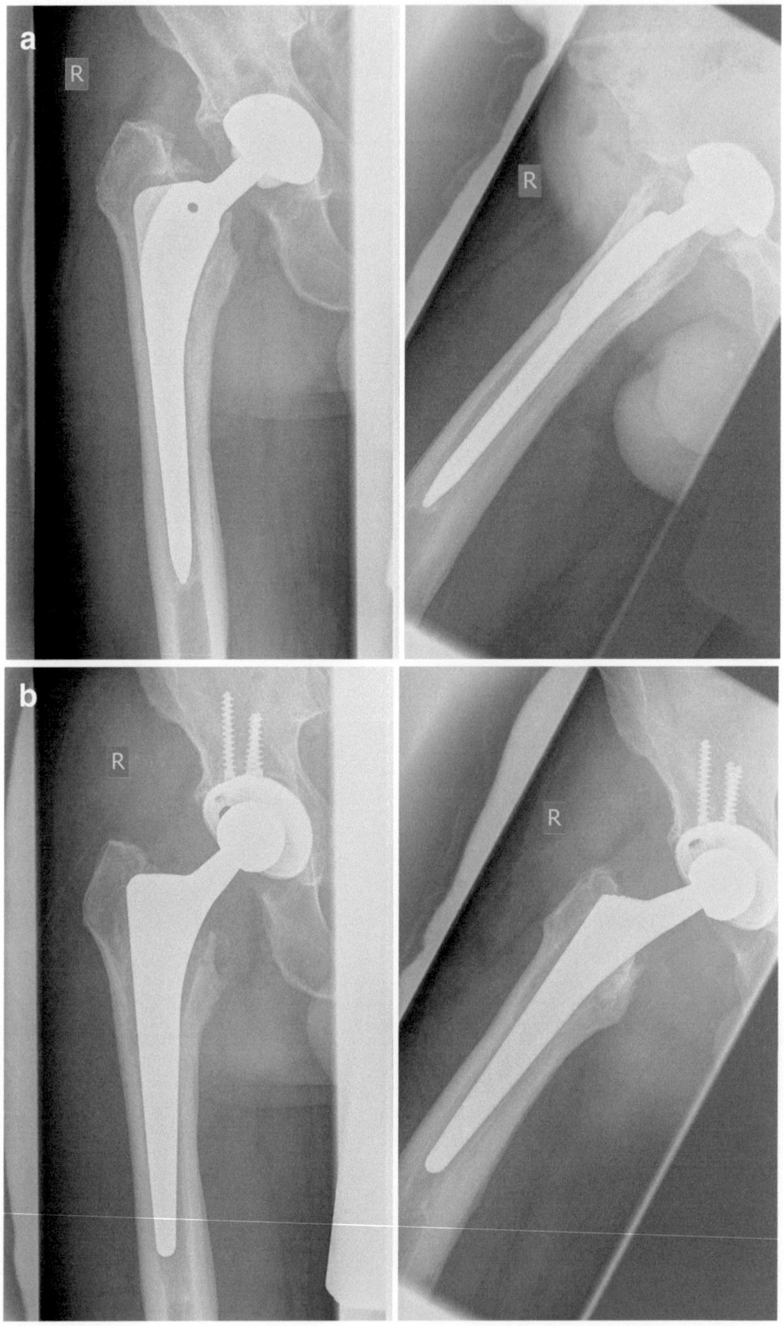

Fig. 11.5 (**a**) Stem loosening of a cementless stem on the right, which has sufficiently stable metaphyseal bone to allow proximal anchoring of a new stem in this case of a minor bone defect (Paprosky type II), and a misaligned cup. (**b**) Prosthesis revision to a cementless standard stem (CLS, Zimmer Biomet, Winterthur, Switzerland) and press-fit cup (Allofit-S, Zimmer Biomet, Winterthur, Switzerland)

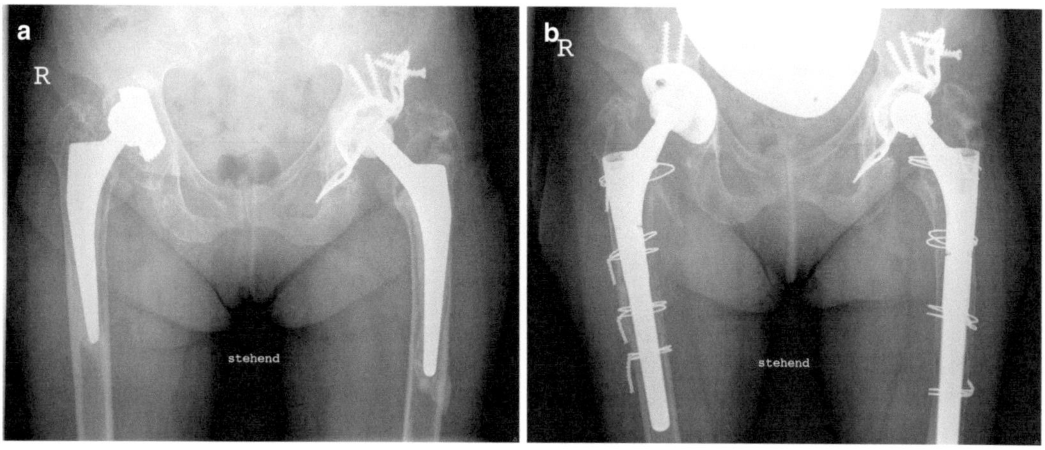

Fig. 11.6 (**a**) Stem loosening on both sides (and cup loosening on the right) with metaphyseal and diaphyseal bone defect (Paprosky type IIIA) and osteopenic metaphyseal bone that no longer permits proximal stem fixation. (**b**) Radiograph after transfemoral stem revision using a Revitan Curved (Zimmer Biomet, Winterthur, Switzerland) 6 months earlier on the left and transfemoral stem and cup revision (using Revitan Curved and Allofit-S) 3 months earlier on the right

and does not exhibit significantly increased curvature in the sagittal plane. In these femurs, however, longer stems can only be implanted without osteotomy in a curved form (Fig. 11.7a–d). Longer straight shafts require transfemoral access, primarily to avoid ventral perforations of the femur with the prosthesis tip. Significant varus deformities and substantial curvature in the sagittal plane require corrective osteotomies for both types of stem (straight and curved); in most cases, a double osteotomy is required (Fig. 11.4a–d).

11.7 Re 5: Selection of the Method of Fixation (Proximal or Distal)

After analyzing the mechanical characteristics of the bone (see 2), the need for osteotomies (see 3), and the choice of prosthesis shape (see 4), the appropriate method of fixation can now be selected. If metaphyseal and diaphyseal bone substance is preserved, and if the femur is straight in the frontal plane and there is no need for an osteotomy, a metaphyseal fixed or distally fixed stem such as a three-surface fixation stem can be selected for endofemoral implantation (Figs. 11.8a, b and 11.9a–c). Otherwise, the implant should be anchored distally using a transfemoral approach (Fig. 11.10a, b). A revision endoprosthesis with distal fixation in the nonfractured distal bone can also be implanted to treat a periprosthetic fracture with a loosened implant (Fig. 11.11, b).

During preoperative planning, not only the type of fixation but also the respective fixation distance is determined in order to gain an impression of the resulting primary stability of the implant.

Distal fixation should be carried out in diaphyseal bone that is as undamaged as possible. The fixation zone is usually located in the isthmus below the old prosthesis bed and involves scratch-fit, cone-in-cylinder, or cone-in-cone fixation. If the cortical bone is of good quality, a fixation distance of 30–50 mm is usually sufficient for transfemoral implantation, depending on the type of

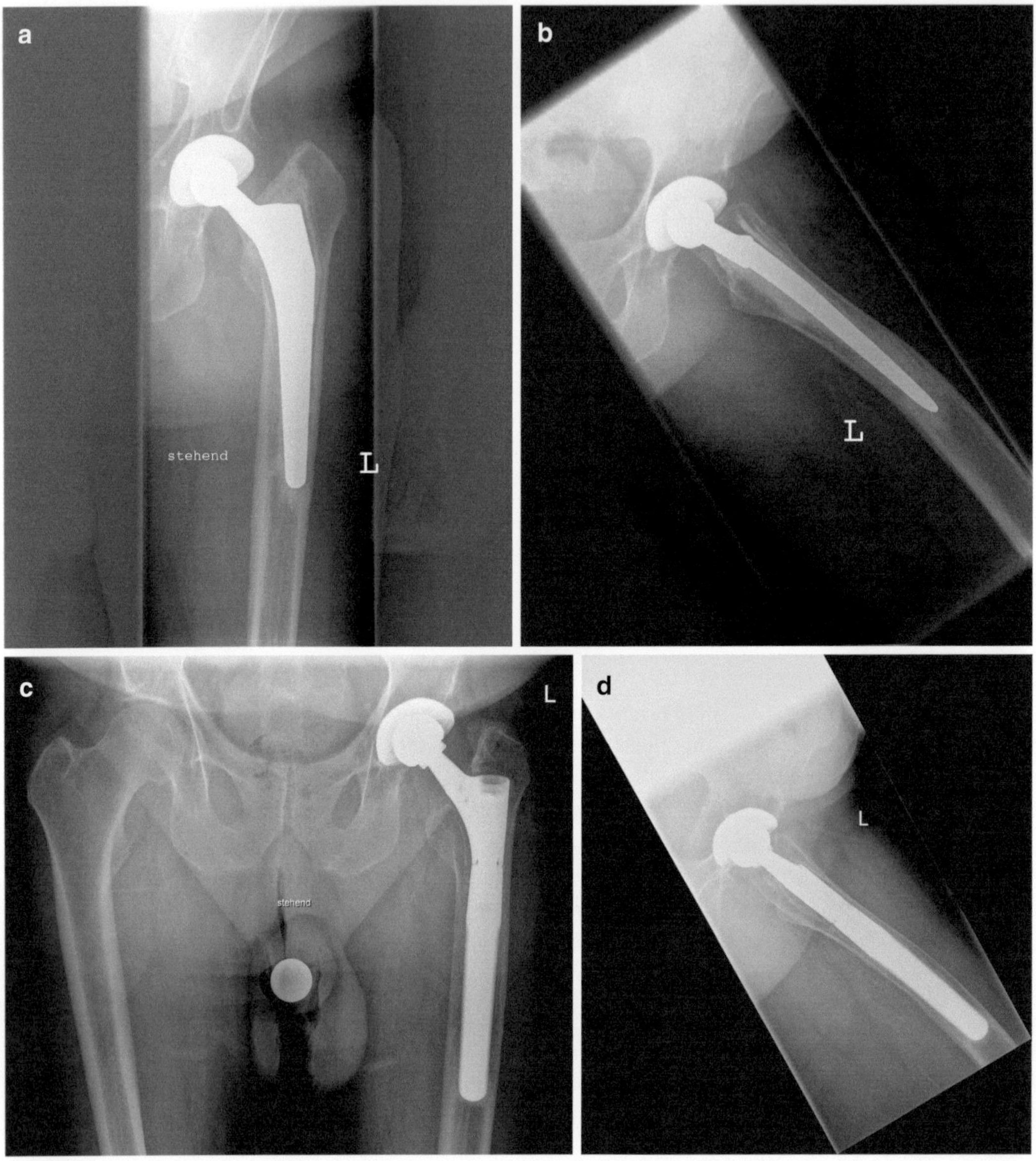

Fig. 11.7 (**a**, **b**) Stem loosening on the left in which endofemoral implantation of a longer curved revision stem appears possible. (**a**) A.p. radiograph, (**b**) Lateral radiograph. (**c**, **d**) Radiograph 1 year postoperatively after endofemoral replacement with the modular revision stem Revitan Curved (Zimmer Biomet, Winterthur, Switzerland). (**c**) Radiograph a.p., (**d**) Lateral radiograph

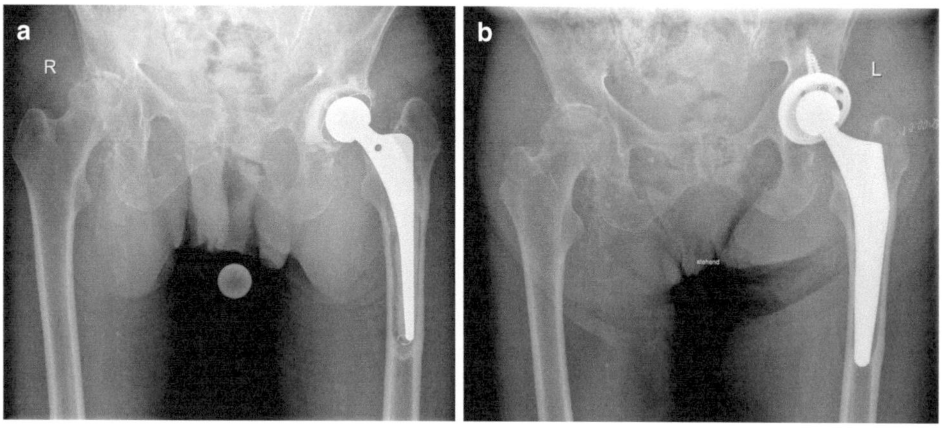

Fig. 11.8 (**a**) Stem loosening with a Paprosky IIIA type bone defect, but still sufficient metaphyseal bone to allow proximal fixation. (**b**) Stem loosening on a metaphyseal anchored, hydroxyapatite-coated standard stem (Exception, Zimmer Biomet, Winterthur, Switzerland)

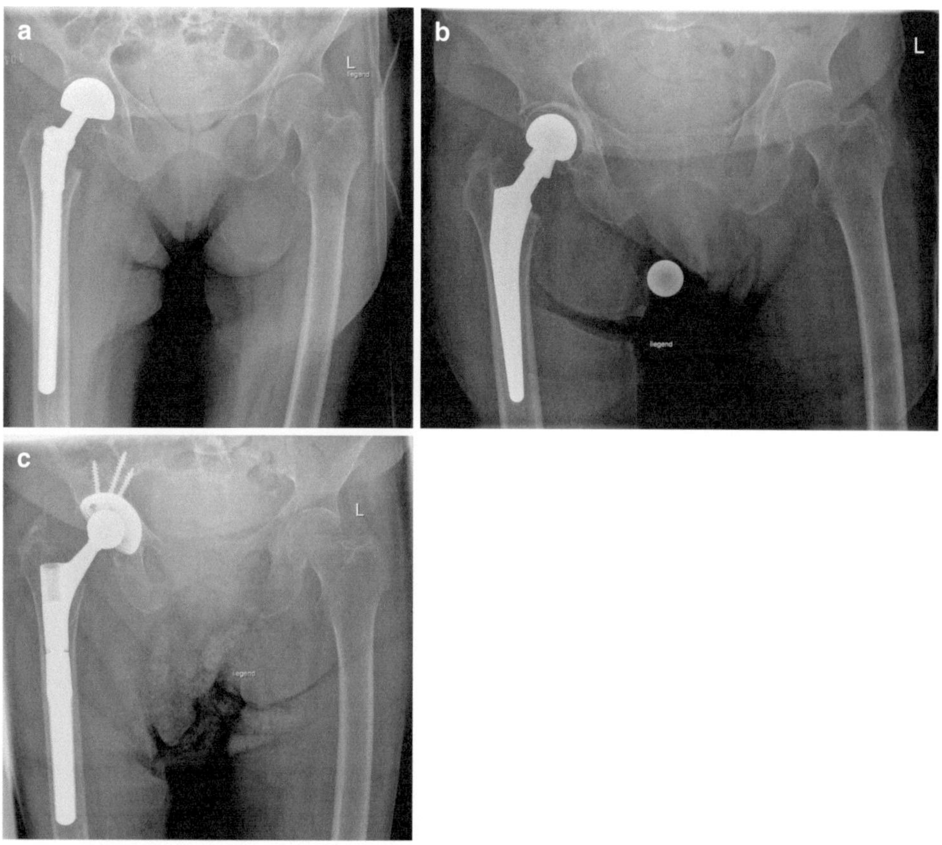

Fig. 11.9 (**a**) Periprosthetic infection of a dual-mobility prosthesis with a modular distal revision stem and a Paprosky II type bone defect. Given the extent of proximal osteolysis and the proximal defect after explantation and insertion of a spacer (**b**), a distally fixed modular revision stem (Revitan Curved, Zimmer Biomet, Winterthur, Switzerland) with endofemoral three-surface fixation was the preferred option. (**c**) Exchange of the spacer with a modular revision stem Revitan Curved anchored with three-surface fixation and press-fit cup Allofit-S (Zimmer Biomet, Winterthur, Switzerland)

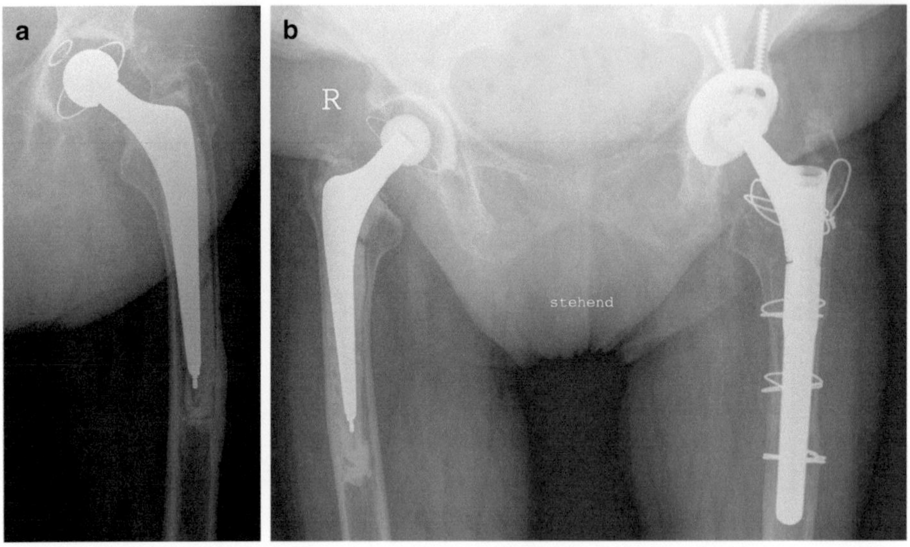

Fig. 11.10 (**a**) Prosthesis loosening with varus of the stem and fracture-prone Paprosky IIIA type bone defect indicating a transfemoral revision. (**b**) Radiograph 9 months postoperatively after transfemoral prosthesis revision to a modular revision stem Revitan Curved and press-fit cup Allofit-S (Zimmer Biomet, Winterthur, Switzerland). The bony flap has already achieved bony consolidation, and proximal bone regeneration has occurred through callus formation

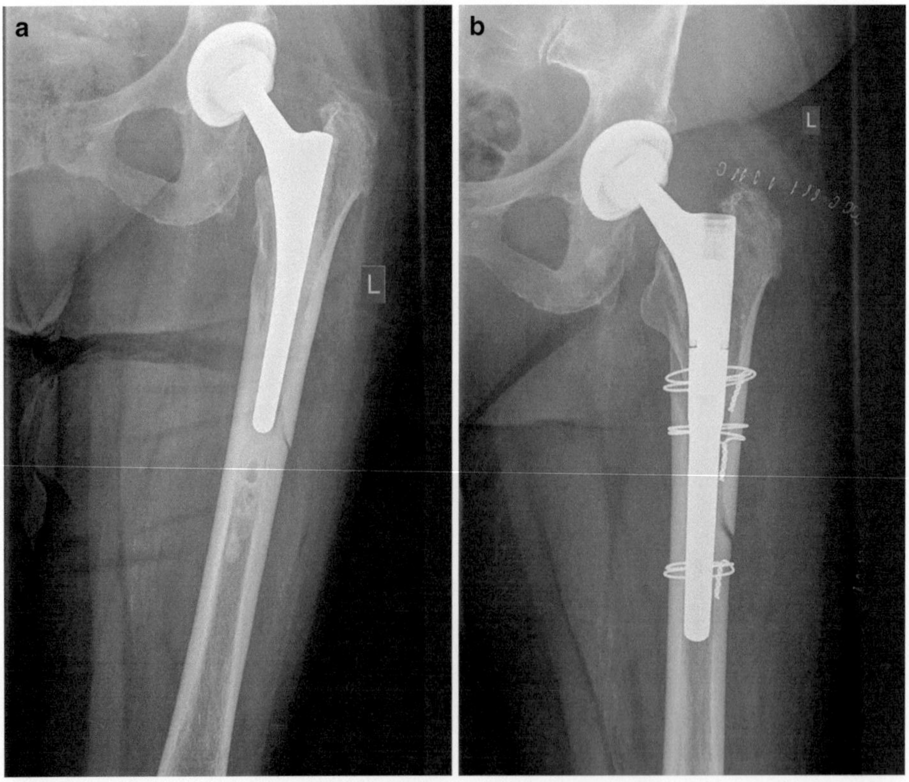

Fig. 11.11 (**a**) Periprosthetic fracture of the Vancouver B2 type. The loosening of the stem was evident during intraoperative testing. (**b**) Postoperative radiograph after transfemoral stem revision with fixation of the modular revision stem Revitan Curved (Zimmer Biomet, Winterthur, Switzerland) below the fracture in the isthmus of the femur

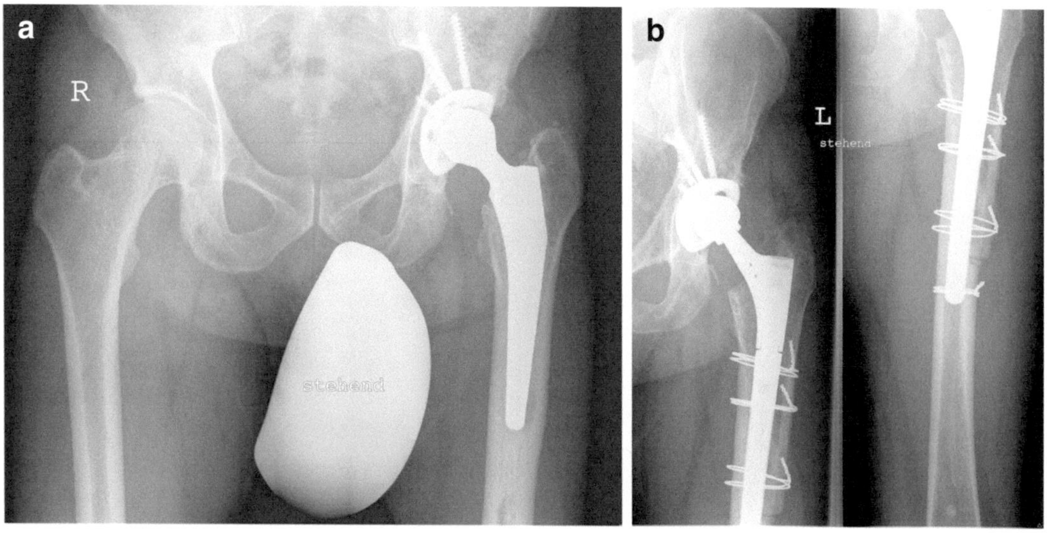

Fig. 11.12 (**a**) Stem loosening with sound cortical bone in the isthmus of the femur. (**b**) Radiograph 6 months after the transfemoral revision procedure with a modular revision stem Revitan Curved (Zimmer Biomet, Winterthur, Switzerland) with a short 3 cm distal fixation in the isthmus of the femur. Partial bony consolidation of the flap

fixation and type of stem (Fig. 11.12a, b). In the case of endofemoral implantation, the overall contact surface of the stem with the cortical bone is larger. For both implantation strategies (endofemoral and transfemoral), a shorter distal component (for modular prostheses) and a short monoblock prosthesis can be used if the isthmus is intact (Fig. 11.13, b). This anchorage area is usually below the tip of the prosthesis to be revised, in the isthmus of the femur. In smaller patients, the isthmus can be quite short.

If the cortex is thin (due to cavitary bone loss caused by loosening or due to osteoporosis), the revision stem requires a correspondingly longer fixation distance (Figs. 11.6a, b and 11.7a, b). If the isthmus is only hinted at Paprosky type IV due to severe osteoporosis or defects in the isthmus, distal fixation can be optimized with some revision stems by additional placement of locking screws (Fig. 11.14a, b). If the isthmus and cortex are affected by osteoporosis, thicker and longer distal components are required. It is desirable for the bony anchorage zone to extend at least 10 mm cranially beyond the most proximal locking hole.

11.8 Re 6: Selection of Component Sizes

Component sizes are determined once the bone morphology and quality have been analyzed in the radiographs, the necessity for a femoral osteotomy has been determined, and the type of fixation and/or implantation has been decided upon.

In the case of distally fixed modular stems, the distal component is selected that achieves a sufficiently long fixation zone in the diaphyseal bone. The proximal component is then selected to achieve the correct leg length, offset, and center of rotation. With curved stems, additional attention should be paid to the localization of the femoral curvature to ensure that the bow of the stem prosthesis matches the medullary canal as closely as possible. Accordingly, shorter or longer proximal components can be selected to ensure that the curved distal component matches the correct femoral curvature or varus. For distal monoblock prostheses, all aspects (fixation zone and leg length, offset, and center of rotation) are

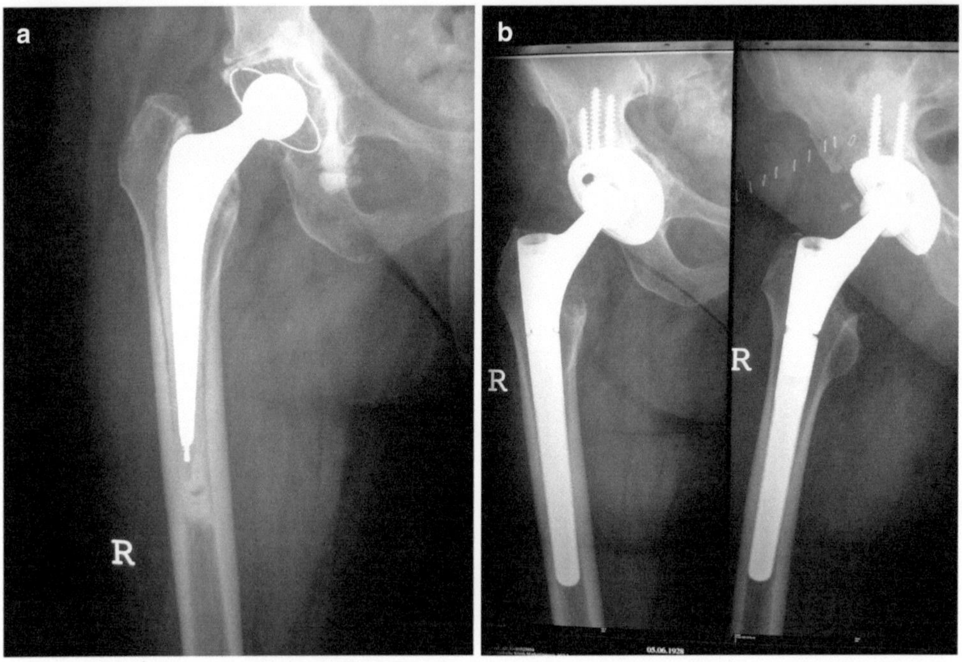

Fig. 11.13 (**a**) Prosthesis loosening with sound cortical bone in the distal femur and a short distal cement plug. (**b**) Endofemoral stem revision with a short modular revision stem Revitan Curved and press-fit cup Allofit-S (Zimmer Biomet, Winterthur, Switzerland)

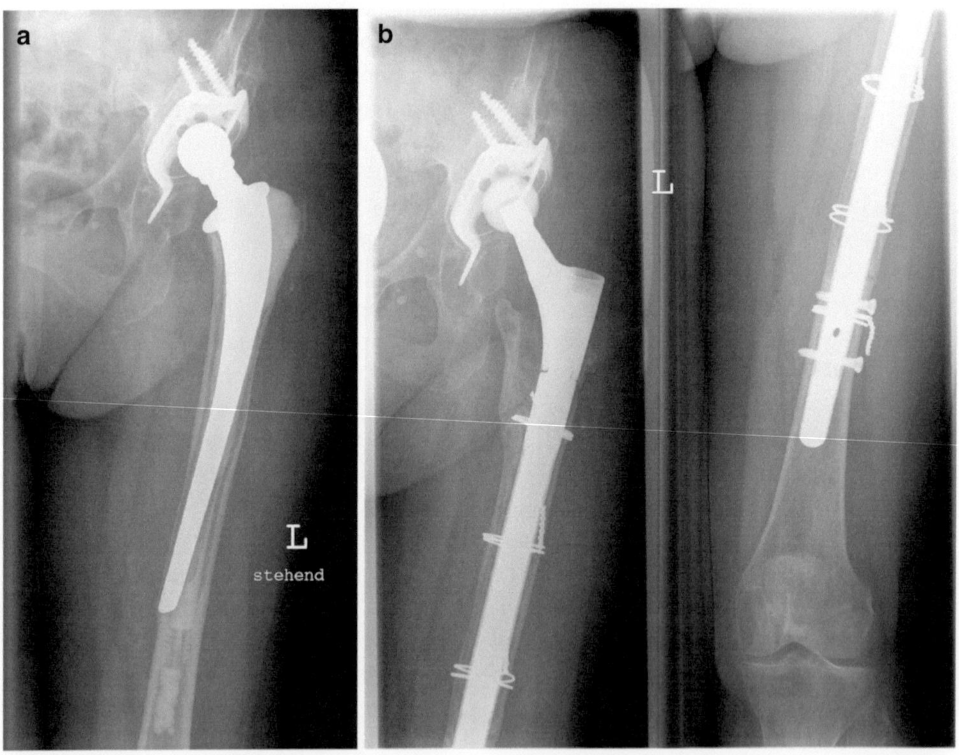

Fig. 11.14 (**a**) Stem loosening with poor cortical bone in a Paprosky IIIB type bone defect. (**b**) Radiograph 6 months after transfemoral revision to the modular revision stem Revitan Curved with distal locking (Zimmer Biomet, Winterthur, Switzerland). The flap shows bony consolidation

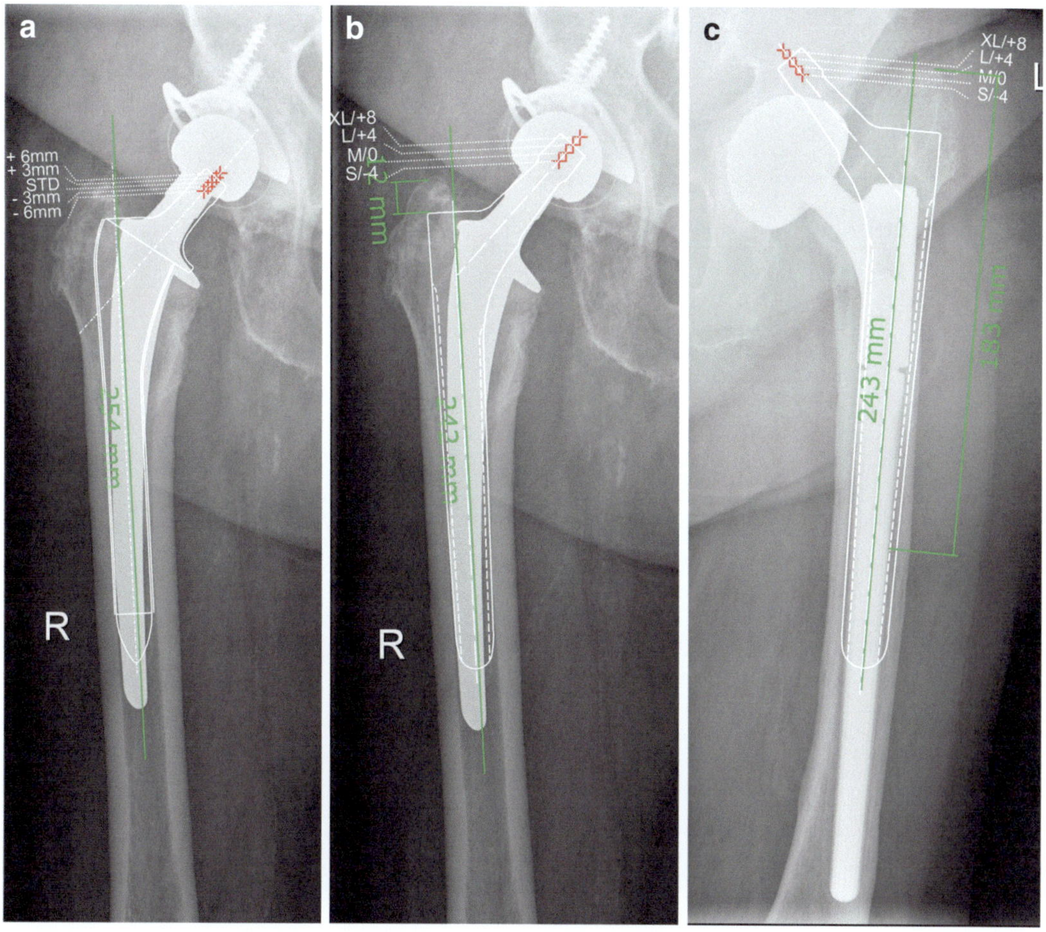

Fig. 11.15 (**a**) Planning a monoblock revision stem with scratch-fit fixation (Arcos Monoblock, Zimmer Biomet, Warsaw, IN, USA). (**b**) Planning a monoblock revision stem (Wagner SL, Zimmer Biomet, Winterthur, Switzerland) with endofemoral implantation and distal cone-in-cone locking. (**c**) Planning a monoblock revision stem (Wagner SL) with transfemoral implantation due to a varus of the stem. The length of the flap is shown on the side

planned with the entire prosthesis (Fig. 11.15a–c). For metaphyseal anchored modular prostheses of the S-ROM type, the central component is planned first, since it can be placed in the femoral diaphysis without establishing complete contact, followed by the proximal sleeve, which enables the corresponding proximal bone contact (Fig. 11.16a, b). For monoblock prostheses, again, everything is planned with the entire prosthesis in one step (Fig. 11.17).

For distal fixation with tapered modular revision stems, a distal component is selected with the thickness and length that will provide a sufficiently effective circular fixation zone in the isthmus region of the femoral diaphysis. If the cortex is of good quality, a fixation zone of 30 to 50 mm is usually sufficient for the transfemoral approach and approx. 40 to 70 mm for the endofemoral approach, depending on the selected type of stem. Accordingly, a shorter distal com-

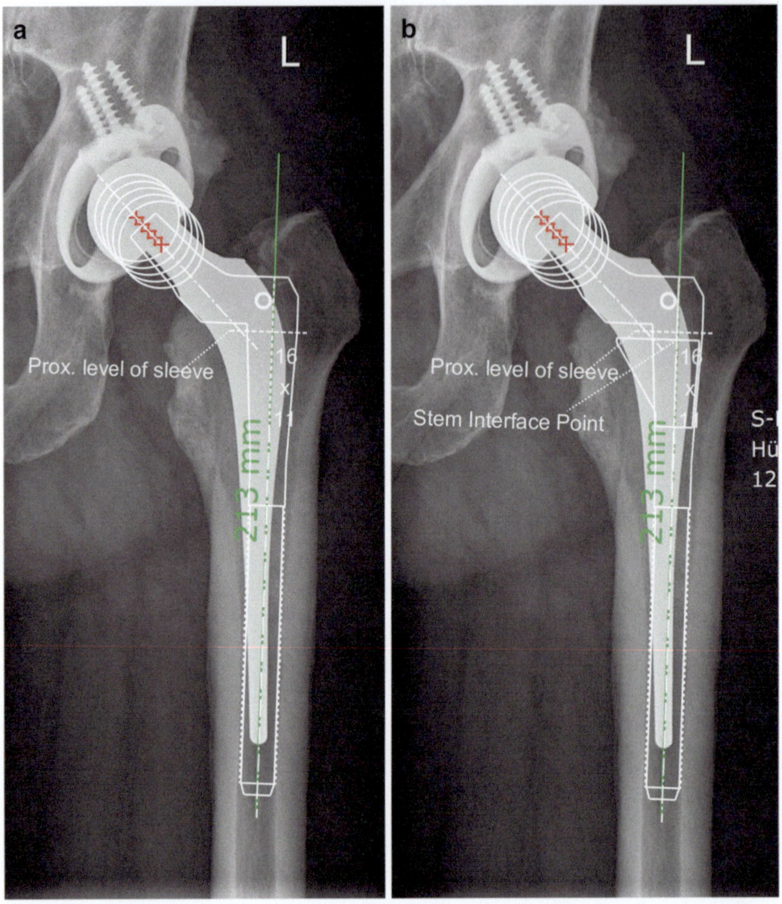

Fig. 11.16 Planning the implantation of the modular revision stem S-ROM (DePuy Synthes, Warsaw, IN, USA). (**a**) Use of the central distal component. (**b**) Use of the proximal sleeve component

ponent can be used (Fig. 11.18a). If the cortex is thin (due to cavitary bone loss caused by loosening or due to osteoporosis), the prosthesis requires a longer fixation distance (Fig. 11.19a). In general, a shorter thicker stem is preferable to a long thinner stem when selecting the thickness of the distal component. If a sufficiently firm circular fixation in the isthmus cannot be achieved distally due to the nature of the isthmus, a longer distal component is selected for revision stems with the option of distal interlocking, in which additional locking screws are inserted distally of the isthmus for supplemental stabilization. The thickness of the stem is determined by the medullary cavity of the femoral diaphysis, with the aim of achieving the best possible, lengthy bone contact with the stem (Fig. 11.20). Fixation with the locking screws alone is not effective.

There are a number of different proximal components (conical, cylindrical, calcar), depending on the type of prosthesis. In this case, the more voluminous proximal components serve to increase the bone–prosthesis contact interface. The possibility of using a particular type of component must be checked preoperatively and intraoperatively to avoid the risk of fracture. If conical proximal components and components with vanes in the direction of the greater trochanter are used, the greater trochanter in particular is at risk of fracture. The length of the chosen component should be such that the center of rotation of the joint can be set correctly and/or which enables the exact leg length

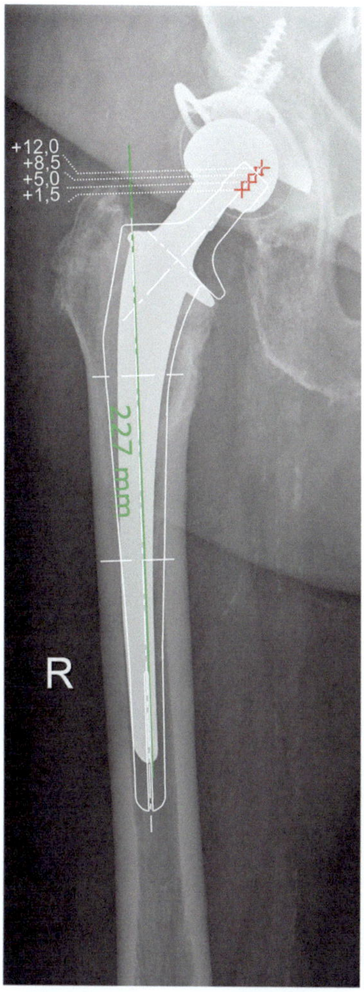

Fig. 11.17 Planning a monoblock revision shaft with metadiaphyseal fixation (CORAIL, DePuy Synthes, Warsaw, IN, USA)

to be achieved (Figs. 11.18b, 11.19b, and 11.20c).

11.9 Preparation of the Preoperative Planning Sketch

The preoperative planning sketch is used to check and document the plausibility of the abovementioned planning points. However, it must be mentioned here that not all points such as bone quality and fixation distance can be determined beyond doubt during preoperative planning. These points can only be determined reliably during surgery. Nevertheless, preoperative planning is essential because it minimizes the uncertainties of revision surgery and thus helps to avoid complications.

11.9.1 Step 1: Mapping the Axes and, Where Necessary, the Osteotomies

The centromedullary axis, which represents the center of the medullary cavity, is marked. The plane of reference for the center of the hip joint is defined and drawn perpendicular to the centromedullary axis at the level of the trochanter major (Fig. 11.21). If the centromedullary axis extends proximally into the greater trochanter, there will be an increased risk of an unintentional fracture of the trochanter or further distally of the femur, if an endofemoral procedure is used (Fig. 11.21). In such cases, the femur should be corrected by an osteotomy during a transfemoral access (extended trochanteric osteotomy). If so, the distal limit of the transfemoral approach and, if necessary, the level of a medial osteotomy (for double osteotomies) should be noted. This determines the height "H1" of the lateral femoral bone flap (from greater trochanter to distal end of the flap) (Fig. 11.22). The distal end of the flap should be at or just above the tip of the prosthesis or at the apex of a varus bow. However, care must be taken to ensure that the isthmus remains sufficiently intact for adequate distal fixation of the revision stem. The planned fixation zones of the stem can now be plotted (Fig. 11.22).

11.9.2 Step 2A: Mapping the Distal Components for Distally Fixed Stems

The distal component is selected. When choosing the thickness, care should be taken to ensure that there is a sufficiently long diaphyseal bone con-

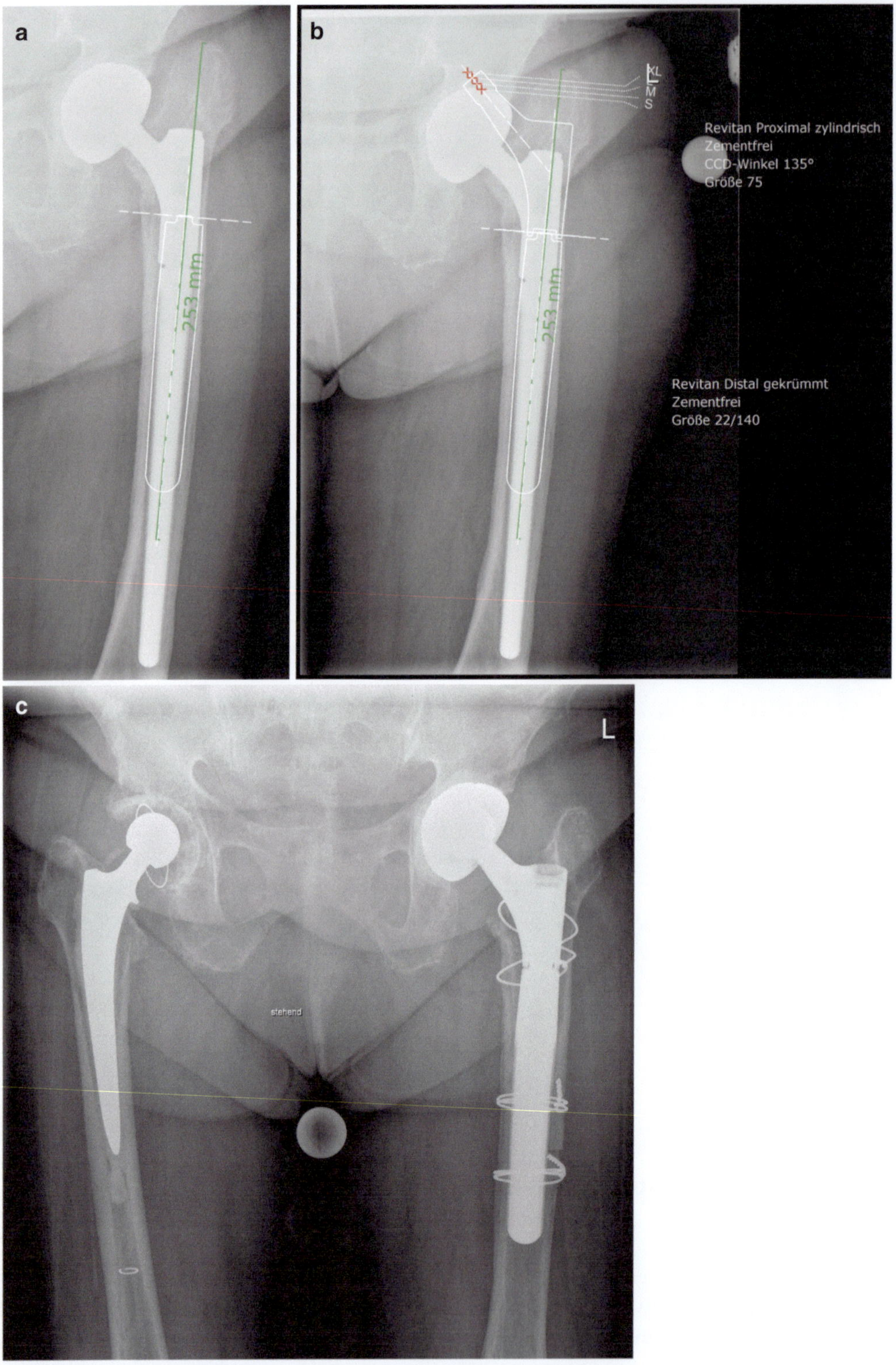

Fig. 11.18 Planning the transfemoral implantation of a modular, distally fixed revision stem with a short fixation distance based on sound cortical bone. (**a**) Planning the distal component. (**b**) Planning the proximal component. (**c**) Radiograph 3 months after surgery

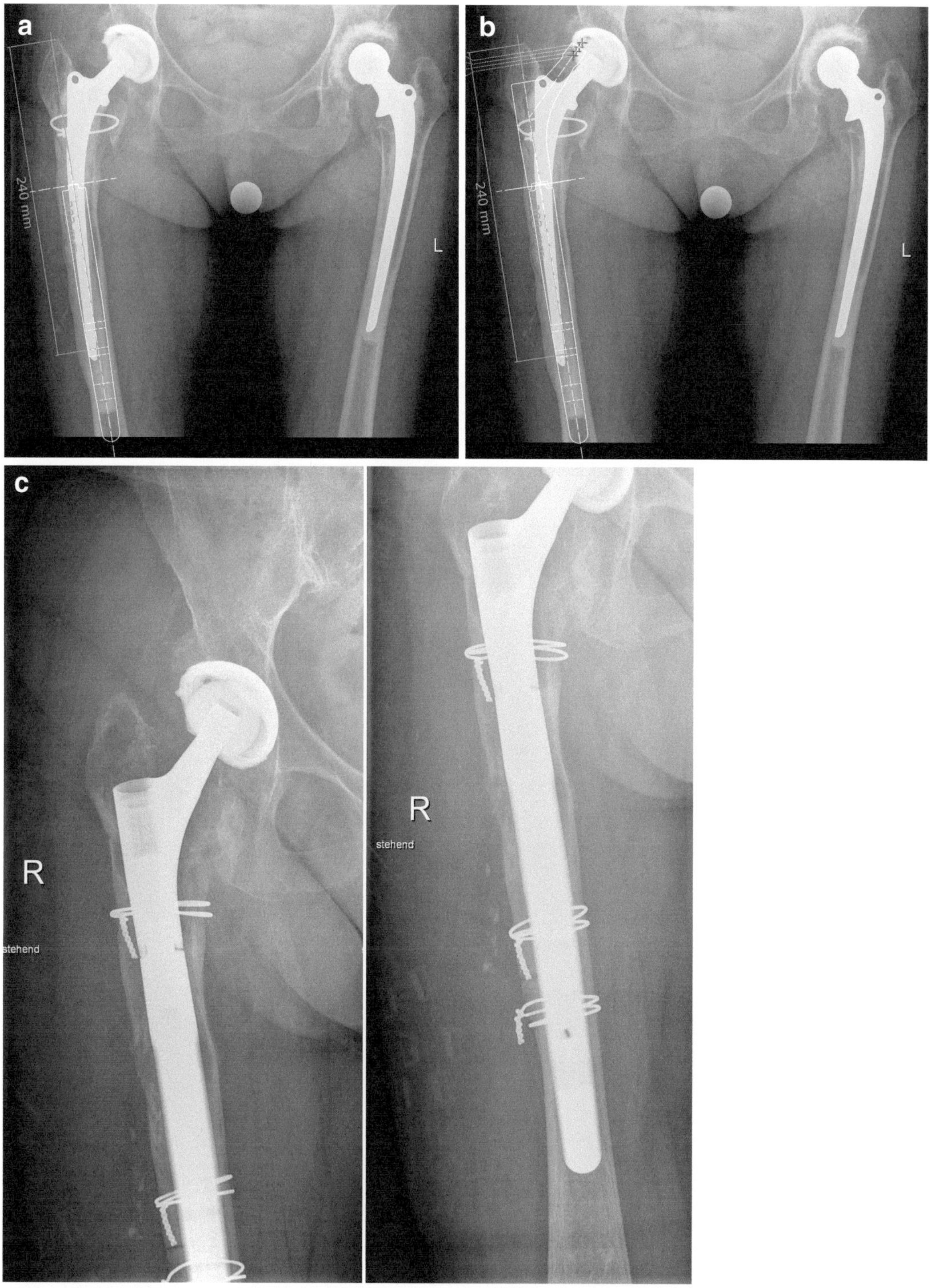

Fig. 11.19 Planning the endofemoral implantation of a modular, distally fixed revision stem with a longer fixation distance due to poor cortical bone. (**a**) Planning the distal component. (**b**) Planning the proximal component. (**c1** and **c2**) Radiograph 3 months after surgery

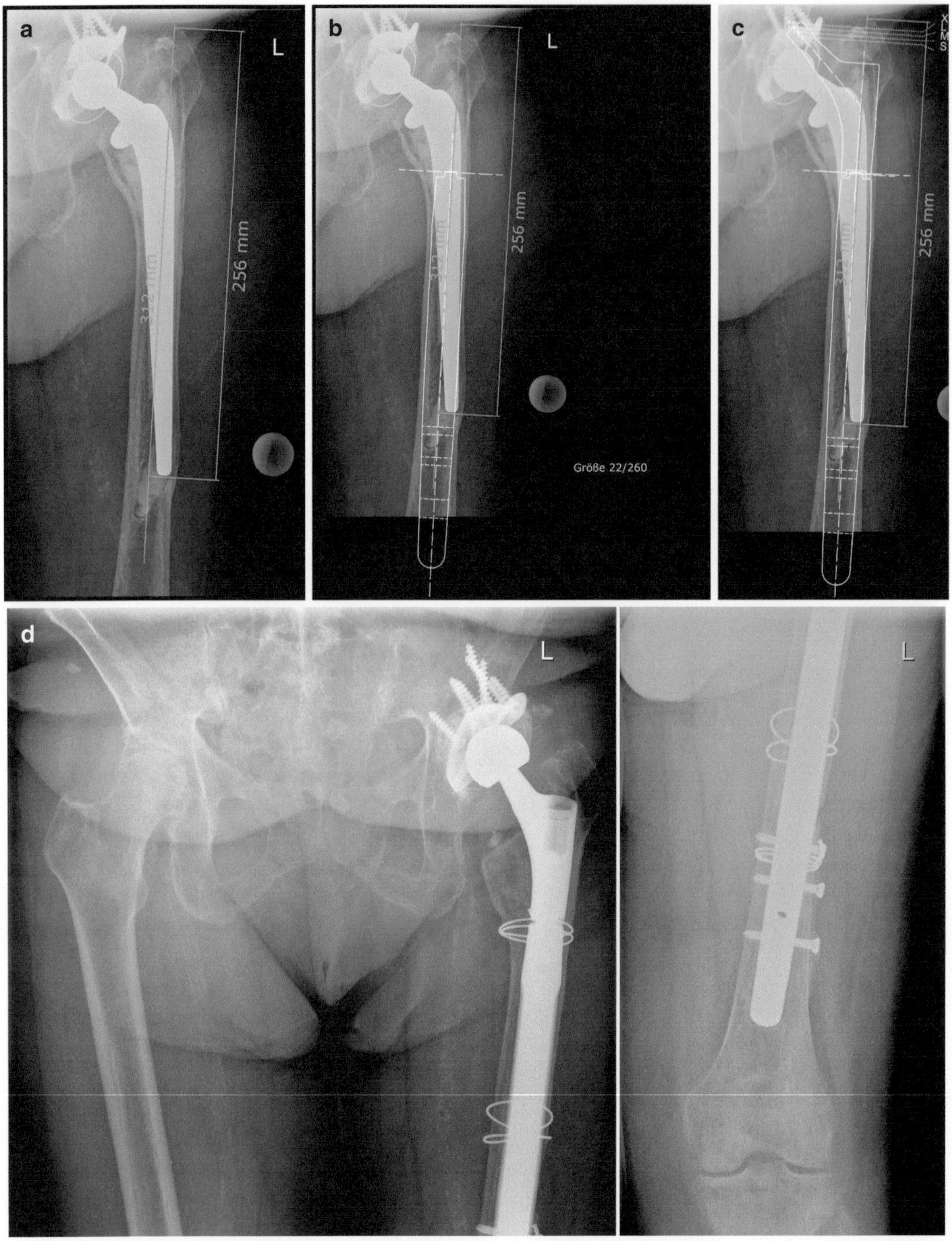

Fig. 11.20 Planning the transfemoral implantation of a modular, distally fixed revision stem with distal locking due to a Paprosky IIIB type bone defect with a fixation distance of less than 3 cm in the residual isthmus. (**a**) Mapping of the centromedullary axis and the planned length of the flap. (**b**) Planning the distal component with distal locking below the flap. (**c**) Planning the proximal component. (**d1** and **d2**) Radiograph 3 months after surgery

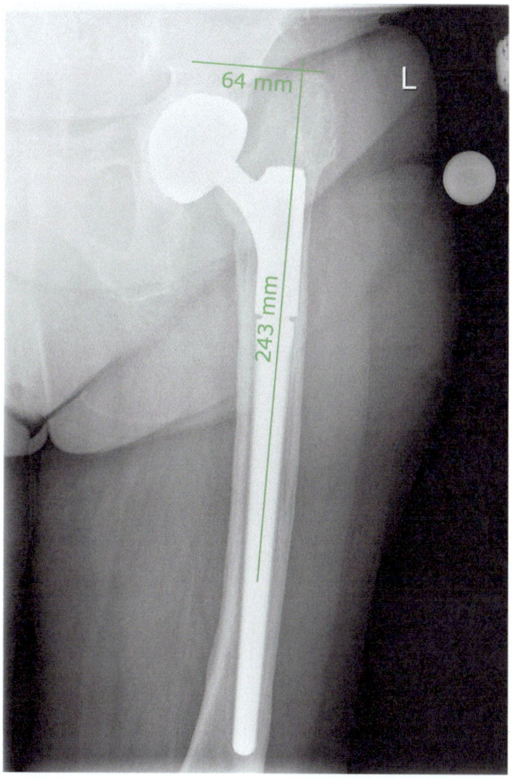

Fig. 11.21 Mapping the centromedullary axis as a reference

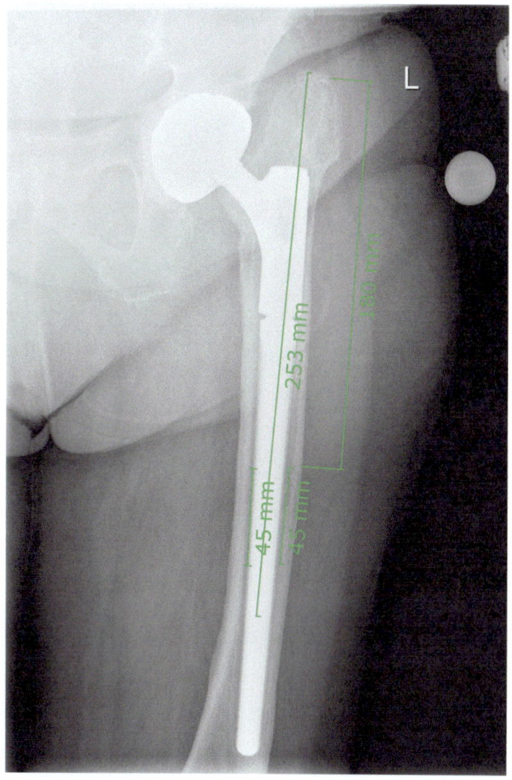

Fig. 11.22 Mapping the planned length of the flap H1 (here 180 mm). Mapping the planned fixation distance in the isthmus

tact in accordance with the stem prosthesis used, in the case of a transfemoral approach, in the isthmus of the femur (Fig. 11.23a). The same procedure is used for monoblock prostheses, but care must be taken to ensure that the leg length and center of rotation are correctly adjusted (Fig. 11.24). If the cortex is of good quality, a fixation distance of 30–50 mm is usually sufficient for transfemoral access, depending on the stem used; if the cortex is thin, the prosthesis requires a longer fixation distance. A three-point fixation (only pointwise contacts over a short distance) must be avoided, as it leads to subsidence. Therefore, a thick, shorter stem is preferable to a long, thinner stem, as the latter is more likely to result in a three-point fixation.

11.9.3 Step 2B: Mapping the Distal Components for Proximally Fixed Stems

The distal or central component is selected. The chosen thickness is the one that provides central alignment in the diaphysis, with incomplete circumferential bone contact (Fig. 11.16a). The same procedure is used for monoblock prosthe-

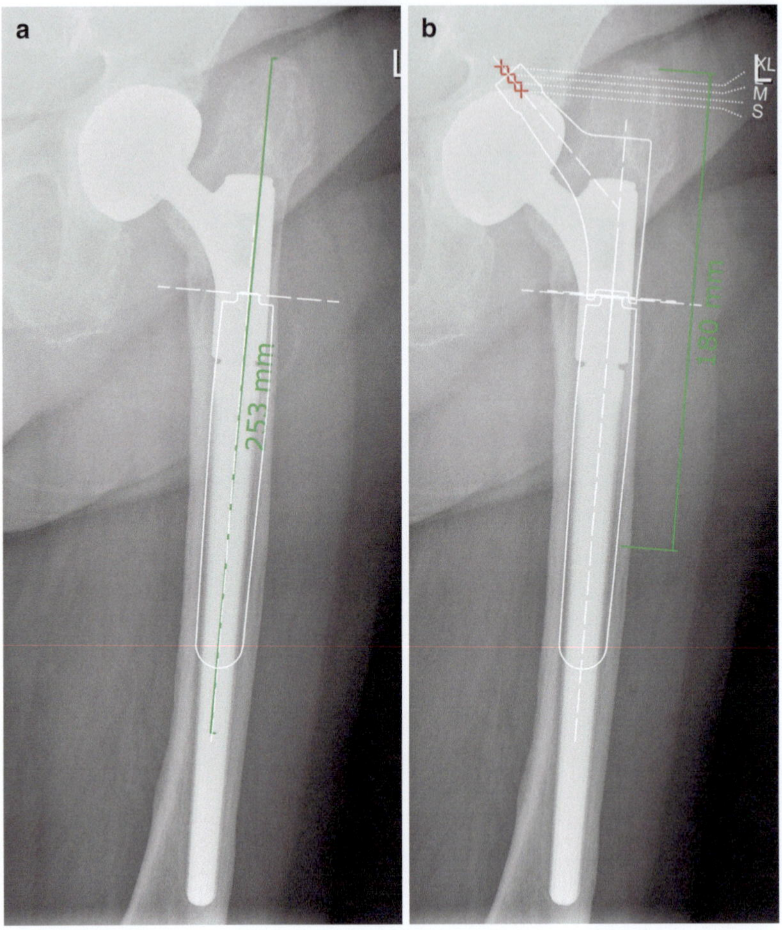

Fig. 11.23 (**a**) Mapping the distal component that achieves fixation in the selected fixation zone of the isthmus. (**b**) Mapping the proximal component that allows reconstruction of the correct leg length and center of rotation

ses, but at the same time care is taken to ensure that a metaphyseal fixation with sufficient bone contact is achieved and that the leg length and center of rotation are correctly adjusted (Fig. 11.25).

11.9.4 Step 3A: Mapping the Proximal Component for Distally Fixed Stems

The proximal component is positioned on the distal component to achieve the correct leg length, offset, and center of rotation (Fig. 11.23b). If several variants of the proximal component are available (conical or cylindrical, calcar), care must be taken to ensure that an endofemoral procedure with the selected component does not compromise the greater trochanter and increase the risk of fracture. It may be necessary to change to a less voluminous component shape (e.g., cylindrical). For monoblock prostheses, the correct adjustment of the leg length and center of rotation is made with the selecting of the correct thickness of the prosthesis stem (Fig. 11.24).

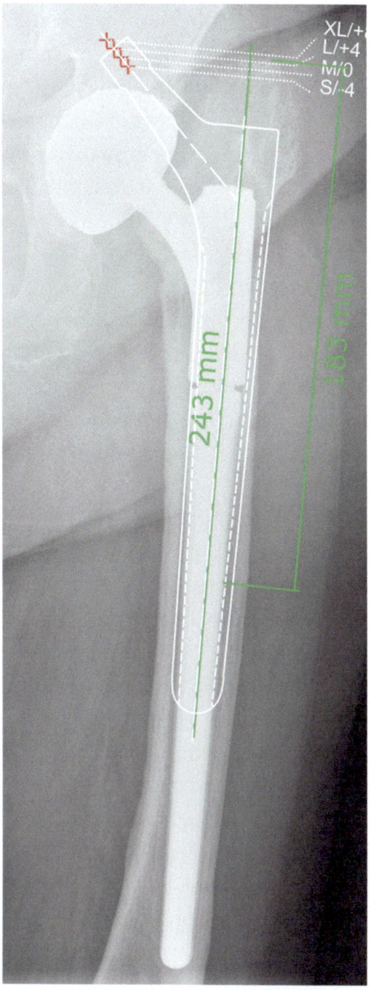

Fig. 11.24 With a monoblock prosthesis, the component of appropriate length and thickness is selected and positioned to achieve fixation in the planned fixation zone and to reconstruct the leg length and center of rotation

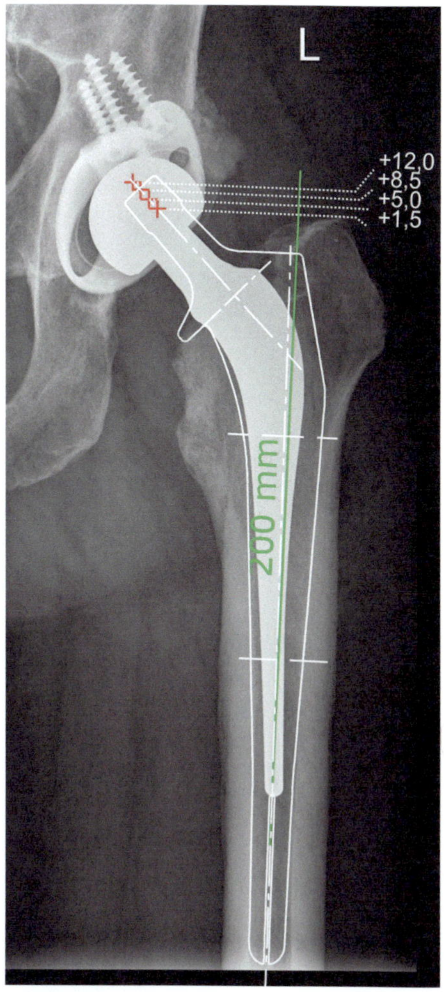

Fig. 11.25 Planning a monoblock prosthesis with proximal metaphyseal fixation (here CORAIL stem, DePuy Synthes, Warsaw, IN, USA)

11.9.5 Step 3B: Mapping the Proximal Component for Proximally Fixed Stems

For modular proximal fixation stems, the proximal component is selected that provides metaphyseal support and enables the correct leg length, offset, and rotation center to be achieved. For modular proximal fixation stems with a proximal prosthesis body (e.g., modular Mallory-Head, Biomet, Warsaw, IN, or their successors Arcos, Zimmer Biomet, Warsaw, IN, USA), we recommend planning the proximal component first and then the distal component. With the S-ROM prosthesis, the central component is selected and then the sleeve through which the central component is inserted is chosen so that the optimum metaphyseal support and/or fixation can be achieved (Fig. 11.16b).

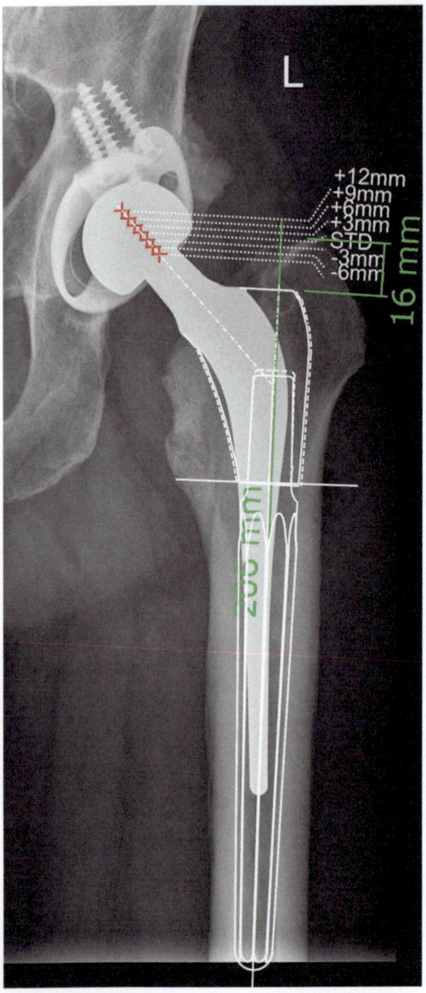

Fig. 11.26 Measurement of the height H2 (here 16 mm) from the lateral prosthesis shoulder to the tip of the greater trochanter (here with an endofemorally planned Arcos stem) (Zimmer Biomet, Warsaw, IN, USA)

11.9.6 Step 4: Mapping Reference Points and Distances

These reference points and distances should help to implement preoperative planning during surgery.

In endofemoral three-surface fixation, the major trochanter is chosen as the reference point. To check the penetration depth of the revision stem, the distance "H2" (greater trochanter to lateral prosthesis shoulder) is drawn and measured (Fig. 11.26). This distance is first checked intraoperatively with the trial prosthesis or the proximal trial component placed on the actual distal component. Depending on the bone quality, however, there may be deviations here because, for example, until the distal prosthesis component is securely fixed in the femur, it has penetrated the femur somewhat deeper than planned. This must then be taken into account when selecting the final implants.

For the transfemoral approach (extended trochanteric osteotomy), the distal end of the femoral flap is selected as the reference point. To check the penetration depth of the revision stem, the distance "H3" (distal end of the femoral flap to the lateral prosthesis shoulder) is drawn and measured (Fig. 11.27). These are first checked intraoperatively with the trial prosthesis or the proximal trial component placed on the actual distal component. Depending on the bone quality, however, there may be deviations here because; for example, by the time the distal prosthesis component is securely fixed in the femur, it has penetrated a few millimeters deeper than planned. This must be taken into account when selecting the final implants.

11.9.7 Step 5: Further Steps in Digital Planning

Digital planning, which is the most common method used today, can be used to simulate leg length correction after digitally removing the femur with the prosthesis (Fig. 11.28a, b).

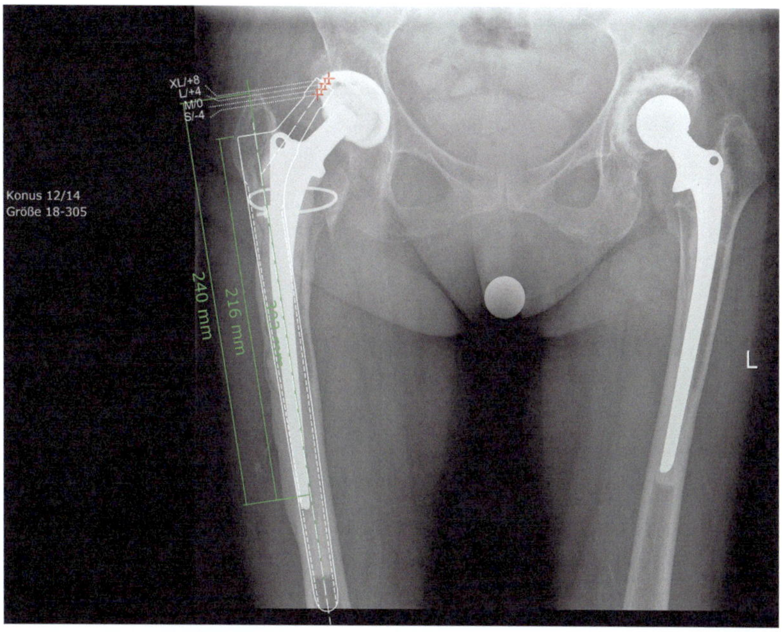

Fig. 11.27 Measurement of height H3 from the end of the flap to the lateral prosthesis shoulder (on the proximal component) (here 216 mm)

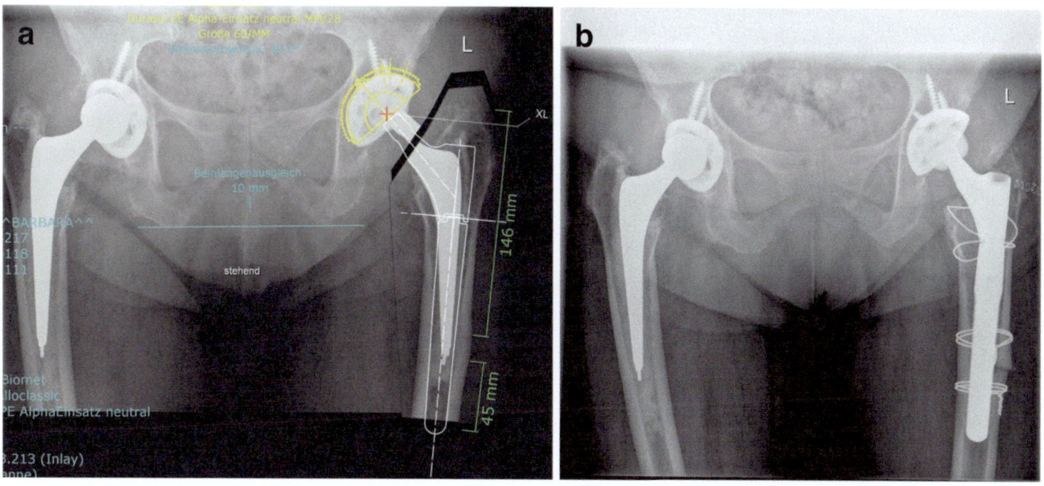

Fig. 11.28 (**a**) Digital excision of the femur with planned prosthesis and simulated repositioning of the prosthesis to adjust the leg length correctly. (**b**) Postoperative radiograph after revision of stem and inlay on the left

References

1. Lanting BA, MacDonald SJ. The painful total hip replacement: diagnosis and deliverance. Bone Joint J. 2013;95-B:70–3.
2. Fink B, Lass R. Diagnostischer Algorithmus für die Fehleranalyse bei schmerzhaften Hüfttotalendoprothesen. Z Orthop Unfall. 2016;154:527–44.
3. Fink B, Makowiak C, Fuerst M, Berger I, Schäfer P, Frommelt L. The values of synovial biopsy and joint aspiration in the diagnostic of late periprosthetic infection of total knee arthroplasties. J Bone Joint Surg. 2008;90-B:874–8.
4. Fink B. Revision of late periprosthetic infections of total hip endoprostheses: pros and cons of different concepts. Int J Med Sci. 2009;6:287–95.
5. Fink B, Gebhard A, Fuerst M, Berger I, Schäfer P. High diagnostic value of synovial biopsy in peri-

prosthetic joint infection of the hip. Clin Orthop Relat Res. 2013;471:956–64.
6. Parvizi J, Tan TL, Goswami K, Higuera C, Della Valle C, Chen AF, Shohat N. The 2018 definition of periprosthetic hip and knee infection: an evidence-based and validated criteria. J Arthroplasty. 2018;33:1309–14.
7. Fink B, Schuster P, Braun R, Tagtalianidou E, Schlumberger M. The diagnostic value of routine preliminary biopsy in diagnosing late prosthetic joint infection after hip and knee arthroplasty. Bone Joint J 2020;102-B(3):329–335.
8. Schäfer P, Fink B, Sandow D, Margull A, Berger I, Frommelt L. Prolonged bacterial culture to identify late periprosthetic joint infection: a promising strategy. Clin Infect Dis. 2008;47:1403–9.
9. Trampuz A, Piper KE, Jacobson MJ, Hanssen AD, Unni KK, Osmon DR, Mandrekar JN, Cockerill FR, Steckelberg JM, Greenleaf JF, Patel R. Sonication of removed hip and knee prostheses for diagnosis of infection. N Engl J Med. 2007;357:654–63.
10. Wolff J. Das Gesetz der Transformation der Knochen. Berlin: Hirschwald-Verlag; 1892.

Choice of the Surgical Approach 12

Contents

12.1 **Factors Influencing the Choice of Access** 152

12.2 **Anterior Approaches** 153

12.3 **The Transgluteal Approach** 153

12.4 **Trans-Trochanteric Access** 155

12.5 **The Posterior Approach** 155

12.6 **Extended Approaches** 157

References 161

There are a number of standard and extended approaches, all of which have their advantages and disadvantages for the revision of hip endoprostheses and which can be used for the exposure and controlled removal of a prosthesis and/or reimplantation of a new prosthesis. Overall, they should allow good visualization and avoid unintentional damage to the bone (especially through devascularization and fractures) and the musculature. The gluteal musculature in particular should be spared, since it plays a decisive role in the function and stability of the hip joint. Disruption of the vasto-gluteal sling, which connects the gluteus medius muscle and the vastus lateralis muscle, should be avoided since, in the event of a trochanteric fracture, the disruption of the vasto-gluteal sling means that the counterpart to the gluteus medius no longer exists and dislocation of the greater trochanter is unavoidable. Thus, all approaches that weaken the gluteal muscles and transect the vasto-gluteal sling are detrimental to maintaining the important function of the gluteal muscles. When selecting an approach, the flexibility of that approach must also be taken into account in the event of any intraoperative complications. The different approaches should be evaluated with regard to their flexibility and the possible disadvantages of having to extend them. Preoperative planning must include a realistic assessment of possible complications and the necessity for an extension of the operation, whereby it is better to think through a "worst-case scenario" than to be unrealistically optimistic.

Supplementary Information The online version contains supplementary material available at [https://doi.org/10.1007/978-3-030-84821-7_12]. The videos can be accessed by scanning the related images with the SN More Media App.

B. Fink, *Femoral Revision Arthroplasty*, https://doi.org/10.1007/978-3-030-84821-7_12

Table 12.1 Exposure of different regions during hip prosthesis revision according to the respective access routes [1]

	Exposure of femur			Exposure of acetabulum		
Approach	Metaphysis	Canal	Lateral cortex	Anterior	Superior	Posterior
Smith–Petersen	++	+	+	+++	++	+
Watson—Jones	++	++	+++	++	+	+
Transgluteal	+++	++	+++	++	+	++
Trans-trochanter	+++	+++	+++	+++	+++	+++
Posterior	+++	++	+++	++	+++	+++

In principle, the approaches can be divided into four types, whereby the distinction is made on the basis of their localization with respect to the gluteus medius and minimus muscles. For a detailed description of the individual standard approaches, please refer to the corresponding literature in, for example, books on surgical approaches.

The anterior (Smith–Petersen) and anterolateral (Watson–Jones) approaches lie ventral to the abductor muscles. The transgluteal approach detaches the anterior part of the gluteus medius and minimus muscle from the greater trochanter. The trans-trochanteric approach involves the osteotomy of the greater trochanter. The posterior or posterolateral approach lies dorsal to the abductor muscles. All have their advantages and disadvantages and allow the different areas to be presented with varying degrees of exposure during revision surgery (Table 12.1). Although femoral revision arthroplasty is the principal topic of this book, the exposure of the various aspects of cup revision will be summarized in tabular form [1] (Table 12.1).

12.1 Factors Influencing the Choice of Access

Various preoperative factors influence the choice of access for revision arthroplasty.

1. The indication for revision surgery: Is only the cup to be replaced or should the stem also be exchanged? Preoperative planning must include an assessment of how certain it is that, for example, a cup revision can be carried out in isolation and that stem revision will not become necessary because of intraoperative problems with the stability of the joint, leg length, offset, or compatibility of the prosthesis components. Conversely, preoperative planning must assess the probability of an additional cup revision during stem revision because of stability problems, for example. In the event of an acute periprosthetic infection, where the implant is to be left in place and only the articulating components are to be replaced, the previous approach can usually be repeated. This is different in the case of a chronic periprosthetic infection that requires the removal of all foreign material (implants and cement). If, at the same time, there are problems in the soft tissues that have to be addressed (e.g., granulomas caused by a metal-on-metal coupling, preexisting rupture of the gluteal muscles, abscesses, fistulas), it is important to ensure that these can be easily reached with the chosen route of access.
2. The quality and shape of the bone: For example, if there is osteolysis in the region or thinning of the greater trochanter, any access should be avoided (anterior, anterolateral) that results in increased pressure on the greater trochanter and thus significantly increases the risk of an unintentional fracture. If axial deviations of the femur have to be corrected during revision, in order to ensure correct implantation of the femoral revision prosthesis, extended approaches should be adopted that allow this to be done effectively and in a controlled manner.
3. The type of prosthesis to be revised: The design of the prosthesis to be replaced influences the choice of the access. What is the extent of the coating of the cementless stem? Are there wings or collars that need to be chiseled out? Where in the cortex is the cementless prosthesis still fitting tightly? How far does the distal cement plug extend distally?

4. Position of the implants: If there is a very small offset with a short distance between the greater trochanter and the bone of the pelvis, the dislocation can be significantly more difficult with a transgluteal approach. Increasing the offset after revision with a transgluteal approach makes reinsertion and healing of the gluteus medius muscle to the greater trochanter more difficult too. The situation is even more critical when a cup is protruded into the pelvis. In this case, the muscle tension of the gluteus medius muscle must be neutralized in order to be sure of joint dislocation and removal of the implants. Therefore, in this special case, the trans-trochanteric approach or the extended trochanteric osteotomy (transfemoral approach) is the most suitable approach.
5. Patient-specific factors: In this case, it is primarily the individual soft tissue status that matters. If there is significant obesity or significant muscle hypertrophy, this can make access to the femur more difficult, especially with anterior approaches, and can significantly increase the pressure on the trochanter region.
6. Experience of the surgeon: On the one hand, the surgeon is happy to choose the access he or she is accustomed to for primary implantation. However, the surgeon ought to be familiar with several other approaches as well. None of the standard approaches are suitable for addressing with certainty all possible problems during a revision. Therefore, the surgeon must also be familiar with extended approaches and, in my opinion, must also master the transfemoral approach.
7. Previously existing access: In my opinion, this only plays a role in a revision due to, for example, an early periprosthetic infection. Otherwise, the choice of access should be based on the options for exposure, protection of bone and muscles, and the problems to be expected, as well as its extendibility in case problems arise. However it makes little sense to revise a hip from the anterior side in order to spare the small external rotators, when it was previously operated on via the posterior approach.

12.2 Anterior Approaches

The paths of the Smith–Peterson anterior approach run between the sartorius muscle and the tensor fasciae latae muscle and between the rectus femoris muscle and the tensor fasciae latae muscle (Fig. 12.1). It is suitable for simple revision of the acetabulum on its own. However, with major acetabular cup revisions, the tensor fasciae latae muscle must be partially or completely detached, which cancels out the advantage of a muscle-sparing approach [2]. The anterolateral Watson–Jones approach and its variations run between the tensor fasciae latae muscle and the gluteus medius muscle (Fig. 12.2). Its use in revision is limited. A proximal extension to the acetabulum is limited by the neurovascular bundle of the tensor fasciae latae, as is the access to the posterior acetabular rim. Access to the femoral canal is made more difficult by the anterior part of the gluteus medius muscle. Thus, the risk of trochanter fractures is increased, especially during revision with anterior approaches, since a direct, straight approach into the femur is not possible [3]. Instead, the femur must be entered in an arc, which increases the force exerted on the trochanter and increases the risk of uncontrolled fracture. Regis et al. [4] reported fracture of the greater trochanter associated with 77.7% (7 of 9) of Wagner SL revision stems implanted via the anterolateral approach. Thus, the anterior approaches are more suitable for cup revision and/or inlay and head replacement alone [5].

12.3 The Transgluteal Approach

The direct lateral, transgluteal approach is used for revision surgery of both the cup and stem (Fig. 12.3). However, it leads directly to a weakening of the abductors if used for a primary total hip arthroplasty. Ugland et al. [6] observed a positive Trendelenburg sign (20% of cases) significantly more often for the lateral approach compared to the anterolateral approach (1.8% of cases). Svennson et al. [7] found that 56% of 97 patients who had undergone a primary total hip arthroplasty via the transgluteal approach exhibited a separation of X-ray markers placed on

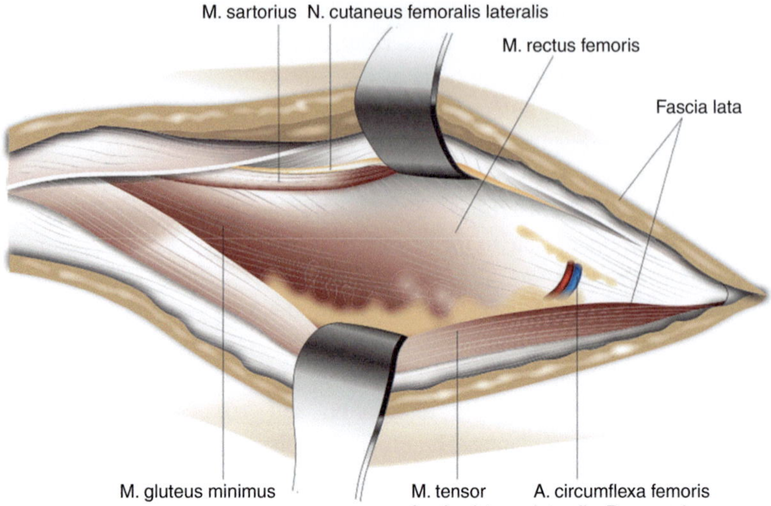

Fig. 12.1 Anatomy of the intermuscular path for the anterior approach (Smith–Peterson approach)

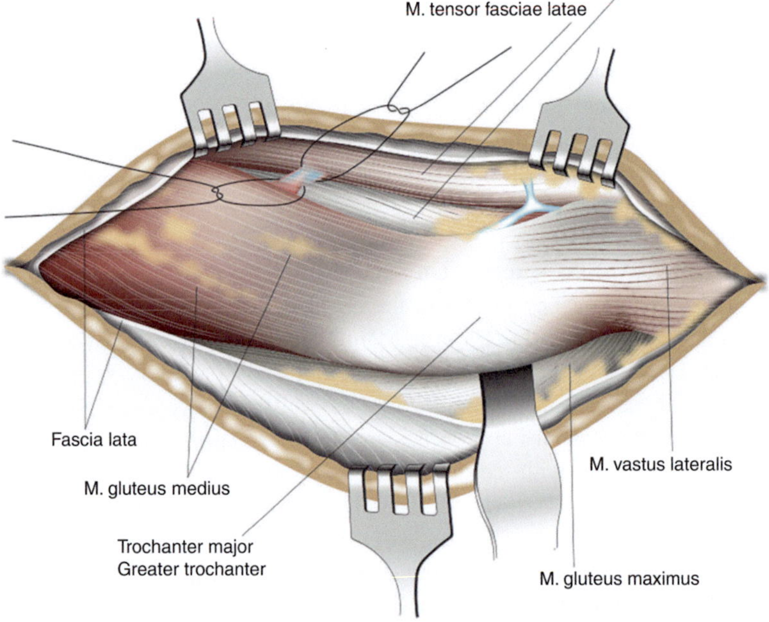

Fig. 12.2 Anatomy of the intermuscular path for the anterolateral approach (Watson–Jones approach)

each side of the transected muscle during reinsertion. The repeated reinsertion of the separated parts of the gluteus medius during prosthesis revision surgery is likely to further weaken the gluteal muscles and complicate functional convalescence. Therefore, transgluteal access for revision appears to be associated with significant functional disadvantages. In addition, the greater trochanter is exposed to increased force and is at risk of fracture. Picado et al. [8] observed unintentional intraoperative fractures of the greater trochanter in 12.5% (3 of 24) of patients with an endofemoral, transgluteal-implanted, modular distal fixation revision stem Restoration (Stryker, Kalamazoo, MG, USA).

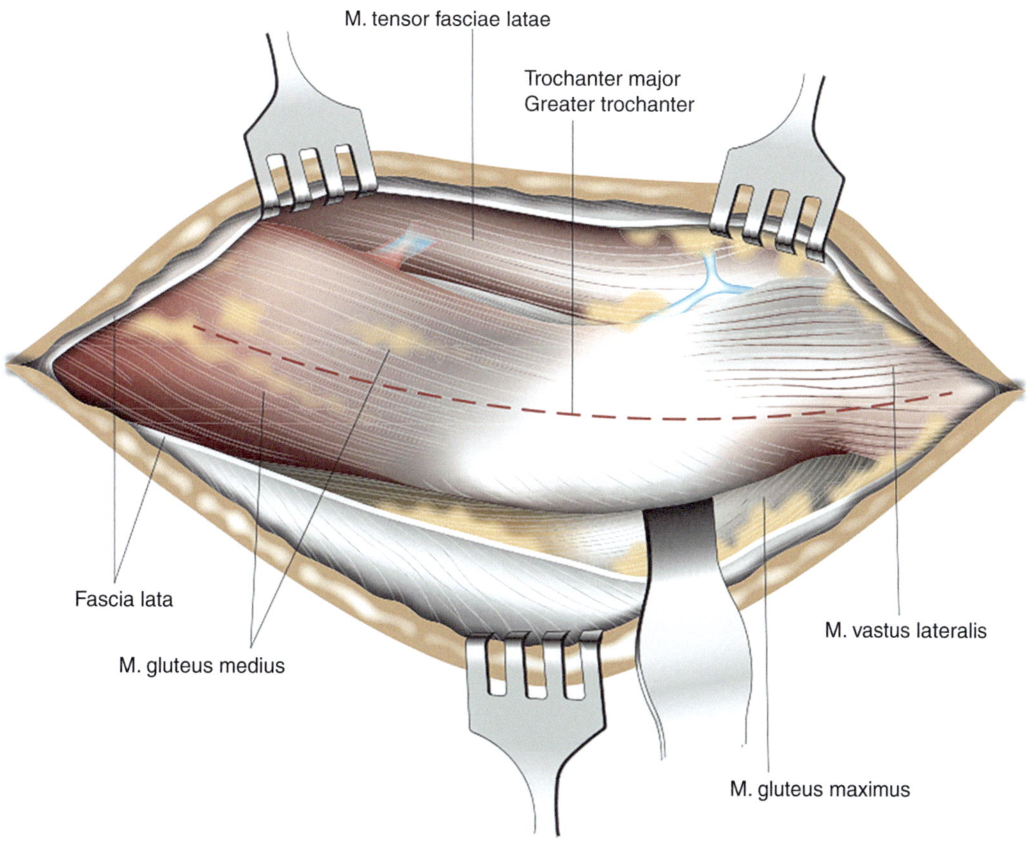

Fig. 12.3 Anatomy of the structures for the transgluteal approach

12.4 Trans-Trochanteric Access

The traditional trans-trochanteric approach provides excellent exposure of the cup and the proximal section of the femur (Fig. 12.4). A sufficiently thick piece of trochanter is required for re-healing after closure with tension band wiring. Hook plates should only be used for closure in exceptional cases where the trochanter has thinned out and a fracture has already occurred, as they are proximally bulky and can cause local irritation and pain. Despite the good cup exposure, the classic trans-trochanteric approach has been largely abandoned with respect to revision arthroplasty because of the high rates of non-union, which are reported to be between 10 and 20% [9, 10].

12.5 The Posterior Approach

The posterior or posterolateral standard approach allows good exposure of the cup and direct straight access to the stem with very good protection of the gluteal muscles (Fig. 12.5, Fig. 12.6 for Video 12.1). However, dislocation rates of 4–20% have been reported after revision surgery [11]. This risk can be reduced to 2% by posterior capsule flap augmentation during the reinsertion of the external rotators [11]. Therefore, at least for the first aseptic revision of the hip joint via the posterolateral approach (if another approach was used for the primary implantation), capsule flaps should be prepared in the form of a capsuloplasty, which can be used for augmenting the reinsertion of the external

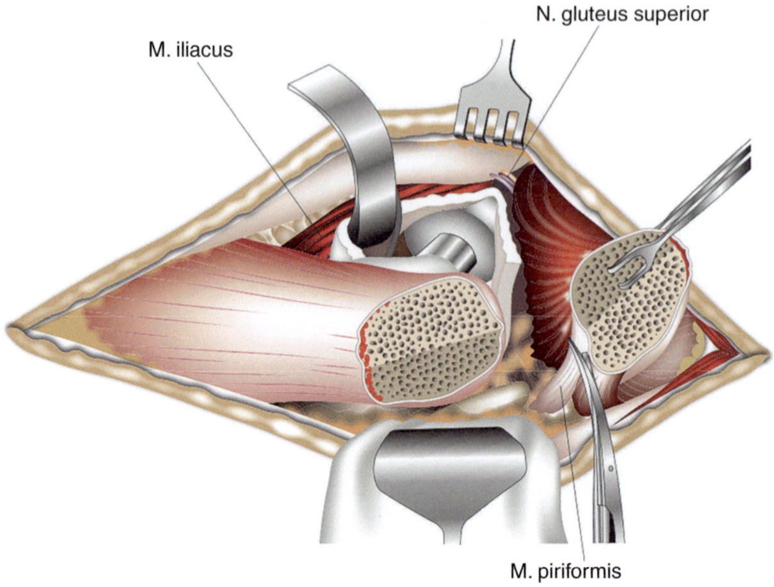

Fig. 12.4 Anatomy of the structures for the trans-trochanteric approach

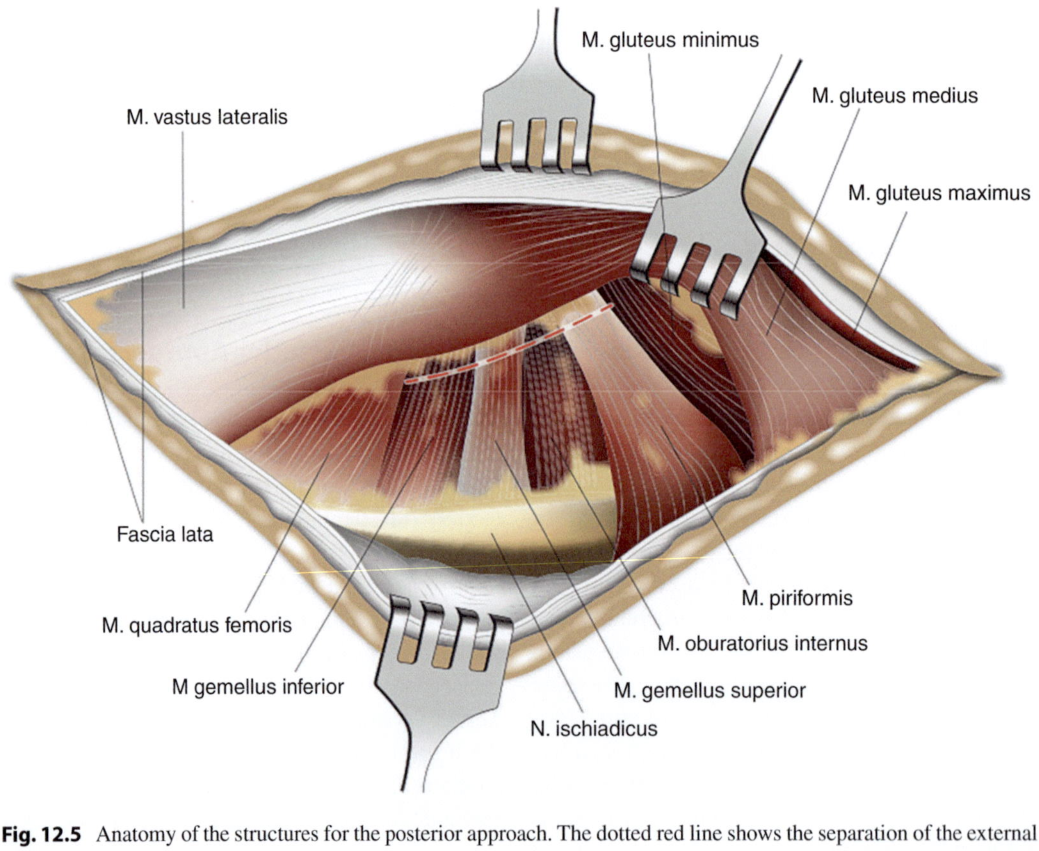

Fig. 12.5 Anatomy of the structures for the posterior approach. The dotted red line shows the separation of the external rotators

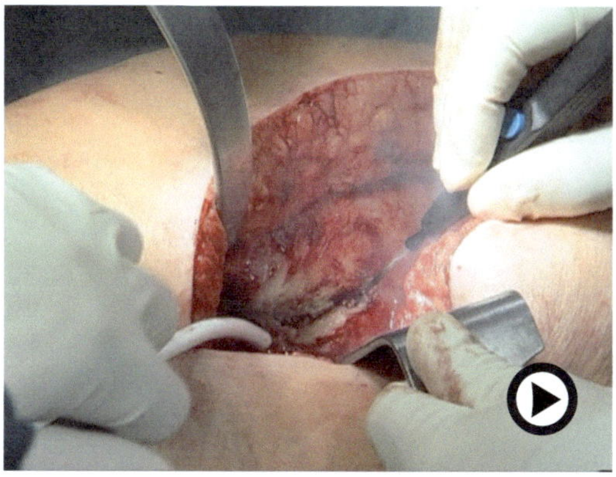

Fig. 12.6 (Video 12.1) Exposing the hip joint via the posterolateral approach (▶ https://doi.org/10.1007/000-4pj)

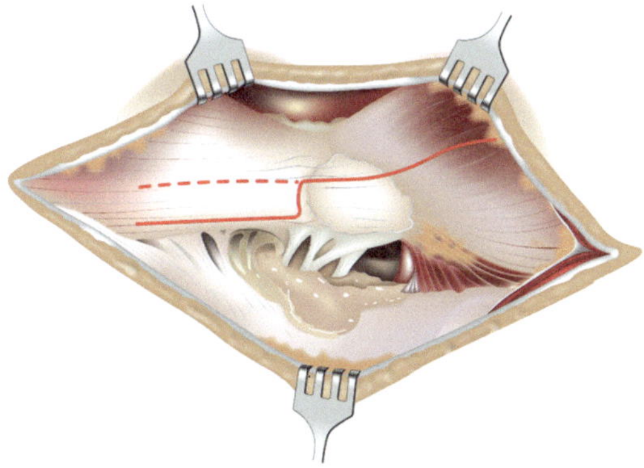

Fig. 12.7 Exposure of the anatomical structures for the vastus slide. The red line shows the path of the incision through the muscles

rotators. Using prosthesis heads with a diameter of 36 mm and, if necessary, inlays with elevated rims can further reduce the risk of dislocation. If the gluteal muscles have already been damaged by the previous operations, so-called dual-mobility cups help to increase the stability of the hip [1]. The posterolateral approach has the decisive advantage during revision that it can easily be extended up to the knee. This approach follows the lateral intermuscular septum and does not damage the vastus lateralis muscle, which is important for vascularization of the femoral bone. This approach can then be further extended into a lateral subvastus approach to the knee joint, which in turn enables the implantation of an extra- or intramedullary total femoral replacement prosthesis. Moreover, this access route can easily be converted into a transfemoral approach at any time (see Chap. 15).

12.6 Extended Approaches

The extended transgluteal approach, known as a vastus slide, extends the normal transgluteal approach distally by proceeding dorsally at the level of the innominate tubercle of the greater trochanter and then continuing distally along the lateral intermuscular septum (Fig. 12.7). It can also be positioned further ventrally as a distal extension of an anterolateral approach. It is used for extended exposure of the proximal femur, for example, to create a ventral bone window for cement removal or to remove embedded osteosynthesis material. The vastus slide has the disadvantage that it involves a more or less pronounced transection of the vasto-gluteal sling, thus weakening it. This creates the risk of an unintentional dislocation of the trochanter if a fracture should occur during revision, since the counterpart of the gluteal muscle (the vastus lateralis muscle) has been separated from it during the approach. When performing a vastus slide, the gluteus medius should not be split more than 4 cm above the original acetabular rim or more than 5 cm cranially from the tip of the trochanter in order to avoid iatrogenic damage to the superior gluteus nerve and the superior gluteal artery [9].

The traditional trans-trochanteric approach can be extended distally in the same way as the vastus slide, thus creating a so-called "sliding trochanteric osteotomy" or "trochanteric slide", which can be used, for example, to fashion a femoral window or to enlarge the exposure of the acetabulum [12] (Fig. 12.8a–c). Furthermore, it is often used for the implantation of an allograft prosthesis composite (APC) of the proximal femur, in which cerclages are used to reattach the trochanter and the muscles to the allograft. The trochanteric slide achieves greater healing rates here than the traditional trans-trochanteric approach [13]. In a modified form (leaving about 1 cm of the posterior greater trochanter in contact with the femur), it also leaves the external rota-

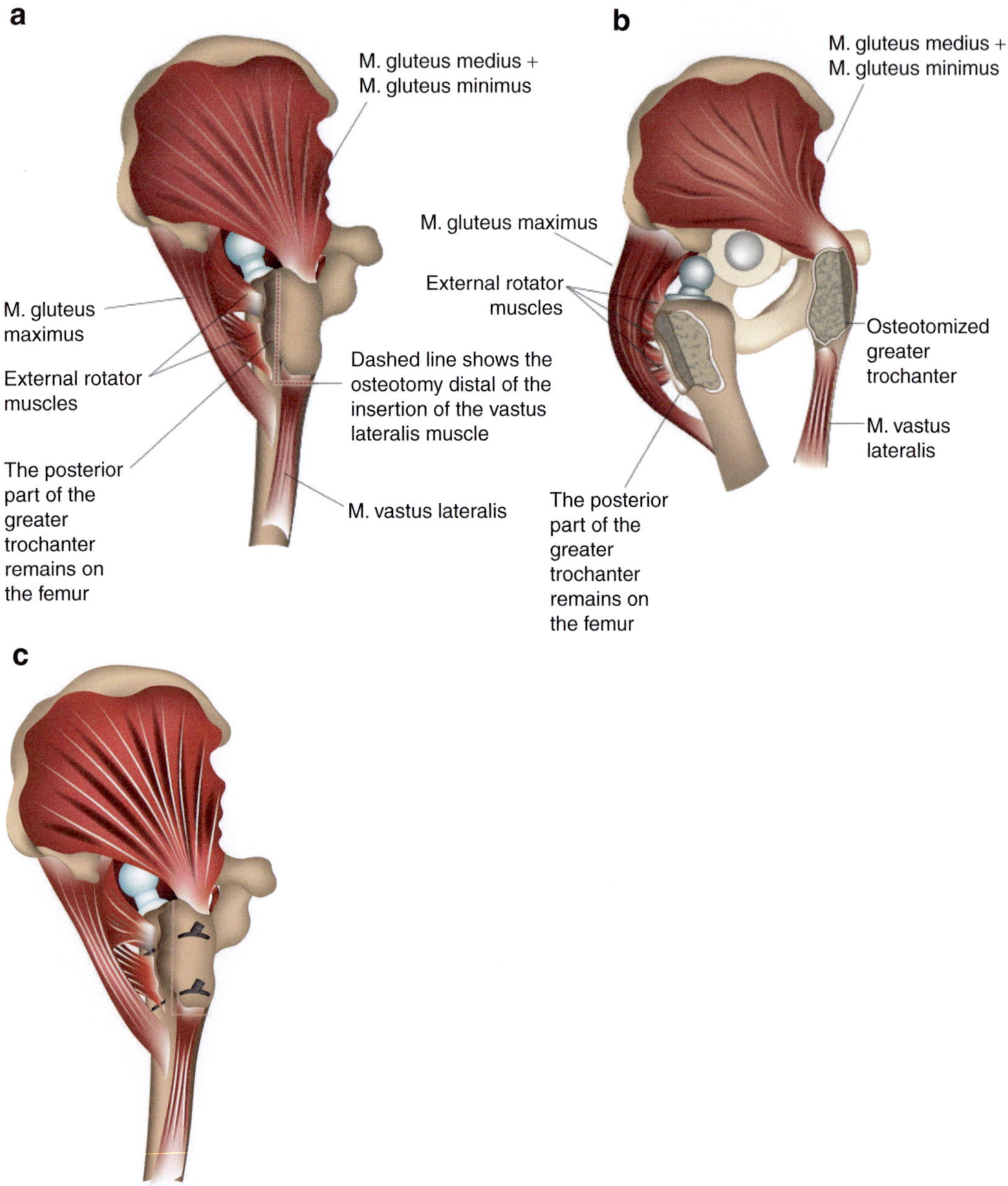

Fig. 12.8 Exposure of the anatomical structures for the trochanteric slide. (**a**) Exposure of the route of the osteotomy. (**b**) Greater trochanter folded back with intact vasto-gluteal sling. (**c**) Reattached greater trochanter

tors untouched. This reduces the tendency to dislocation. The patient is positioned on his side, and a longitudinal incision is made above the greater trochanter. After cutting the fascia latae above the middle of the vastus lateralis muscle, the latter is repositioned slightly from posterior to anterior. The dorsal end of the gluteus medius muscle is identified, and the piriformis muscle is palpated. The path of the osteotomy of the trochanter runs from dorsal–distal to proximal–ventral and begins between the gluteus medius and minimus anterior and the piriformis muscle and the external rotators posterior (Fig. 12.8a). The greater trochanter is osteotomized lengthwise from its tip to the insertion of the vastus lateralis muscle. This maintains the union between the greater trochanter, the abductors, and the vastus lateralis muscle with the vasto-gluteal sling. Here, too, care must be taken to ensure that the trochanteric fragments are sufficiently thick for subsequent healing and to avoid fragmentation of the trochanter. The thickness of the fragment is usually about 2 cm. In the case of a cup revision with the stem left in place, however, some bone must be left at the prosthesis shoulder for better healing. The trochanter is then moved ventrally with the muscle complex, which allows very good exposure of the joint (Fig. 12.8b). Two double cerclages are usually used for subsequent reinsertion (Fig. 12.8c). After surgery, the patient should not perform active abduction for 6 weeks in order not to endanger the healing of the trochanter. In a follow-up examination of 83 trochanteric slide osteotomies, Lakstein et al. [13] found bony healing of the trochanter in 84.4%, fibrotic healing in 10.8%, and nonunion in 4.8%. He observed trochanteric fragmentation in 15.6%, persistent trochanteric problems in 15.6%, and weakness of the abductors in 7.2% of cases.

Because of the relatively common problems associated with the “trochanteric slide,” our favored extended approach is a modification of the transfemoral approach (extended trochanteric osteotomy) described by Heinz Wagner [14–17] (Fig. 12.9). In our opinion, it is indicated for hip prosthesis revisions in cases of broken endoprosthesis stems, axial deviation of the femur, a significantly thinned bone at risk of fracture, a stable cement mantle, a partially fixed cementless prosthesis stem (especially for stems with rough surfaces), and for periprosthetic fractures. The advantages of stem revision via a transfemoral approach, or the so-called extended femoral osteotomy, include direct access to the distal canal of the femur for removal of distal cement and effective preparation of the new prosthesis fixation bed, avoidance of intraoperative fractures and perforations of the femur, more reliable healing of the osteotomy compared to trans-trochanteric osteotomy, reduced operating time for difficult implant removal, protection of the vasto-gluteal sling, and new bone formation through callus formation [12, 18–25] (Fig. 12.10a–e). The transfemoral approach allows the controlled removal of firmly seated stems and the cement mantle, e.g., in septic prosthesis revision of firmly osseointegrated cementless prosthesis stems with a coarse surface structure or a stable cement mantle with bony osteolysis [26]. In addition to the removal of all foreign material, a radical debridement of the prosthesis bed and osteolysis can be successfully achieved [26, 27]. If performed correctly, a reproducibly effective healing of the bony flap can be achieved (Tables 15.1, 15.2, and 15.3). The disadvantages of the transfemoral approach, on the other hand, certainly include the greater technical complexity, the size of the access with potentially greater blood loss, and the slightly longer rehabilitation time until the Trendelenburg signs become negative [28, 29]. The transfemoral approach is discussed in more detail in a separate chapter (see Chap. 15).

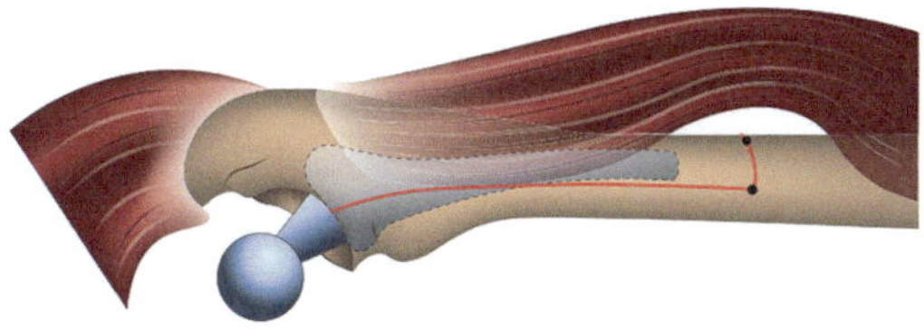

Fig. 12.9 Exposure of the anatomical structures for the transfemoral approach. The red line shows the path of the osteotomy

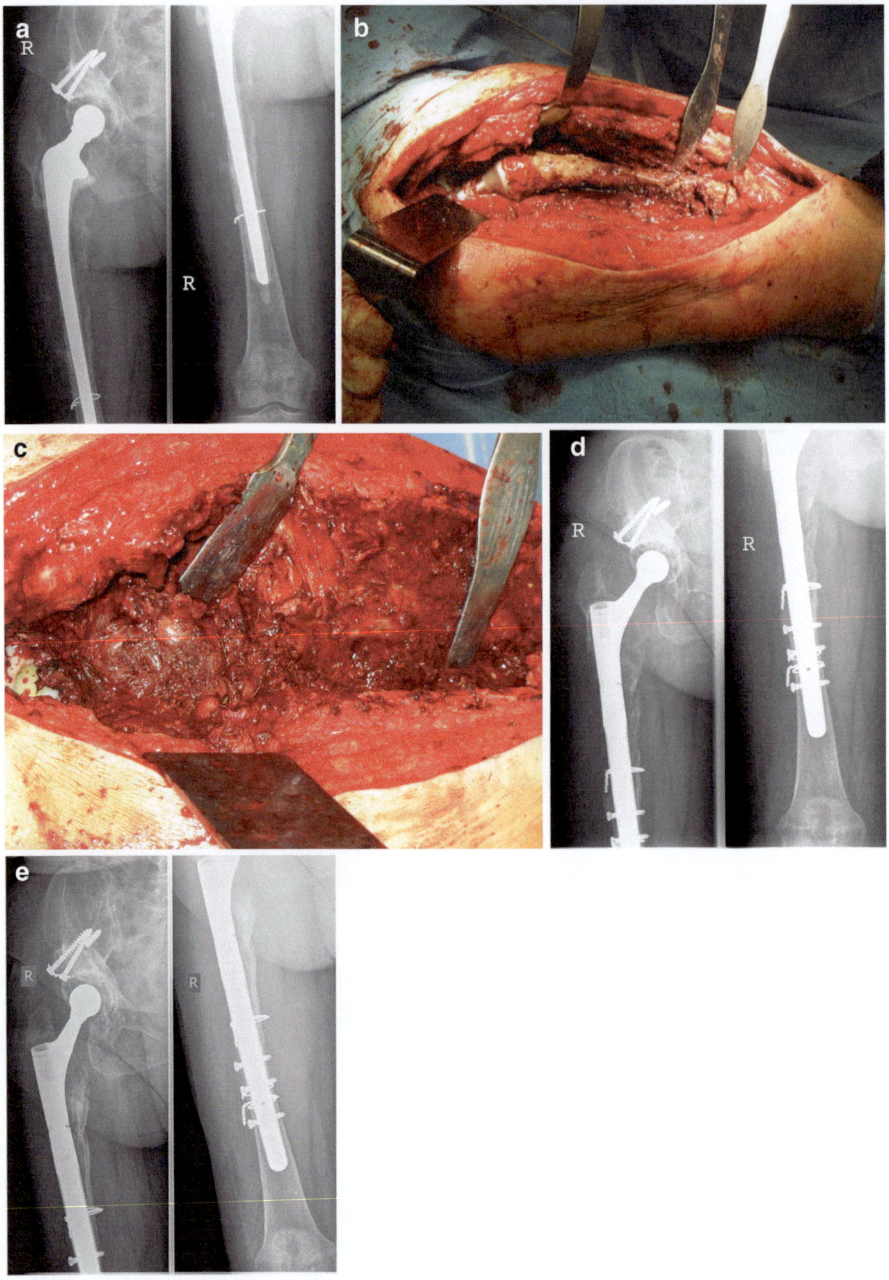

Fig. 12.10 Transfemoral revision of a cemented revision stem 10 years after implantation showing pronounced abrasion-induced osteolysis and defects. A periprosthetic infection was ruled out before and during surgery. (**a**) Preoperative radiograph with stem loosening and pronounced osteolysis in the stem region. (**b**) Intraoperative status with exposure of the stem via a transfemoral approach. The greater trochanter is folded ventrally with the residual bone of the lateral femur and the attached musculature, and the vasto-gluteal sling is preserved. (**c**) Intraoperative status after removal of the stem. The periprosthetic membrane associated with stem loosening contains hemosiderin and has not yet been removed. The residual lateral femur bone is folded up ventrally with the attached muscle. (**d**) Radiograph 2 weeks after surgery for revision to the modular revision stem Revitan Curved with distal locking (Zimmer Biomet, Winterthur, Switzerland). The greater trochanter was fixed with fiber wire through the holes of the proximal shaft component. (**e**) Radiograph 2 years after surgery showing distal osteointegration of the stem with no change in position, medial bone regeneration, and virtually unchanged position of the greater trochanter. The latter has been achieved by using the transfemoral approach to preserve the vasto-gluteal sling

References

1. Kerboull L. Selecting the surgical approach for revision total hip arthroplasty. Orthop Trauma Surg Res. 2015;101:S171–8.
2. Nogler M, Mayr E, Krismer M. The direct anterior approach to the hip revision. Oper Orthop Traumatol. 2012;24:153–64.
3. Fink B. Extended approach in hip revision and preservation of the muscles. Is that possible? Z Orthop Unfall. 2013;151:243–7.
4. Regis D, Sandri A, Bonetti I, Graggion M, Bartolozzi P. Femoral revision with Wagner tapered stem. A ten-to 15 year follow-up study. J Bone Joint Surg Br. 2011;93-B:1320–6.
5. Halser J, Flury A, Dimitriou D, Finsterwald M, Helmy N, Antoniadis A. Is revision total hip arthroplasty through the direct anterior approach feasible? Arch Orthop Trauma Surg. 2020;140(8):1125–32. https://doi.org/10.1007/s00402-020-03469-5.
6. Ugland TO, Haugeberg G, Svenningsen S, Ugland SH, Berg OH, Pripp AH, Nordsletten L. High risk of positive Trendelenburg test after using the direct lateral approach to the hip compared with the anterolateral approach. A single-centre, randomized trial in patients with femoral neck fracture. Bone Joint J. 2019;101-B:793–9.
7. Svensson O, Sköld S, Blomberg G. Integrity of the gluteus medius after the transgluteal approach in total hip arthroplasty. J Arthroplasty. 1990;5:57–60.
8. Picado CHF, Savarese A, dos Santos Cardamoni V, Sugo AT, Garica FL. Clinical, radiographic, and survivorship analysis of a modular fluted tapered stem in revision hip arthroplasty. J Orthop Surg. 2019;28:1–8.
9. Masri BA, Campbell DG, Garbuz DS, Duncan CP. Seven specialized exposures for revision hip and knee replacement. Orthop Clin North Am. 1998;29:229–40.
10. Jando VT, Greidanus NV, Masri BA, Garbuz DS, Duncan CP. Trochanteric osteotomies in revision total hip arthroplasty: contemporary techniques and results. Instr Course Lect. 2005;54:143–55.
11. Suh KT, Roh HL, Moon KP, Shin JK, Lee JS. Posterior approach with posterior soft tissue repair in revision total hip arthroplasty. J Arthroplasty. 2008;23:1197–203.
12. Glassman AH. Exposure for revision: total hip replacement. Clin Orthop Relat Res. 2004;(420):39–47.
13. Lakstein D, Kosashvili Y, Backstein D, et al. Modified trochanteric slide for complex hip arthroplasty: clinical outcomes and complication rates. J Arthroplasty. 2010;25:363.
14. Wagner H. Revisionsprothese für das Hüftgelenk bei schwerem Knochenverlust. Orthopäde. 1987;16:295–300.
15. Wagner H. Revisionsprothese für das Hüftgelenk. Orthopäde. 1989;18:438–53.
16. Wagner H, Wagner M. Femur-Revisionsprothese. Z Orthop. 1993;131:574–7.
17. Wagner H, Wagner M. Hüftprothesenwechsel mit der Femur-Revisionsprothese. Erfahrungen von 10 Jahren. Med Orth Tech. 1997;117:138–48.
18. Chen WM, McAuley JP, Engh CA Jr, Hopper RH Jr, Engh CA. Extended slide trochanteric osteotomy for revision total hip arthroplasty. J Bone Joint Surg Am. 2000;82-A:1215–9.
19. Della Valle CJ, Berger RA, Rosenberg AG, Jacobs JJ, Sheinkop MB, Paprosky WG. Extended trochanteric osteotomy in complex primary total hip arthroplasty. A brief note. J Bone Joint Surg Am. 2003;85-A:2385–90.
20. Huffman GR, Ries MD. Combined vertical and horizontal cable fixation of an extended trochanteric osteotomy site. J Bone Joint Surg Am. 2003;85-A:273–7.
21. Mardones R, Gonzalez C, Cabanela ME, Trousdale RT, Berry DJ. Extended femoral osteotomy for revision of hip arthroplasty: results and complications. J Arthroplasty. 2005;20:79–83.
22. Miner TM, Momberger NG, Chong D, Paprosky WL. The extended trochanteric osteotomy in revision hip arthroplasty: a critical review of 166 cases at mean 3-year, 9-month follow-up. J Arthroplasty. 2001;16:188–94.
23. Paprosky WG, Weeden SH, Bowling JW Jr. Component removal in revision total hip arthroplasty. Clin Orthop Relat Res. 2001;(393):181–193.
24. Peters PC Jr, Head WC, Emerson RH Jr. An extended trochanteric osteotomy for revision total hip replacement. J Bone Joint Surg Br. 1993;75-B:158–9.
25. Younger TI, Bradford MS, Magnus RE, Paprosky WG. Extended proximal femoral osteotomy. A new technique for femoral revision arthroplasty. J Arthroplasty. 1995;10:329–38.
26. Fink B, Grossmann A, Fuerst M, Schäfer P, Frommelt L. Two-stage cementless revision of infected hip endoprostheses. Clin Orthop Relat Res. 2009;467:1848–58.
27. Lim SJ, Moon YW, Park YS. Is extended trochanteric osteotomy safe for use in 2-stage revision of periprosthetic hip infection? J Arthroplasty. 2011;26:1067–71.
28. Fink B, Grossmann A, Schubring S, Schulz MS, Fuerst M. A modified transfemoral approach using modular cementless revision stems. Clin Orthop Relat Res. 2007;462:105–14.
29. Fink B, Grossman A, Schubring S, Schulz MS, Fuerst M. Short-term results of hip revisions with a curved cementless modular stem in association with the surgical approach. Arch Orthop Trauma Surg. 2009;129:65–73.

Removal of the Old Stem 13

Contents

13.1 **Instrumentation** ... 166

13.2 **Techniques of Stem Removal** ... 166

13.3 **Advanced Special Techniques** ... 166
13.3.1 Longitudinal Femoral Osteotomy ... 166
13.3.2 Extended Trochanteric Osteotomy (ETO) and/or Transfemoral Access ... 169
13.3.3 Ventral Bone Window ... 170

13.4 **Removal of Broken Stems** ... 170

References ... 172

Removal of the femoral component and/or cement can be difficult. The primary goal is to achieve removal with minimal loss of surrounding bone, to avoid unintentional fractures, and to preserve the muscles important for bone function and vascularization. In the preoperative planning stage, this surgical step and possible difficulties in this regard must be analyzed and options for augmenting the procedure in case of difficulties and complications must be considered. The following points should be addressed during preoperative planning:

1. It is necessary to analyze the bone for thinning, osteolysis, and axial deviation in order to avoid unintentional fractures.
2. If the stem is to be removed endofemorally, care must be taken to avoid possible hindrances in its path proximally out of the femur. This is especially true for the greater trochanter, which can be located above the entry point of the stem and can fracture if the stem is extracted without due care and attention.
3. The surface structure of the stem to be removed must be assessed. Smoothly polished cemented stems can usually be knocked out of the cement mantle easily. This may be more difficult with roughened cemented stems. Cemcentless stems in particular must be assessed with regard to their ease of removal. The surface structure plays a major role in this respect. Roughly structured stems (e.g., ESKA stems, ESKA, Lübeck, Germany; Solution stems, DePuy Synthes, Warsaw, IN, USA) are difficult if not impossible to remove

---

Supplementary Information The online version contains supplementary material available at [https://doi.org/10.1007/978-3-030-84821-7_13]. The videos can be accessed by scanning the related images with the SN More Media App.

B. Fink, *Femoral Revision Arthroplasty*, https://doi.org/10.1007/978-3-030-84821-7_13

endofemorally, whereby the extent of the rough surface structure is critical here. Proximal coarse-structured stems are easier to remove than stems with a coarse surface structure along the entire stem or hydroxyapatite-coated stems.
4. The design of the prosthesis stem to be removed should be considered. Cementless stem prostheses with collars preclude the medial entry of chisels at the calcar of the femur. Curved stems (e.g., customized prostheses) are difficult to chisel endofemorally. Straight stems without collars, on the other hand, allow the circumferential use of narrow chisels to loosen the stem.
5. The removal of additional components such as screws or plates must be included in the procedure for extracting the stem.
6. Planning for cemented stems must include the removal of the cement and especially the distal cement plug below the tip of the stem and, if necessary, the cement stopper. Long cement plugs that extend into or even beyond the isthmus of the femur cannot be removed endofemorally from the proximal side without a significant risk of perforation or even fracture (see Chap. 14).

The stem undergoing removal should be clearly identified before surgery and the following points clarified preoperatively, if necessary, with the appropriate representative of the prosthesis supplier:

1. Identification of the name or type of stem and the manufacturer.
2. Presence of a screw thread in the stem for a stem-specific extractor.
3. Stem with or without collar.
4. Modular head versus monoblock prosthesis.
5. Length of the stem: short stem, standard length, long stem.
6. Surface of the stem (smooth polished, rough, grit-blasted, coarse-textured).
7. Integrity of the stem (exclusion of stem breakage).

If a cementless stem is to be removed, the following points should also be considered:

1. Localization of the structured surface that allows osteointegration of the stem.
2. Extent of the structured surface.
3. Modularity of the stem.

A loosened prosthesis stem can usually be removed easily from the proximal side using the endofemoral approach and appropriate extraction instruments. Some stems have a specially threaded socket in the shoulder for the attachment of a corresponding extraction tool. Otherwise, special instruments can be placed around the neck of the prosthesis and then fastened to it (Fig. 13.1 and Fig. 13.2 for Video 13.1). If the prosthesis stems have a collar and/or hole in the shoulder, they can also be used to facilitate removal (Fig. 13.3).

Firmly seated cemented and cementless stems are much more difficult to remove and may require special techniques. Firmly fixed stems require a planned removal in the event of:

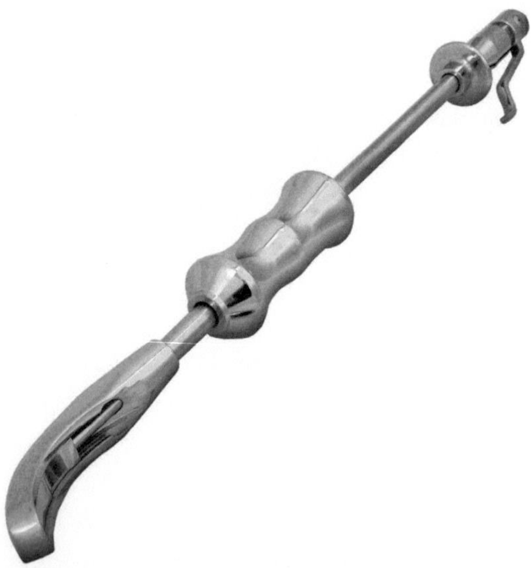

Fig. 13.1 Impaction instruments for a prosthesis stem (ABC tool, endocon, Neckargemünd, Germany)

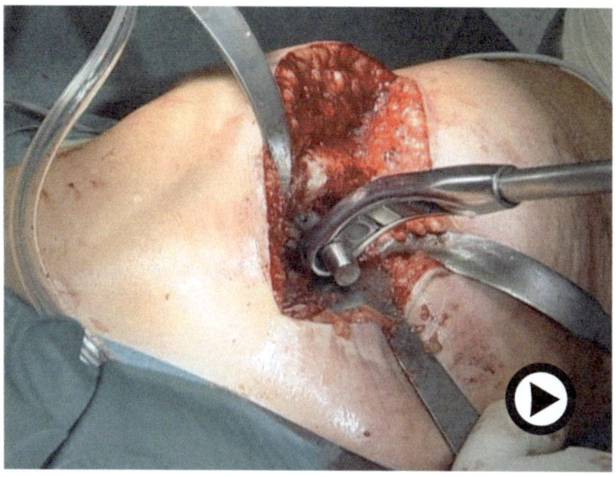

Fig. 13.2 (Video 13.1) Removing a loosened cemented stem with the aid of the ABC Tool (endocon, Neckargmünd, Deutschland) (with permission of Zimmer Biomet, Winterthur, Switzerland) (▶ https://doi.org/10.1007/000-4pm)

1. A periprosthetic late infection: Here, all foreign material (prosthesis and where applicable cement) must be removed and the infected prosthesis bed radically debrided. The transfemoral approach allows this to be done in a controlled and effective manner.
2. A failure of the prosthesis stem forcing the complete removal of the implant (Fig. 13.4): As an exception, after exclusion of a periprosthetic infection, a short, cementless, or cemented stem can be implanted above a stem that has broken distally at the tip after removal of the proximal part of the prosthesis.
3. Damage to the neck of the prosthesis stem caused by a long-standing ceramic head breakage that no longer permits the use of a head sleeve adapter (e.g., BioBall, Merete Medical, Berlin, Germany). Here, the possibility of using the sleeve adapter is tested intraoperatively with the trial adaptor. If significant movement is detected during the test fitting, the stem itself must be replaced.
4. An old monoblock stem with an integrated head, where the exchange of the cup alone does not lead to sufficient stability of the joint.

An unplanned removal of a firmly fixed stem is necessary in cases of:

1. In the course of a cup revision where it becomes apparent intraoperatively that the required leg length or stability of the joint cannot be achieved without a stem revision.
2. A malrotated stem that only becomes apparent during surgery and leads to an unavoidable instability of the joint and/or impingement of the stem.
3. An incompatibility of the stem with the new prosthesis head. This situation can be avoided by an adequate preoperative acquisition of information about the inserted stem, although this can sometimes be very time-consuming.

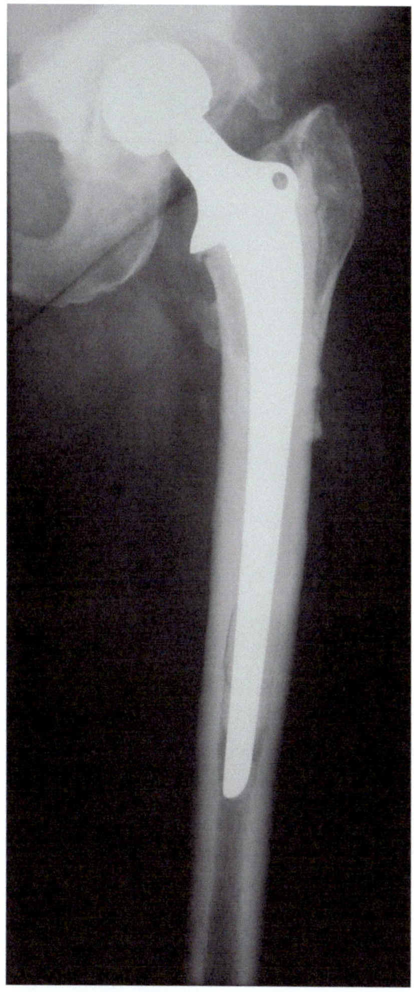

Fig. 13.3 Partially loosened cemented stem with collar and hole in the prosthesis shoulder

The removal of firmly attached stems requires, on the one hand, good direct access to the femoral canal from the proximal side and, on the other hand, the possibility of a safe enlargement of the

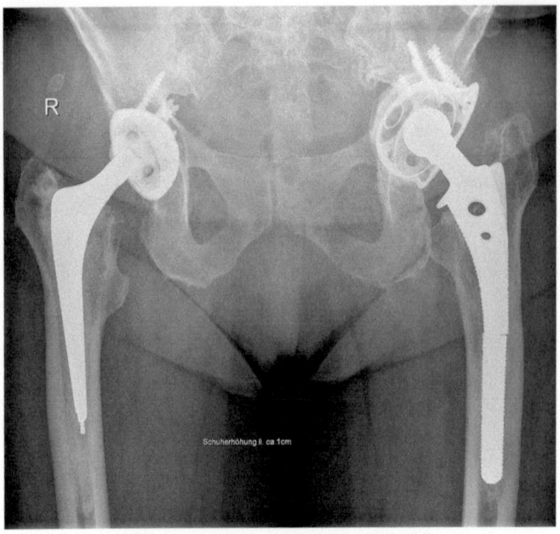

Fig. 13.4 Broken MECRON stem on the left and cup loosening of a Müller ring (Zimmer Biomet, Winterthur, Switzerland)

access without damaging the musculature, the vasto-gluteal sling, and the risk of an unintentional fracture. Of all the possible approaches (see Chap. 12), we prefer the posterolateral route.

13.1 Instrumentation

Revision arthroplasty requires a number of special instruments, which must be considered in the preoperative planning. Special implant-specific instruments or general removal instruments (e.g., pneumatic chisels) may have to be ordered. A wide range of different chisels, drills, and corkscrews is required for cement removal (see Chap. 14). But also the removal of cementless stems requires a number of thin flexible chisels, all of which must be sharp (Fig. 13.5). The pneumatic chisel system (OrthoClast, endocon, Neckargemünd, Germany) allows very good endofemoral removal of proximal cementless straight stems that do not have a collar (Fig. 13.6a, b). Kirschner wires can be drilled past the stems to loosen them, and thin saw blades are also helpful. In cases of broken prostheses, a distal round prosthesis component can be drilled around and loosened with hollow reamers (trephines), if necessary after visualization via a transfemoral approach [1, 2] (Fig. 13.7).

13.2 Techniques of Stem Removal

First, all scar tissue and bone above the shoulder are removed that could inhibit the removal of the stem proximally from the femur. This reduces the risk of an unintentional trochanteric fracture. An overly vigorous, forceful procedure should be avoided in order not to increase the risk of fracture.

Once the proximal entry point of the stem has been cleared, the surgeon can now carefully chisel along the stem with thin narrow chisels. Thin flexible chisels can be guided distally past the prosthesis and loosen the stem from its proximal bed (Fig. 13.8). Kirschner wires can then loosen the prosthesis further distally at the tip (Fig. 13.8). Alternatively, a pneumatic chisel (OrthoClast, endocon, Neckargemünd, Germany) can be used, the thin, flexible, long chisel of which can be guided to the tip of the stem. In this case, it must be ensured that the chisel runs along the prosthesis according to the markings on the blade of the chisel (Fig. 13.6b).

If the greater trochanter is at risk of fracture due to its position above the prosthesis shoulder or because of osteolysis-related thinning of the bone, the unintentional fracture of the greater trochanter should be avoided by employing a well-controlled transfemoral approach with a larger bony flap and preservation of the vasto-gluteal sling.

13.3 Advanced Special Techniques

13.3.1 Longitudinal Femoral Osteotomy

If the removal of the prosthesis from the fixation bed is not possible using a chisel, a longitudinal femoral osteotomy can be performed as the first step in the revision of a cementless prosthesis stem that has a proximal coating or a structured surface. As with the transfemoral approach, the procedure involves access via the lateral intermuscular septum, reaching the femur slightly above the linea aspera. This is continued to

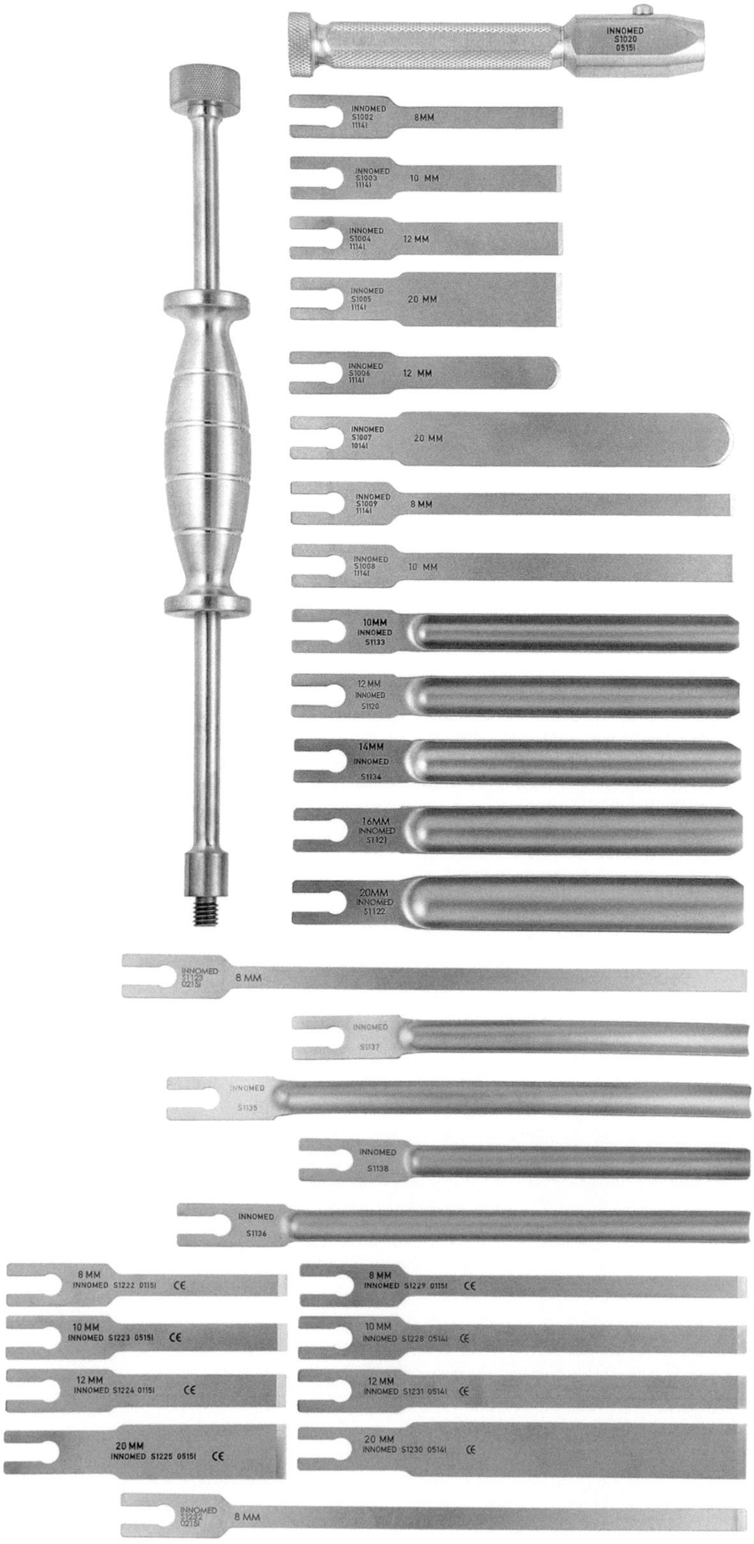

Fig. 13.5 Set of thin chisels for removing cementless stems (endocon, Neckargemünd, Germany)

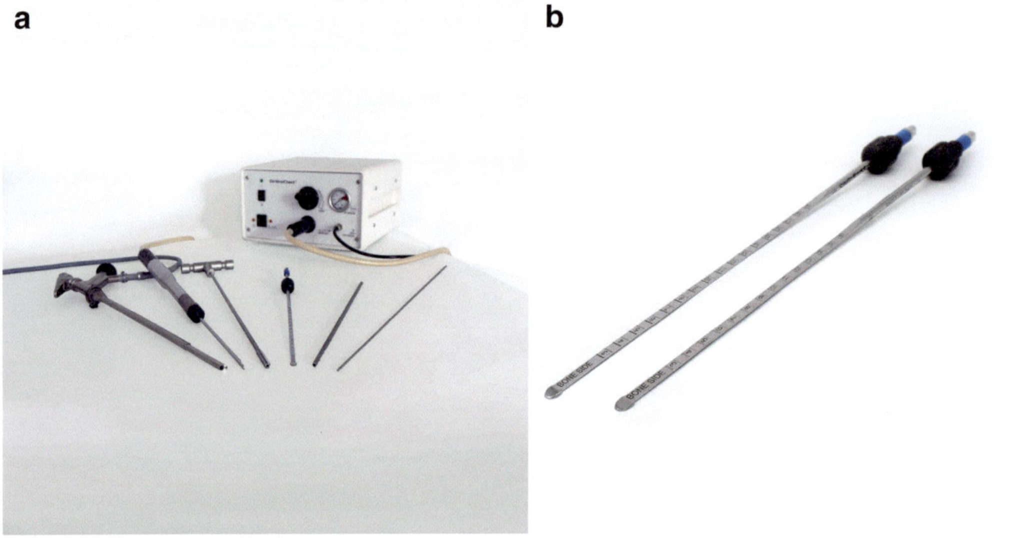

Fig. 13.6 (**a**) Pneumatic flexible chisel (Osteoclast, endocon, Neckargemünd, Germany). (**b**) Blade of the long flexible osteoclast chisel

Fig. 13.7 Reaming of the distal part of a broken prosthesis stem endofemorally with a trephine (hollow reamer)

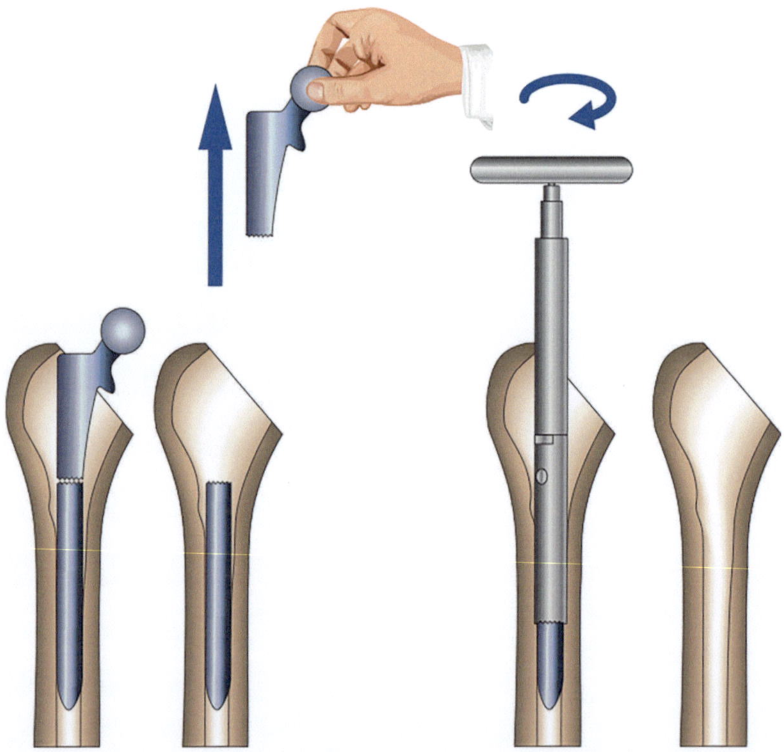

slightly proximal of the tip of the prosthesis (see Chap. 15). An osteotomy is cut proximally along this line with an oscillating thin saw blade (0.7 mm), cooled with Ringer's solution, extending proximally in a slight arc to dorsal (Fig. 13.9). The course of the osteotomy can be marked beforehand with small drill holes (Fig. 13.9). Subsequently, chisels are carefully inserted in an attempt to open up the femur a little. Then, narrow chisels are again introduced from proximal

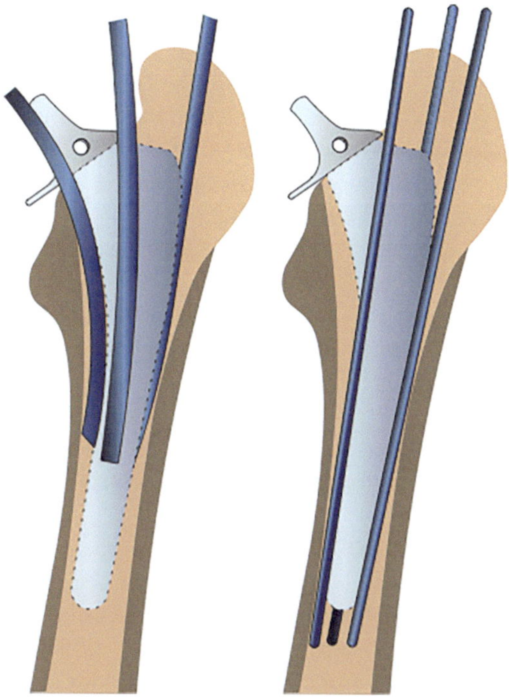

Fig. 13.8 Chiseling of the proximal stem and reaming of the distal stem with K wires

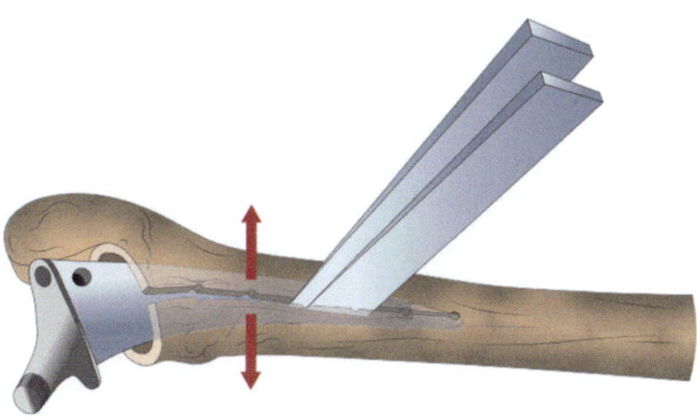

Fig. 13.9 Longitudinal femoral osteotomy

to distal, and an attempt is made to drive out the stem with a set of impaction tools. If this fails again, the surgeon should switch from the longitudinal osteotomy to a transfemoral approach (see Chap. 15). Piyakunmala et al. [3] did not observe any complications with this technique in 19 patients. Nagoya et al. [4] were able to show in 16 cases that even longer standard stems of the Zweymüller type could be used after such a longitudinal osteotomy. The resulting callus formation along the osteotomy promoted the osteointegration of the new prosthesis stem [4].

13.3.2 Extended Trochanteric Osteotomy (ETO) and/or Transfemoral Access

The transfemoral approach is suitable for the removal of firmly seated stems (see Chap. 15), in particular:

- Broken stems.
- Stems with rough surface structure over the entire stem.
- Fracture-prone, thin bone.
- Axis deviations of the femur.
- Obvious subsidence of the stem.
- Pronounced periarticular soft tissue ossification.
- Periprosthetic late infection.
- If a cup requiring revision is found to protrude significantly into the lesser pelvis.

It permits safe stem removal while avoiding unintentional fractures and protecting the musculature (especially the vasto-gluteal sling). The length of the flap depends on the structure of the stem to be removed:

- For stems with a coarsely structured surface: flap extends to the tip of the stem.
- For stems with microporous surface over the whole stem: flap up to 3–4 cm shorter than the prosthetic stem.
- For stems with partial proximal microporous coating: flap to the end of the surface coating.
- For cemented stems: flap to approx. 3–4 above the end of the distal cement plug.

If a firmly fixed, coarsely structured stem is present, it often has to be sawn out of the medial femur ventrally after carefully chiseling out and folding up the lateral bony flap. A thin, narrow saw blade bent lengthwise can be used for this purpose (Fig. 13.2 for Video 13.1 and Fig. 13.10 for Video 13.2).

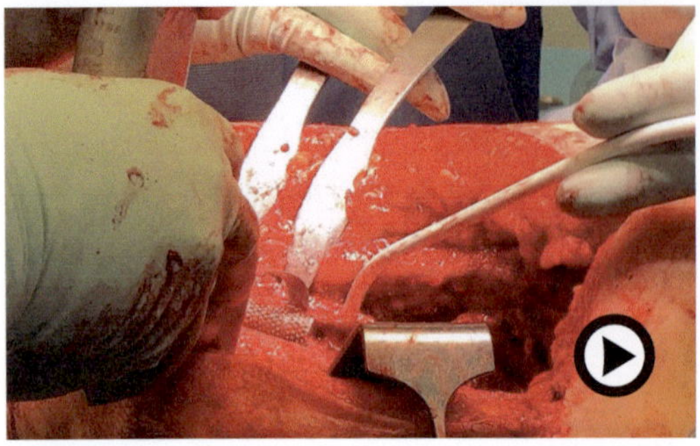

Fig. 13.10 (Video 13.2) Removing a broken distal prosthesis stem component using a bowed saw blade via the transfemoral approach (▶ https://doi.org/10.1007/000-4pk)

13.3.3 Ventral Bone Window

With anterior, anterolateral, and lateral approaches from ventral, a ventral bone window can be created distal to the level of the greater trochanter in order to loosen proximal fixation stems from their fixation bed. However, this is only possible on the ventral side facing the bony flap. Such a window can also be used to remove the cement mantle of a cemented stem. In my opinion, however, the cement in this area can usually be removed from proximally and the removal of the distal cement plug is not really made any easier with this window.

The proximal ventral bone is separated from the muscle located on it, which in turn separates the window bone from the tissue that is important for the vascularization of this bone. Holes are drilled at the 4 corners of the bony flap, and then, these 4 holes are linked together to form the bone window by making converging angled cuts with a thin saw blade under cooling. The convergence prevents the window from falling in during subsequent closure. The window is lifted and removed by chisels (Fig. 13.11). After removal of the old stem and, if necessary, cement, the window is closed again with a double cerclage or cable and a new cementless or cemented stem is inserted [5]. With cemented stems, the bone window is more distal and usually extends further into the femur than with proximal fixation cementless stems (see Chap. 14).

Park et al. [6] reported 75 revision surgeries with such a ventral window via a lateral access and reimplantation of a cementless distal fixation stem. 2% of these procedures resulted in nonunion of the window, 8.9% in stem subsidence, 3.6% in intraoperative fracture, and a 10-year stem survival rate of 91.1%.

We prefer a transfemoral approach in these situations because it avoids the devascularization of the bony flap and the unpredictability of safely loosening a cementless stem through the window and/or safely removing the distal bone cement.

13.4 Removal of Broken Stems

1. The removal of broken stem prostheses is a special challenge for the surgeon. The proximally loosened part of the stem can usually be removed proximally without difficulty. However, proximal scarring and bony overgrowths in the area of the greater trochanter must also be removed to prevent unintentional fractures of the trochanter when the stem is knocked out. Special techniques are required to remove the firmly seated distal stem portion. The distal component must first be reached. If the prosthesis stem breaks proximally, the distal portion can be reached endofemorally. If the femur is straight and the stem is cylindrical, the distal portion can be reamed with a trephine (Fig. 13.7). The trephine should be 0.5 mm or 1 mm larger than the diameter of the stem at its thickest point [2]. The hollow reamers can become blunt relatively quickly. Care should therefore be taken when cutting to ensure that the hollow reamer is not blunt, which could result in excessive heat generation and damage to the bone.

   A transfemoral approach or a larger, ventral bone window is recommended for noncylindrical stems, axial deviations of the femur, and stems that are broken further distally. We prefer the transfemoral approach technique because of the better access to the distal part of the stem. When selecting the length of the flap,

Fig. 13.11 Creating a proximal ventral bone window

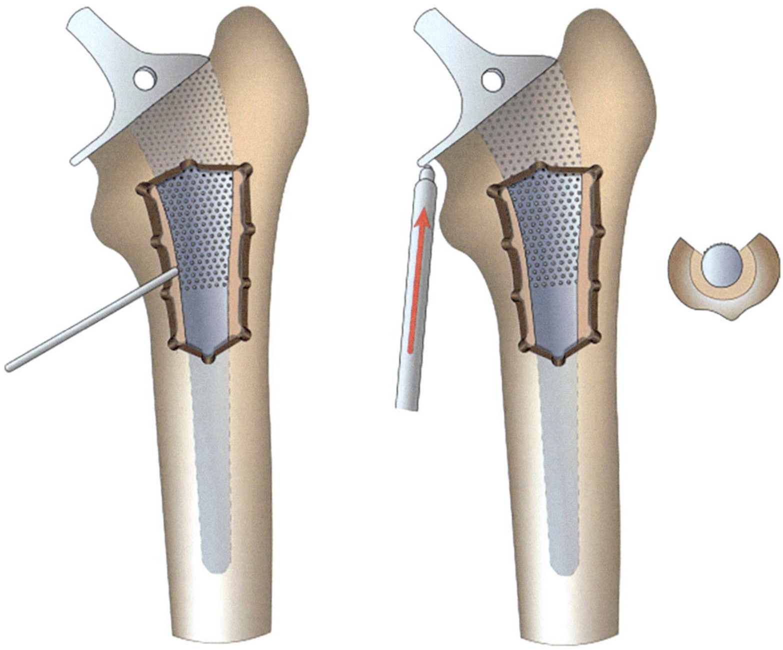

Fig. 13.12 Trephine (hollow reamer) for removal of a distally fractured cylindrical prosthesis stem via the transfemoral approach

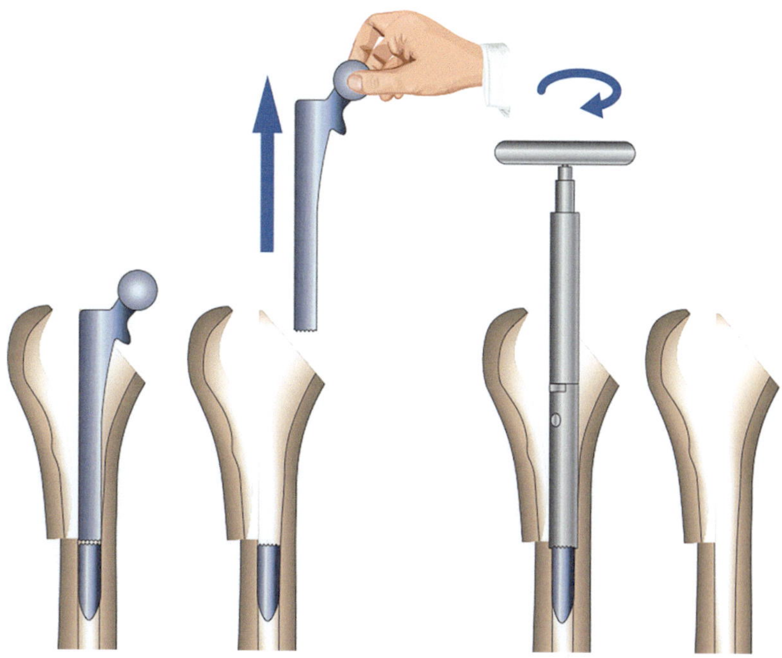

care must be taken to ensure that sufficient fixation distance remains in the isthmus for the selected distally fixed stem. The distal portion of the fractured prosthesis can be loosened and removed with a variety of techniques:

2. The distal portion can be reamed using a hollow reamer (trephine) (Fig. 13.12). The trephine is 0.5 mm or 1 mm larger than the diameter of the stem at its thickest point [2]. This reaming should be performed under visual control, which is why a ventral window or, even better, a transfemoral approach is necessary.

3. The cementless portion, which is still firmly seated distally, is sawn around with a thin saw blade curved along its length (Fig. 13.10 for Video 13.2). Kim et al. [5] reported more than 30 applications of this technique without any problems. The rest that still has to be removed from the isthmus can then be loosened with a thin, flexible blade chisel or a pneumatic chisel.
4. I cannot recommend knocking out the distally fixed segment via perforation holes created on the ventral side of the femur or via a window. The force to be applied here is great and leads to an increased risk of fracture of the femur.

References

1. Paprosky WG, Weeden SH, Bowling Jr JW. Component removal in revision total hip arthroplasty. Clin Orthop Relat Res. 2001:181–193.
2. Pierson JL, Jasty M, Harris WH. Techniques of extraction of well-fixed cemented and cementless implants in revision hip arthroplasty. Orthop Rev. 1993;22:904–16.
3. Piyakunmala K, Sangkomkamhang T, Chareonchonvanitch K. 'Rail road' proximal femoral osteotomy: a new technique to remove well-fixed femoral stem or cement mantle in revision total hip arthroplasty. J Med Assoc Thai. 2009;92(Suppl 6):152–5.
4. Nagoya S, Okazaki S, Tateda K, Kosukegawa I, Kanaizumi A, Yamashita T. Successful reimplantation surgery after extraction of well-fixed cementless stems by femoral longitudinal split procedure. Arthroplast Today. 2020;6:123–8.
5. Kim YM, Lim ST, Yoo JJ, Kim HJ. Removal of a well-fixed cementless femoral stem using a microsagittal saw. J Arthroplasty. 2003;18:511–2.
6. Park CH, Yeom J, Park JW, Won SH, Lee YK, Koo KH. Anterior cortical window technique instead of extended trochanteric osteotomy in revision total hip arthroplasty: a minimum 10-year follow-up. Clin Orthop Surg. 2019;11:396–402.

Removal of the Cement 14

Contents

14.1 **Endofemoral, Proximal Techniques** ... 174

14.2 **Extended Techniques for Removal of Cement** ... 175

References ... 179

When a cemented stem becomes loose, the planned revision procedure determines the extent to which the existing cement mantle has to be removed. For aseptic revision surgery, a cemented stem can be implanted as a cement-in-cement revision if the remaining cement mantle is predominantly solid and intact. In this case, only the loosened proximal cement portions must be removed. In an aseptic situation, even a distally well-seated cement tip can be left in place and serve as a new cement plug provided it does not hinder the implantation of the new cemented stem. In general, all loosened cement portions must be removed. For the implantation of cementless revision stems, as with infected cemented hip prostheses, it is essential that all cement be removed from the femur. Techniques should be selected that allow this goal to be achieved without increasing the risk of unintentional fracture of the greater trochanter or perforation of the femur. In addition, the fixation bed of the new prosthesis should not be weakened by the chosen technique for cement removal.

In preoperative planning, it is therefore important when analyzing the radiographs to devise a strategy for the removal of the distal cement in particular. If, for example, there is a firmly seated elongated distal cement mantle in the isthmus of the shaft, it cannot be removed from proximal using the endofemoral route by drilling or chiseling without a high risk of ventral perforation of the femur with the straight instruments. In addition, the planning procedure should consider whether instruments that might be helpful for removing the cement are available or indeed should be ordered. A large assortment of different chisels with different bevels and cutting directions is just as helpful as an assortment of long ball gouges, drills, sharp curettes, and taps (Fig. 14.1). A number of special instruments have been developed for removal of the cement that can also be helpful. For example, the OSCAR system (endocon, Neckargemünd,

Supplementary Information The online version contains supplementary material available at [https://doi.org/10.1007/978-3-030-84821-7_14. The videos can be accessed by scanning the related images with the SN More Media App.

B. Fink, *Femoral Revision Arthroplasty*, https://doi.org/10.1007/978-3-030-84821-7_14

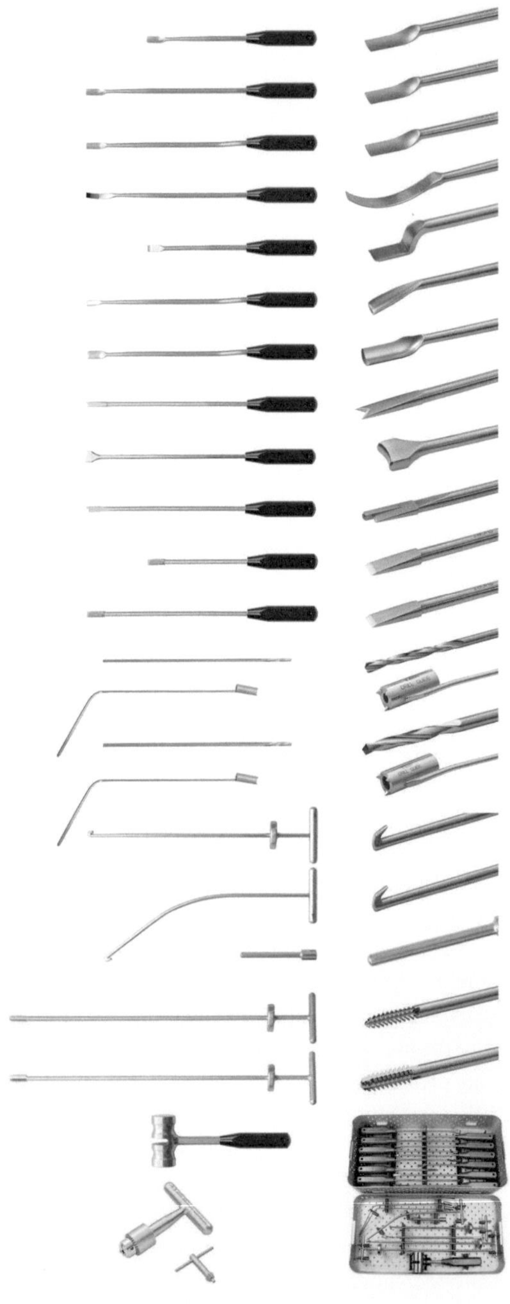

Fig. 14.1 A selection of instruments for removing cement (Innomed, Cham, Switzerland)

Germany) uses ultrasound technology for bone cement removal. The oscillating instrument tip emits ultrasonic waves that soften the cement locally and enable it to be scraped away (Figs. 14.2 and 14.3).

14.1 Endofemoral, Proximal Techniques

Before the cemented stem is removed, all proximal cement around the shoulder and the proximal area of the prosthetic stem must be removed to minimize the risk of trochanteric fracture when the stem is knocked out. The subsequent removal of the cemented stem with an extraction device, which is, for example, fixed around the neck of the stem, is usually straightforward (Fig. 13.1 and Fig. 13.2 for Video 13.1). The proximal cement mantle located in the metaphysis of the shaft can usually be chiseled out easily. The cement mantle is split longitudinally and radially using a sharp chisel with a tip ground on both sides (e.g., nose chisel), and the individual cement pieces are then detached from the bone in pieces using a chisel ground on one side (Fig. 14.4 and 14.5, Fig. 14.6 for Video 14.1). The individual pieces are separated from the bone by tilting the chisel into the femur or rotating the chisel (Fig. 14.5). In order to avoid fractures, swiveling the chisel against the bone is not recommended.

More difficult is the removal of the distal, diaphyseal cement mantle, which is usually more firmly seated than the proximal, metaphyseal one. There are a number of techniques with different functionalities that depend on the stability of the distal cement mantle.

The distal cement mantle can be drilled stepwise. An intramedullary guide may be used for drilling to ensure that the drill is centered (Fig. 14.7). A tap is then screwed into this drill hole. The thickest possible tap that can be screwed in is always used. Hammer blows against the head of the tap can then remove the attached cement ring. The tap should not be screwed in too deeply. Removing smaller cement pieces step by step is better and less risky than trying to remove a large, firmly seated cement piece, which would require considerably more force (Fig. 14.6, Fig. 14.8 for Video 14.2). This method only works with an intact cement mantle. If the cement mantle is partially open at one point, the tap could be pushed against the softer bone and may damage it during further proceedings. Alternatively,

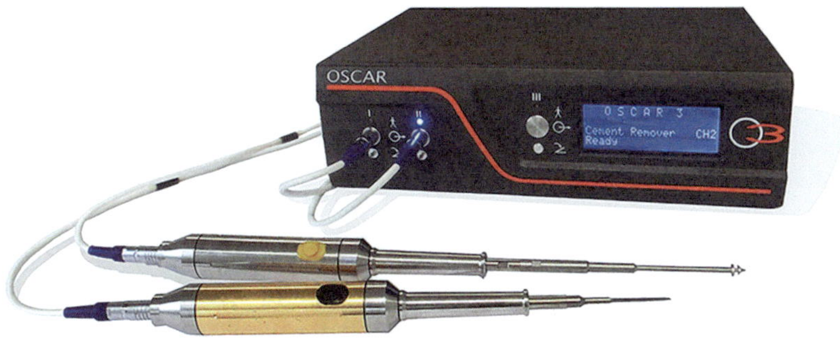

Fig. 14.2 OSCAR system for ultrasonic cement removal (endocon, Neckargemünd, Germany)

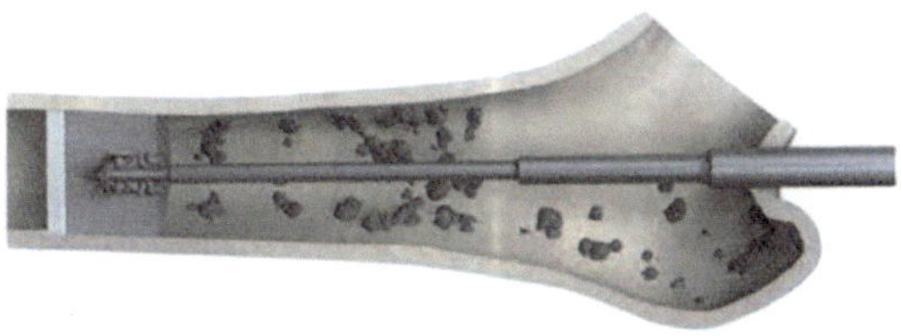

Fig. 14.3 Softening of the cement with the oscillating probe of the OSCAR system (endocon, Neckargemünd, Germany)

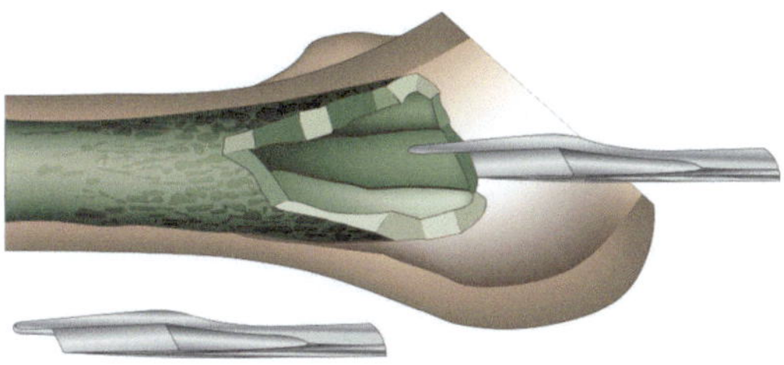

Fig. 14.4 Longitudinal radial splitting of the proximal cement mantle with, for example, a nose chisel

the cement mantle can be made thinner by means of a long ball gouge, after which the thinner cement is usually easier to chisel out (Fig. 14.9).

An easily accessible, short distal piece of cement can be drilled through completely, and the hole can be enlarged slowly with thicker and thicker drills. In this case, we start with a long 4.5-mm drill, followed by 6-mm and 8-mm diameter drills. A retrograde chisel can then be passed through this hole, which then allows cement pieces to be knocked out in a retrograde direction (Figs. 14.7 and 14.10).

Another method is to remove the distal cement mantle using the OSCAR system (endocon, Neckargemünd, Germany). The distal cement mantle is gradually softened by ultrasound and can then be scraped off in a series of gradual steps (Figs. 14.2 and 14.3). Alternatively, the cement is softened and broken up into spaghetti-like strips, which are then allowed to harden again around the ultrasonic probe and be driven out with the probe using a slotted hammer.

Once the cement has been removed, it is important to check that the femur has not been perforated. For this purpose, a sensor can be inserted into the femur and the inner wall was scanned (Fig. 14.7).

14.2 Extended Techniques for Removal of Cement

If the cement cannot be removed with the techniques mentioned above, an extended technique or another procedure must be carried out. Two or three methods have been described for this:

1. On the one hand, a window can be created in the femur. First, the exact location of the residual cement to be removed is determined. For this purpose, the length of the old prosthesis that has already been removed can be used or a fluoroscope. After accessing the femur through the soft tissues, the corners of the window are established by drilling a 3.2-mm hole at each corner and the flap is formed with an oscillating saw, cutting at a slant under cooling (Fig. 14.11). The slightly tapered edges improve bone contact during subsequent closure of the window. The bone window covers 1/4 to 1/3 of the femoral circumference. The window can then be opened using thin chisels, and the bone flap is removed. In this way, the cement can also be

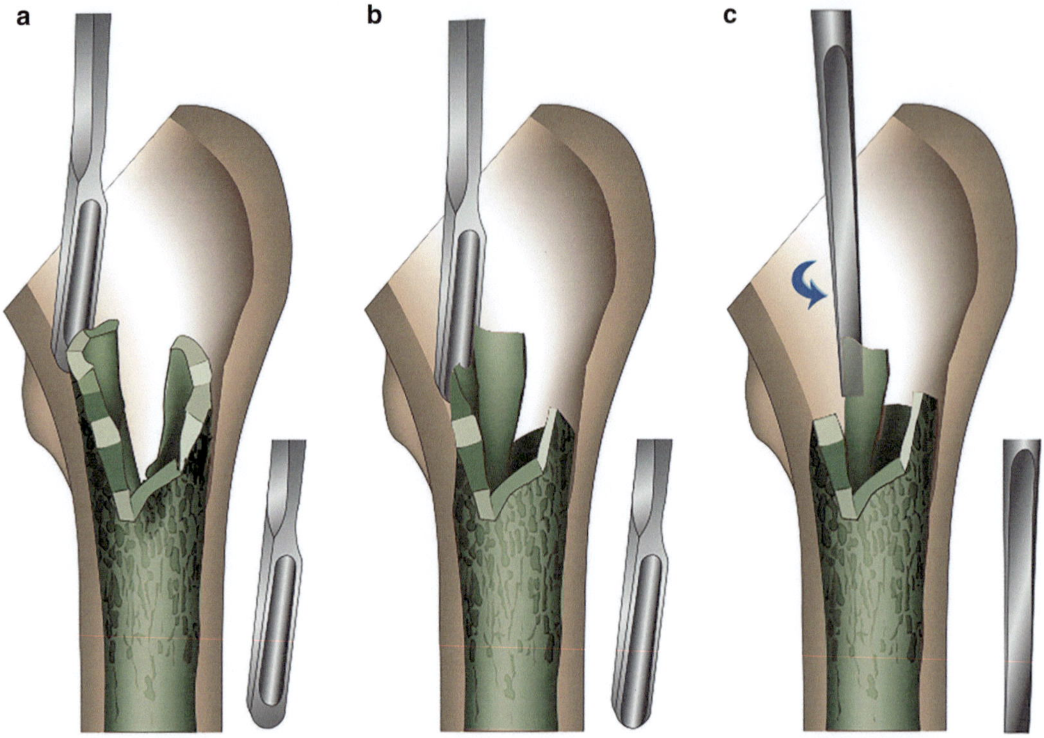

Fig. 14.5 Detaching the individual cement pieces from the bone using a chisel ground on one side by tilting or swiveling the chisel

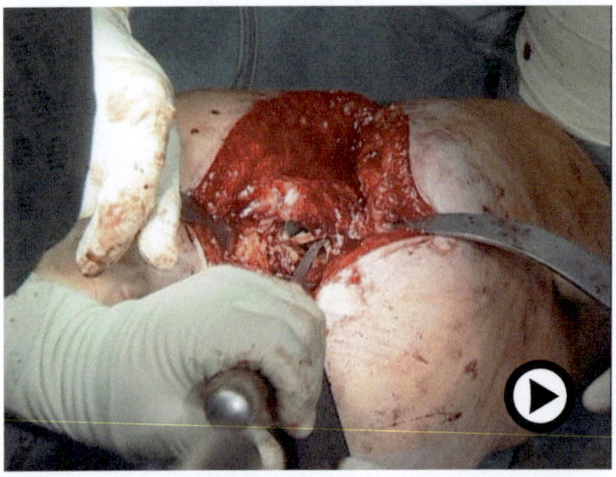

Fig. 14.6 (Video 14.1) Disintegration of the proximal cement mantle by radial chiseling with a nose chisel (with permission of Zimmer Biomet, Winterthur, Switzerland) (▶ https://doi.org/10.1007/000-4pp)

removed around a still firmly seated, cemented stem with appropriate chisels, thus releasing the stem itself. After removal of the cement and, if necessary, of the stem, the window can then be closed again with cerclages. In my opinion, the window should not be placed at the level of the isthmus of the femur, as suggested by Mumme et al. [1] for implantation of the distally fixed, modular revision stem MRP (Peter Brehm, Weisendorf, Germany). This weakens the fixation area of the modular revision stem. In addition, the window area must then be bridged with a sufficiently long (usually 2 diaphyseal widths) cementless revision stem, which makes the implantation of long revision stems necessary [2]. Moreland et al. [3] state that a bridging distance of 5–6 cm is sufficient. If the bony window is not placed at the level of the isthmus of the femur but positioned proximal to it, it should be long enough for the distal cement to be reached at an angle and then removed. If, however, firmly seated cement is located a long way distal of the isthmus, in the region where the femur is widening again, it cannot be brought proximally through the narrower isthmus of the femur without frac-

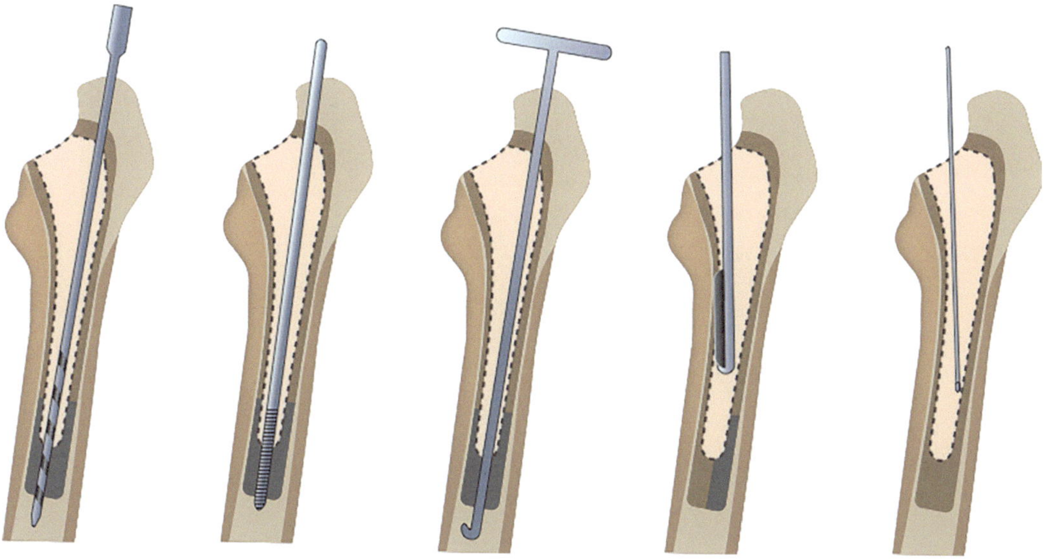

Fig. 14.7 Different methods for removing firmly seated distal cement: From left to right: drilling through the cement, removal with a thread tap or a chisel, and scanning the medullary canal to rule out a perforation

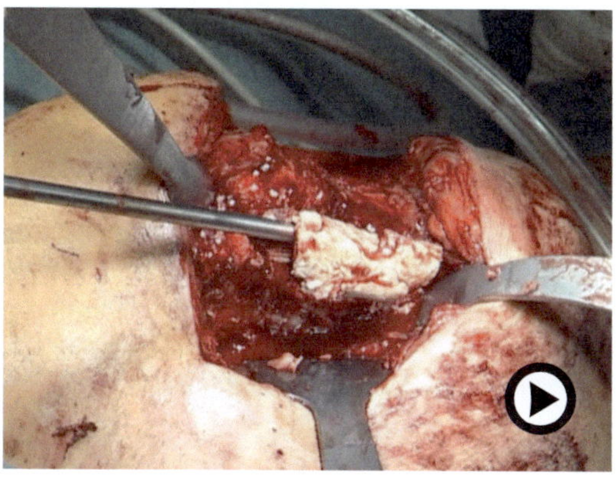

Fig. 14.8 (Video 14.2) Removal of pieces of cement with a tap (corkscrew) (with permission of Zimmer Biomet, Winterthur, Switzerland). Removal of annular cement pieces by means of a tap (corkscrew) (▶ https://doi.org/10.1007/000-4pn)

turing the isthmus. In this case, a suitable bone window distal to the isthmus must be created in order to remove the cement. The revision stem must then be selected accordingly and implanted in such a way that it achieves a secure fit in the isthmus of the shaft and also bridges the distal bone window sufficiently. The distal fixation of the stem is thus achieved at some distance proximal to the tip, an aspect that must be carefully planned preoperatively and checked intraoperatively (using a fluoroscope if necessary).

2. The alternative is to change the procedure to a transfemoral approach (extended trochanteric osteotomy). This is then extended to just above the distal cement piece that still has to be removed, whereby an adequately long section of the isthmus must remain for fixation of the distal stem. As a rule, it is sufficient to extend the flap of the transfemoral access to just above the isthmus (Fig. 14.12). After opening the flap, the residual distal cement can be drilled and removed under visual control as described above (Fig. 14.12).
3. Sydney and Mallory [4] described the controlled perforation of the femur for cement removal, whereby a series of round or oval holes is created in the ventral femur. These holes should be approximately 9 mm in diameter and spaced a minimum of 2 diaphyseal widths apart in order to alleviate the risk of fracture [2, 5]. Sydney and Mallory [6] studied 219 cases treated in this manner and observed a postoperative fracture at the tip of the new stems in 9 cases (4.1%). On the one hand, these holes allow light to enter the med-

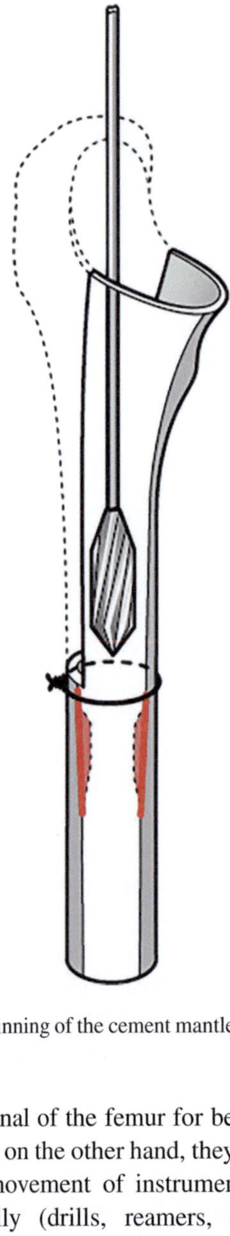

Fig. 14.9 Thinning of the cement mantle caused by a ball gouge

ullary canal of the femur for better visualization, and on the other hand, they allow control of the movement of instruments introduced proximally (drills, reamers, chisels, etc.). However, the ventral femur must be extensively exposed and thus separated from the muscles that are important for its vascularization. This alteration of the musculature and the limitation of the view through the holes compared to the window or transfemoral approach make this procedure of historical interest only.

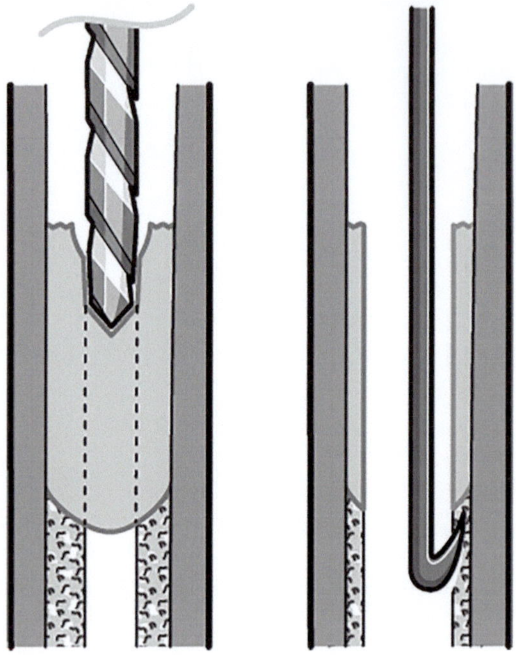

Fig. 14.10 Removal of distal cement pieces by drilling and retrograde chiseling

In the context of the difference between the first two techniques, consideration should be given to which of the two can safely achieve the goal of removing the cement without risking unintentional fractures. In my opinion, the transfemoral approach is more advisable because it allows the distal cement to be removed under visual control and the bony flap remains vascularized because of the muscles attached to it. The latter is not the case with the window, and the removal of cement distal to the window can also be problematic because of the angled access. Lerch et al. [7] compared revision surgery of cemented stems with and without transfemoral access and found 14% of unintentional periprosthetic fractures in the endofemoral approach compared to 0% in the transfemoral approach.

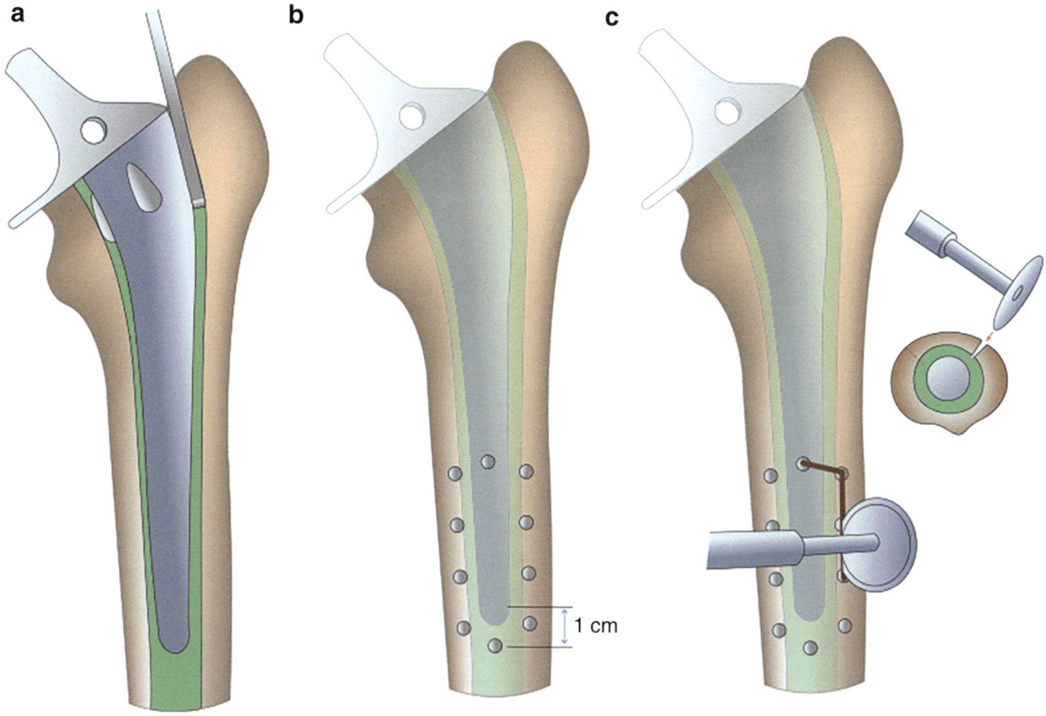

Fig. 14.11 Positioning a bone window for removal of the distal cement

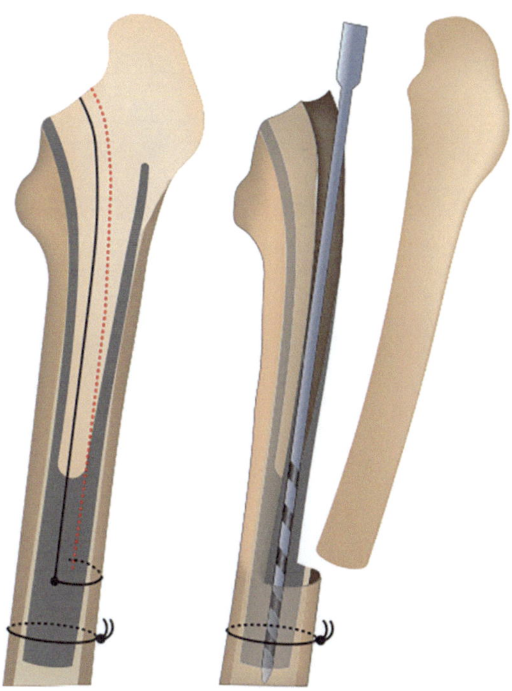

Fig. 14.12 Removal of the distal cement via a transfemoral approach

References

1. Mumme T, Müller-Rath R, Andereya S, Wirtz DC. Uncemented femoral revision arthroplasty using the modular revision prosthesis MRP-Titan revision stem. Oper Orthop Traumatol. 2007;19:56–77.
2. Lombardi AV Jr. Cement removal in revision total hip arthroplasty. Semin Arthroplasty. 1992;3:264–72.
3. Moreland JR, Marder R, Anspach WE Jr. The window technique for the removal of broken femoral stems in total hip replacement. Clin Orthop Relat Res. 1986;(212):245–249.
4. Sydney SV, Mallory TH. Controlled perforation—a safe technique of cement removal from the femoral shaft. Surg Round Orthop. 1988;17:21–8.
5. Mallory TH. Surgical exposure and cement removal in revision total hip arthroplasty. Semin Arthroplasty. 1992;3:257–63.
6. Sydney SV, Mallory TH. Controlled perforation. A safe method of cement removal from the femoral canal. Clin Orthop Relat Res. 1990;(253):168–171.
7. Lerch M, van Lewinski G, Windhagen H, Thorey F. Revision of total hip arthroplasty: clinical outcome of extended trochanteric osteotomy and intraoperative femoral fracture. Technol Health Care. 2008;16:293–300.

Technical Implementation of the Transfemoral Approach

15

Contents

15.1 **Indications for Transfemoral Access** ... 181
15.1.1 Broken Prosthetic Stem ... 182
15.1.2 Thin Bone Prone to Fracture ... 182
15.1.3 Long Cement Mantle ... 183
15.1.4 Firmly Fixed or Only Partially Loosened Cementless Stem ... 184
15.1.5 Axial Deviation of the Femur ... 185
15.1.6 Periprosthetic Fracture of the Femur (Vancouver B2 or B3 Type) ... 186
15.1.7 Periprosthetic Infection with Firmly Seated Implant or Cement or Hard-to-Reach Osteolyses ... 187
15.1.8 Cup Protruding into the Lesser Pelvis ... 189

15.2 **Transfemoral Access Technique** ... 190

15.3 **Variations** ... 198
15.3.1 Double Osteotomy ... 198
15.3.2 Osteotomy Through the Femur After Prior Removal of the Implanted Stem ... 199
15.3.3 Extended Trochanteric Osteotomy ... 199

15.4 **Complications** ... 200

15.5 **Outcomes** ... 200

References ... 206

15.1 Indications for Transfemoral Access

In my view, there are clear indications for a transfemoral approach, which we routinely check during preoperative planning. We will carry out a transfemoral approach if one of the indications listed below is present. If we are certain after the planning phase that we can proceed endofemorally (without osteotomy) without increasing the risk of unintentional fractures, we will perform the operation in that way. If there is any uncertainty during planning, we choose the transfemoral approach, as this has the advantage of avoiding such unintentional fractures, all of which can make the operation significantly more difficult and the outcome less reproducibly predictable. I consider a transfemoral approach to be appropriate for the following indications, all of

Supplementary Information The online version contains supplementary material available at [https://doi.org/10.1007/978-3-030-84821-7_15]. The videos can be accessed by scanning the related images with the SN More Media App.

B. Fink, *Femoral Revision Arthroplasty*, https://doi.org/10.1007/978-3-030-84821-7_15

which are the subject of review at each preoperative planning and can be present in combination:

15.1.1 Broken Prosthetic Stem

In the case of a broken prosthetic stem (Fig. 15.1a, b) the challenge is to remove the broken distal piece in a controlled manner without the risk of unintentional fractures of the femur. The transfemoral approach allows direct access to the distal segment of the prosthesis, which can then be loosened by reaming with a hollow reamer (trephine) or by chiseling with thin narrow chisels or a pneumatic chisel. The transfemoral access then extends either to the beginning of the fractured distal prosthesis segment or to above the isthmus of the femur (Fig. 15.1b). We consider a window at the level of or below the inserted distal prosthesis segment to be less suitable, since the distal segment cannot be chiseled out from it reproducibly. In addition, a window below the prosthetic stem would usually partially or even completely involve the isthmus of the femur, thus weakening the fixation zone of the new stem and requiring very long revision stems in order to bridge the window.

15.1.2 Thin Bone Prone to Fracture

If the femur exhibits thin bone at risk of fracture, either due to loosening of the stem being revised or generally due to osteoporosis (rheumatoid arthritis for example), there is a high risk of fracture during revision surgery (Fig. 15.2a, b). This fracture can affect the greater trochanter and a surgical approach that has altered the vasto-gluteal sling will result in a proximalization of the trochanter. This in turn makes it unlikely that a reproducibly good outcome for the function of the hip joint will be achieved after revision. The other type of fracture in these cases is a spiral fracture that runs into the isthmus of the femur, i.e., where the new prosthesis is to be fixed. The secure distal fixation of the prosthesis becomes more problematic, so that the degree of difficulty of the whole operation is significantly increased. The transfemoral approach avoids these unintentional fractures by creating what might be called a "controlled fracture" with preservation of the greater trochanter and vasto-gluteal sling for function and the isthmus of the femur for fixation of the new stem.

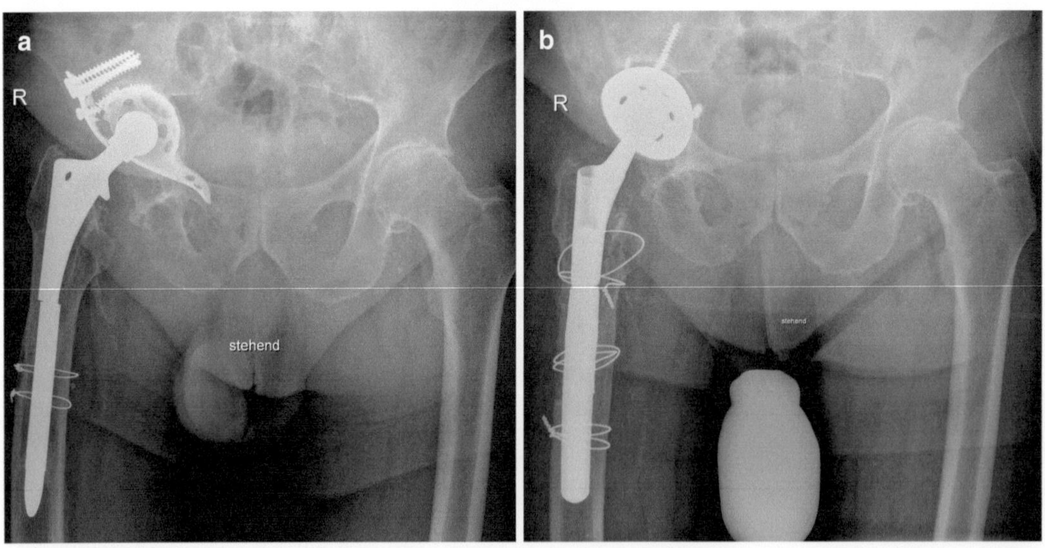

Fig. 15.1 (**a**) Broken nonmodular revision stem Solution (DePuy Synthes, Warsaw, IN, USA) and cup loosening of a Burch–Schneider cage (Zimmer Biomet, Winterthur, Switzerland). (**b**) Radiograph 6 months after prosthesis revision via a transfemoral approach to a modular revision stem Revitan Curved and TMT Multiwhole press-fit cup (Zimmer Biomet, Warsaw, IN, USA)

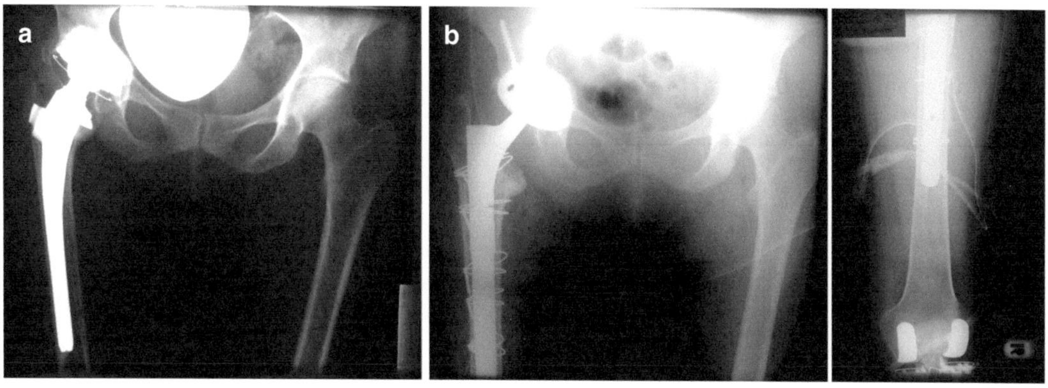

Fig. 15.2 (**a**) 64-year-old female patient with rheumatoid arthritis and prosthesis loosening of a cementless Thabe screw cup (Waldemar Link, Hamburg, Germany) and a cementless stem (Ribbed prosthesis, Waldemar Link, Hamburg, Germany) with thin bone at risk of fracture. (**b-Left** and **Right**) Postoperative radiograph after transfemoral revision to a modular revision stem Revitan Curved and press-fit cup Allofit-S (Zimmer Biomet, Winterthur, Switzerland)

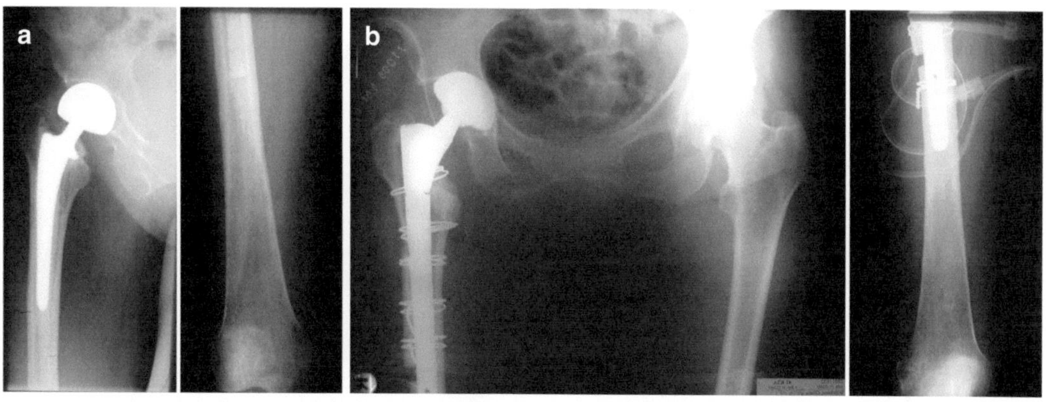

Fig. 15.3 (**a-Left** and **Right**) Loosened dual-mobility prosthesis with a long cement mantle. (**b-Left** and **Right**) Postoperative radiographs after transfemoral prosthesis revision with a modular revision stem Revitan Curved and Allofit press-fit cup (Zimmer Biomet, Winterthur, Switzerland)

15.1.3 Long Cement Mantle

If the cement mantle of the cemented stem under revision extends into the isthmus of the femur (Fig. 15.3a) and a distal fixation revision stem is to be used, it is not possible to drill or chisel the distal cement mantle endofemorally from the proximal side without a high risk of ventral distal perforation. Fenestration of the femur at the level of the isthmus would weaken the isthmus for fixation of the new stem. In the case of a window above the isthmus, the firmly seated distal cement must be removed from around a comer, which is usually difficult and not predictably successful. The transfemoral approach is extended to above the isthmus and then, after the flap is folded back, allows a technically straightforward removal of the proximal cement and direct access to the isthmus (Fig. 15.3b). Since the isthmus itself is straight, the distal cement can now be drilled directly and the residual cement removed with corkscrews or retrograde chisels (see also Chap. 14). Lerch et al. [1] compared revision surgery of cemented stems with and without transfemoral access (extended trochanteric osteotomy) and found 14% of unintentional perforations and fractures associated with the endofemoral approach, but none of these complications with the transfemoral approach.

15.1.4 Firmly Fixed or Only Partially Loosened Cementless Stem

Cementless stems with a coarse surface structure (e.g., ESKA, MECRON, Solution, Judet, Lord) and sometimes a proximal prosthesis collar, which do not enable proximal access to the distal stem area, are an indication for a transfemoral approach (Fig. 15.4a). The coarsely structured stems cause pain when loosened, but cannot be easily removed proximally due to their surface structure. If an attempt is made nevertheless, there is a risk of unintentional fractures of the proximal femur and especially of the greater trochanter. In the case of other stems that are firmly seated and have to be removed due to a periprosthetic infection, for example, an attempt can first be made to loosen them from the proximal side by chiseling or reaming with Kirschner wires. If this is unsuccessful or if it becomes apparent during the procedure that the risk of fracture or perforation is increasing, a transfemoral approach should be implemented (Fig. 15.4b). Even long revision stems, which have to be removed due to a periprosthetic infection, can be removed in this way (Fig. 15.5a). In this case, a long flap is required for transfemoral access to loosen the revision stem. The flap then extends to the area where only a brief chiseling of the prosthesis from its fixation bed in the isthmus is necessary (Fig. 15.5b). However, some residual isthmus should definitely be retained for later fixation of the new prosthesis, e.g., during two-stage septic replacement (then using special techniques such as distal locking; see corresponding Chap. 19) (Fig. 15.5c).

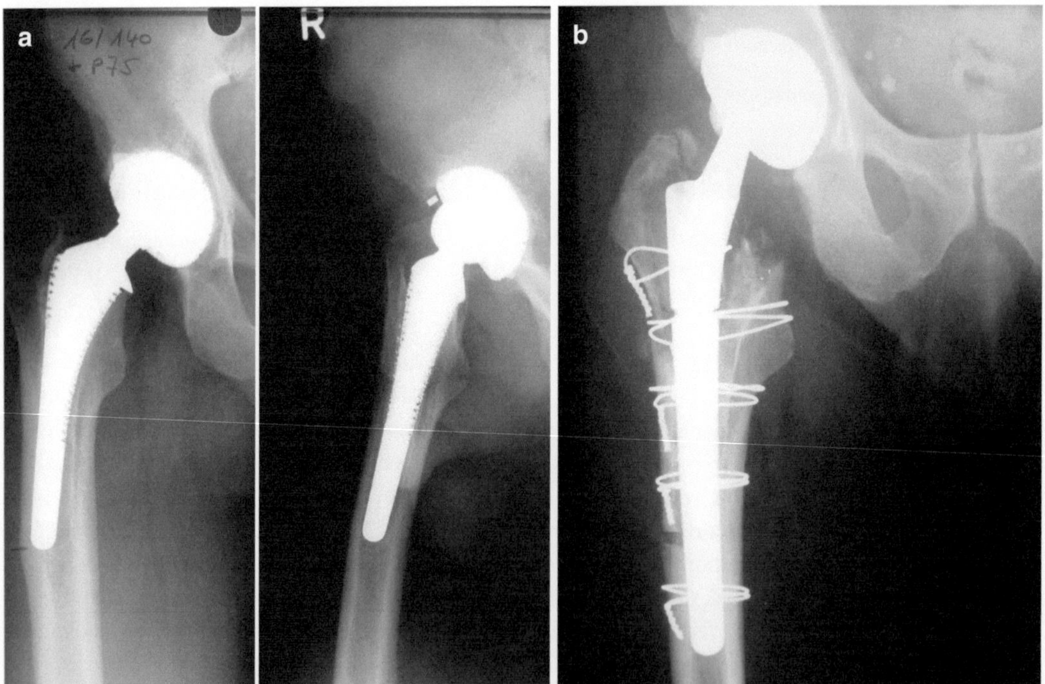

Fig. 15.4 (**a**) Varus deviated, partially loosened, coarsely structured prosthetic stem (ESKA, Lübeck, Germany). (**b**) Radiograph 3 months after transfemoral stem revision to a modular revision stem (Revitan Curved, Zimmer Biomet, Winterthur, Switzerland)

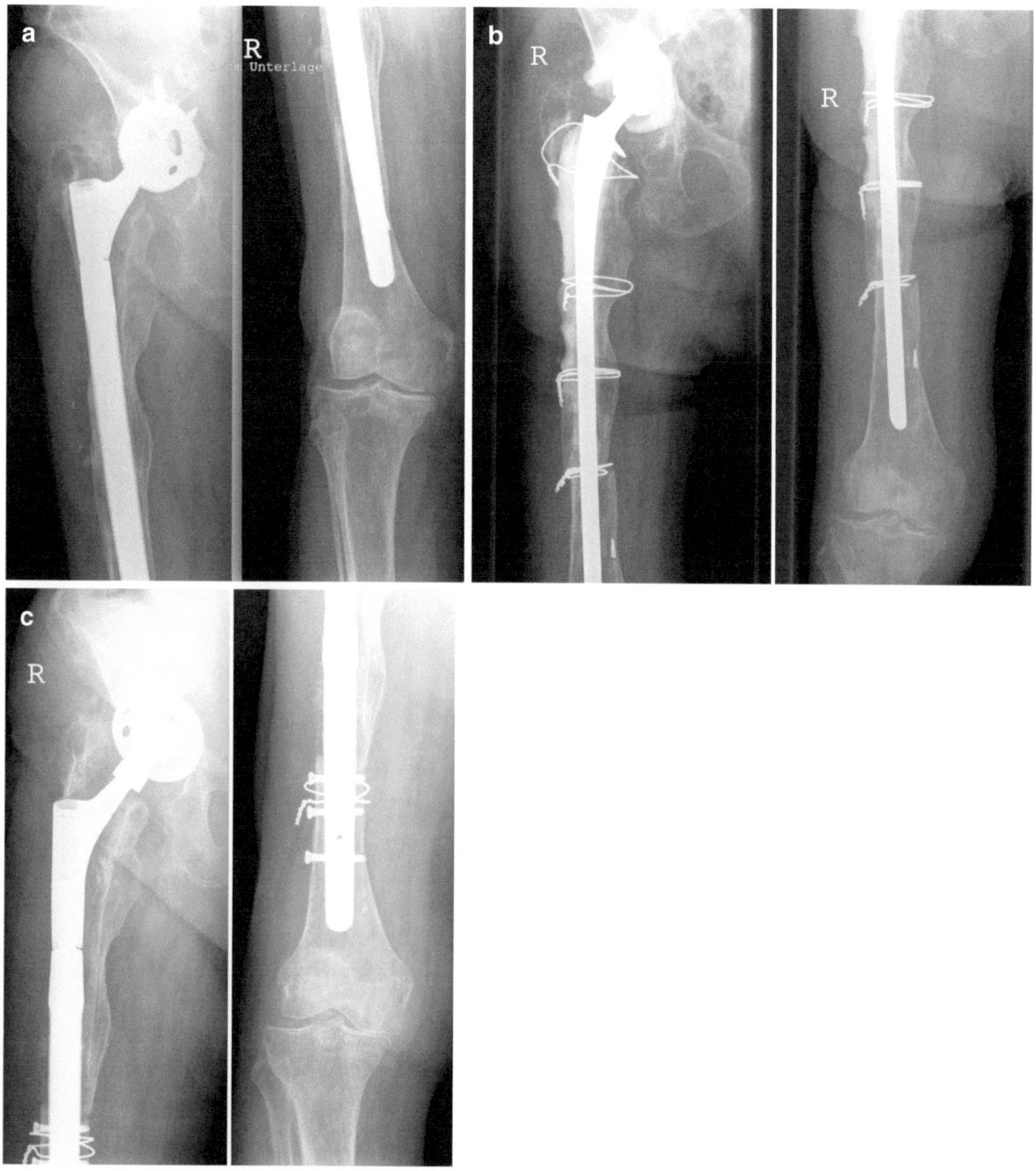

Fig. 15.5 (**a**) Long modular revision stem and coarsely structured cup with a late periprosthetic infection. (**b-Left** and **Right**) Radiograph after removal of the implants via an extended transfemoral access and insertion of an intentionally poorly cemented interim prosthesis as a spacer. (**c**) Radiograph 6 months postoperatively after replacement with a cementless modular revision prosthesis with distal locking (Revitan Curved) and a cementless press-fit cup Allofit-S (Zimmer Biomet, Winterthur, Switzerland)

15.1.5 Axial Deviation of the Femur

During the loosening process of the stem, the force applied to the prosthesis head causes varus alignment of the stem. The bone will follow the stem according to Wolff's remodeling law [2] (Fig. 15.6a, b). This results in a varus deviation of the femur, which must be

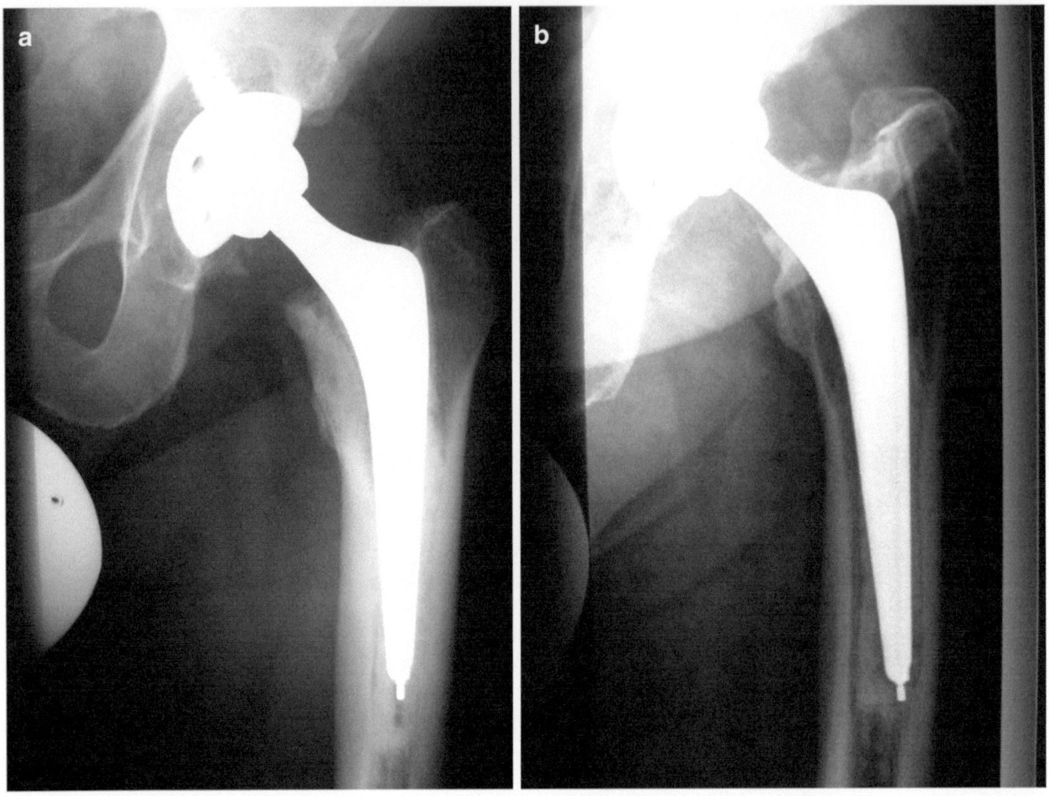

Fig. 15.6 (**a**) Radiograph 3 months postoperative after implantation of a hybrid total endoprosthesis in the left hip. (**b**) Radiograph 10 years after surgery with loosening and varus of the prosthetic stem and varus alignment of the femur

corrected during revision surgery, otherwise perforations and unintentional fractures can occur (Fig. 15.7a, b). The necessity for transfemoral access is recognized during preoperative planning. When the prosthesis is placed in position, it lies in the proximal region of the greater trochanter or even outside the bone (Fig. 15.8). These axial deviations due to stem loosening are not uncommon. In studies by MacDonald et al. [3], 31.1% of revision surgeries involved an axial deviation of the femur that had to be corrected by osteotomy; in a study by Paprosky and Martin [4], the incidence was 30%, and in our own study 37% [5]. The flap for the transfemoral approach extends to the apex of the deformity, where the correction of the axis must then be performed. If there is a severe axial deviation, a double osteotomy is recommended for correction of the femur axis (see below).

15.1.6 Periprosthetic Fracture of the Femur (Vancouver B2 or B3 Type)

A periprosthetic fracture at the level of the stem in conjunction with prosthesis loosening (type Vancouver B2 or B3) requires a stem revision (Fig. 15.9a–c). The fixation of the new stem must be below the fracture; i.e., the stem with its fixation zone must bridge the fracture. This can only be reliably carried out by flapping back the proximal fracture fragment after an osteotomy. This provides direct access to the distal fixation bed and allows the fixation zone to be prepared under visual control. The path of the fracture determines the distal end of the flap. Without osteotomy, i.e., without transfemoral access, there is a risk that the new stem will have its fixation zone in the area of the fracture, which would lead to subsidence or early loosening of the new stem.

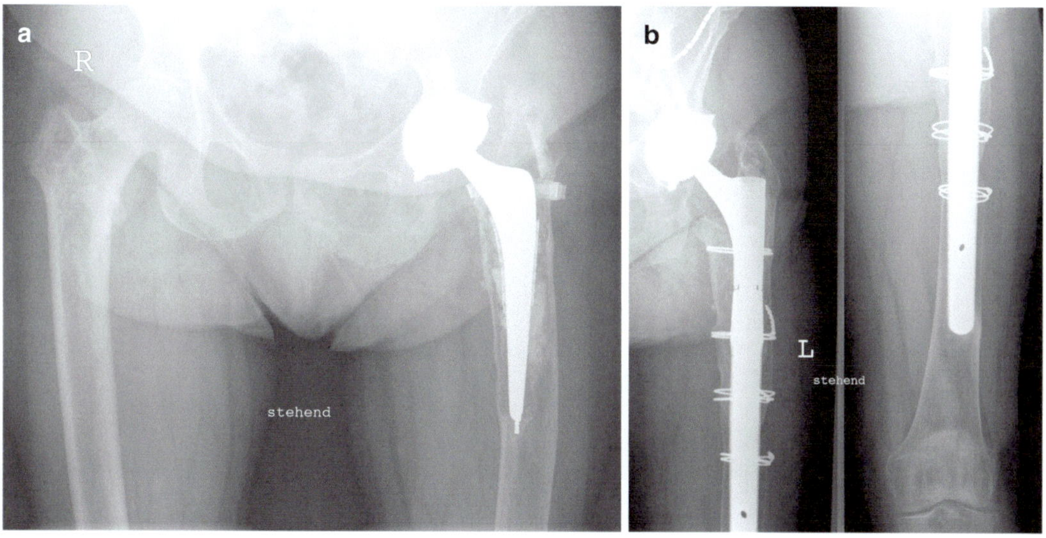

Fig. 15.7 (**a**) Prosthesis loosening with a varus deviation of the loosened stem and femur 6 years after stem revision with impaction grafting. (**b**) Radiograph 6 months after transfemoral prosthesis revision with axial correction of the femur using the modular revision stem Revitan Curved (Zimmer Biomet, Winterthur, Switzerland)

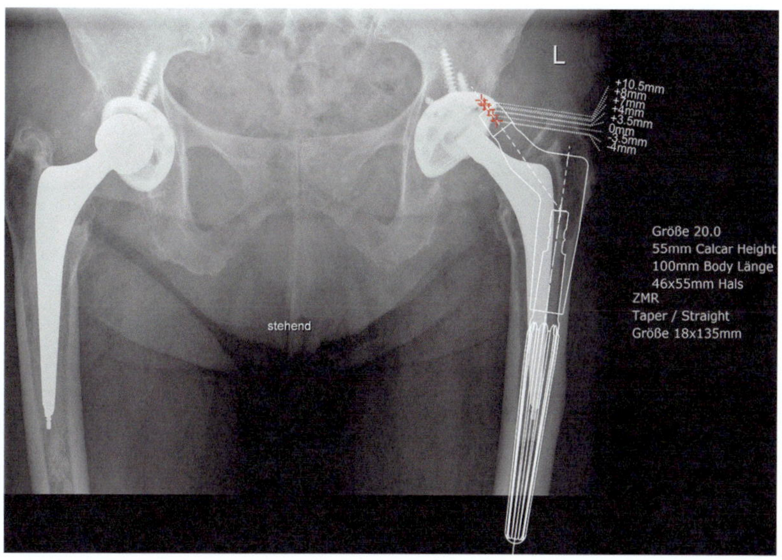

Fig. 15.8 Preoperative planning of a left stem revision to a modular revision stem ZMR (Zimmer Biomet, Warsaw, IN, USA). The planning shows the proximal component inside and partially outside the greater trochanter, indicating the need for axial correction of the femur via a transfemoral approach

15.1.7 Periprosthetic Infection with Firmly Seated Implant or Cement or Hard-to-Reach Osteolyses

In the case of late periprosthetic infections (more than 4–6 weeks after implantation), the bacteria have been able to form a biofilm on the implant, which can no longer be penetrated adequately by the immune defenses and antibiotics [6]. Therefore, all foreign materials (implants and cement) must be removed and the infected prosthesis bed debrided. The challenge here is to perform this adequately and radically without unnecessarily traumatizing major muscles and (especially the gluteus medius muscle and vasto-

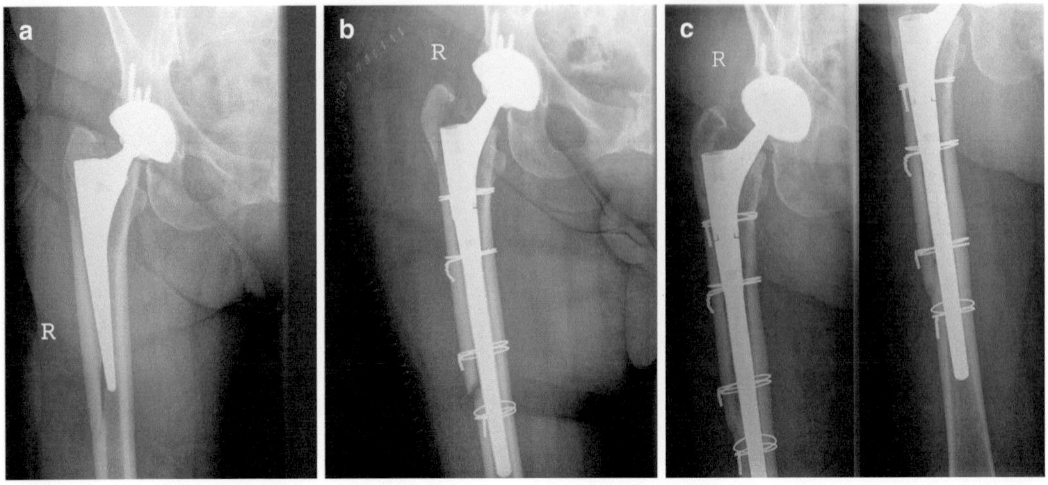

Fig. 15.9 (**a**) Periprosthetic fracture of the Vancouver B2 type with additional fracture of the greater trochanter. (**b**) Radiograph 7 days postoperative after transfemoral stem revision. (**c**) Radiograph 3 months postoperative with healed fractures and osteotomy

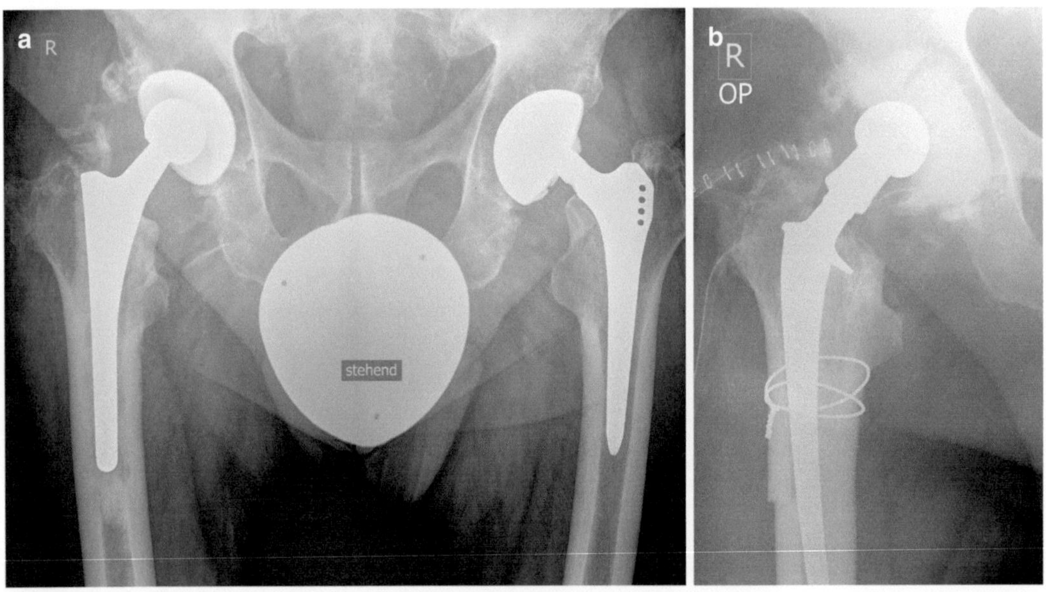

Fig. 15.10 (**a**) Periprosthetic infection of a right total hip arthroplasty with osteolysis in the medial region of the stem. (**b**) Postoperative radiograph after removal of the infected prosthesis via a transfemoral approach and insertion of an interim prosthesis and temporary closure of the flap with double cerclages

gluteal sling) and bone. Especially, the complete debridement of the osteolyses is very difficult endofemorally. The transfemoral approach helps to remove firmly seated implants and cement and to debride osteolyses in the stem region (Fig. 15.10a). After removal of all foreign material, if a spacer is used the flap must be bridged by this spacer over a sufficiently long distance. To do this, after creation of a cup spacer, we introduce double cerclages with the flap open and a longer cemented prosthesis stem is coated with antibiotic-containing bone cement (6 min after mixing the cement). This construct is then inserted into the distal femur and the flap closed by tightening the double cerclages. Any excess cement is removed, and the cement is allowed to harden (Fig. 15.10b). The delayed application of the cement serves to facilitate removal when a new prosthesis is installed, which we do 6 weeks after the first stage. The prosthesis stem can be smeared with blood before coating with cement, which impairs the bond of the prosthesis stem with the cement and thus facilitates removal during the second step of the two-stage septic prosthesis revision. In the second step of the two-stage septic replacement, we reopen the transfemoral access after removal of the double cerclages, perform a new debridement and lavage with an antiseptic solution (e.g., Ocinesept (Schülke & Mayr GmbH, Norderstedt, Germany) or LavaSurge (B.Braun Melsungen, Germany)), and implant the new cementless revision stem while the flap is raised. If a modular revision stem is used, it is assembled in situ and then the flap is closed again with double cerclages. Postoperatively, systemic antibiotics are administered again for 6 weeks (2 weeks intravenously and 4 weeks orally). The implantation of a cemented stem prosthesis is not advisable in my opinion, since on the one hand cement can penetrate into the osteotomy areas and compromise the secure bony consolidation of the flap, and on the other hand, the quality of the cementation is impaired following osteotomy.

15.1.8 Cup Protruding into the Lesser Pelvis

If a cup is loosened and has protruded into the pelvis, the muscle tension of the gluteal muscles must be neutralized in order to remove it in a controlled manner (Fig. 15.11a, b). This can be done by means of a trans-trochanteric approach, the so-called trochanteric slide, or by a transfemoral approach. This osteotomy prior to hip dislocation can avoid the risk of acetabular or even pelvic fracture, but also trochanteric fracture during the dislocation process [7]. The extended osteotomy in the transfemoral approach has the advantage of better healing of the osteotomy compared to the trans-trochanteric approach and the trochanteric slide. In addition, the risk of trochanteric dislocation is lower compared to the trans-trochanteric approach because the vastus lateralis muscle remains on the bony flap to counteract the traction of the gluteal muscle. However, the transfemoral approach then also requires the replacement of the stem (Fig. 15.11b). The trochanteric slide is recommended if a distally stable prosthetic stem is to be left in place (see Chap. 12).

Advantages of transfemoral access:

The advantages of transfemoral access for the listed indications as compared to alternative techniques are [8]:

- The predictably better healing of the flap when compared to the trans-trochanteric approach and the trochanteric slide.
- The lower risk of trochanteric dislocation due to the preservation of the vasto-gluteal sling and the retention of the vastus lateralis muscle on the flap as a counterpart to the muscle force of the gluteus medius muscle that would dislocate the greater trochanter when compared to the traditional trans-trochanteric approach and the extended ventral approaches.
- Minimizing the risk of unintentional fractures and perforation when compared to the endofemoral approach.
- Direct access to the distal femur for removal of the distal cement and controlled preparation of the fixation bed for the distally fixed revision stem under visual control.
- The ability to adjust the tension of the abductor muscles by moving the flap during closure.
- The reduction in the operating time for difficult implant removal.
- Bone regeneration by means of a controlled, elongated femoral osteotomy in which callus formation occurs via the hematoma of the fracture. This leads to the formation of new bone and growth of bone on the newly implanted cementless revision prosthesis with osteointegration of the same. This results in additional proximal prosthesis fixation.

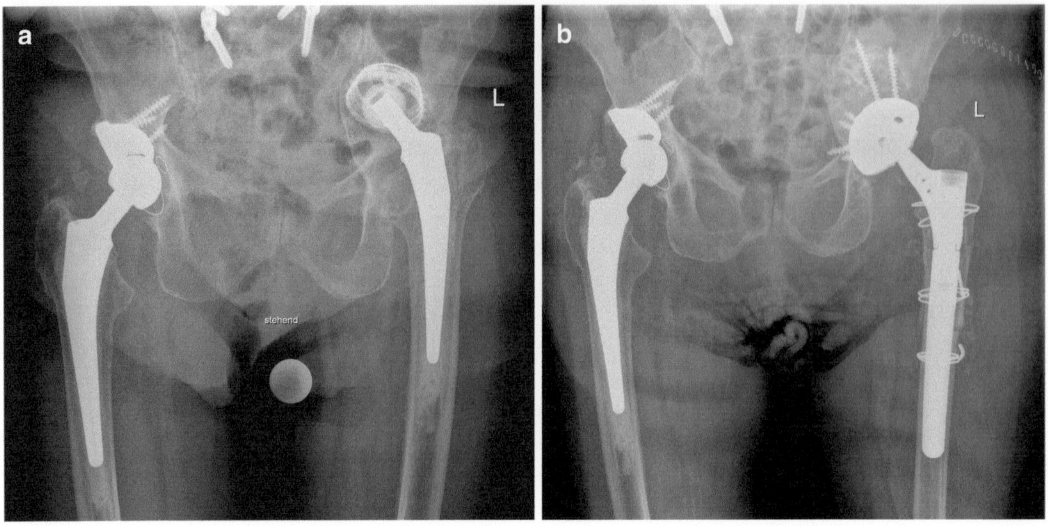

Fig. 15.11 (**a**) Loose cup migrated into the lesser pelvis in a Paprosky IIIB type cup defect. (**b**) Postoperative radiograph with cup exchange via a transfemoral approach to get access to the migrated cup with prevention of unintentional fractures. Therefore, stem exchange to a distally fixed revision stem was also necessary

Meek et al. [9] reported unintentional trochanteric fracture in 30% of a large series of revision surgeries when a transfemoral approach (extended trochanteric osteotomy; ETO) was not performed. Park et al. [10] compared 30 stem revisions without and 32 with transfemoral access (ETO) to a distally fixed modular straight revision stem and found a significantly higher incidence of stem subsidence of more than 5 mm and of femoral perforations in the group without transfemoral access. In addition, McInnis et al. [11] observed 55% subsidence and 24% intraoperative femoral fracture/perforation in 70 stem revisions to a modular, distally fixed straight revision stem, where all but 2 patients were endofemorally implanted.

15.2 Transfemoral Access Technique

In the transfemoral approach, the aim is to osteotomize a bony flap with as little trauma as possible according to the preoperative planning. In principle, several techniques are possible, all of which must be evaluated in terms of reproducibility in achieving the goals. These goals are as follows:

- Variability in the size of the flap (long flaps for the revision of long revision stems must also be possible).
- Minimal traumatization of the muscles on the flap (musculus vastus lateralis), which is important for the vascularity of the flap and thus ensures subsequent bony healing of the flap.
- Integrity of the vasto-gluteal sling (the complex of the M. gluteus medius and musculus vastus lateralis), which is important for the function of the hip joint. In particular, it helps to minimize the risk of unintentional proximalization of the greater trochanter in fractures of the bony flap.
- Good opportunity to manage potential complications with this approach.
- Reproducibly good results in terms of bony consolidation of the flap and clinical outcomes.

These aims make the vastus slide, which transects the vasto-gluteal sling from ventral to dorsal, less suitable. If the flap is fractured during surgery, e.g., due to osteolysis, there is a risk of unintentional trochanter major proximalization with negative consequences for function (Trendelenburg gait).

Working directly through the vastus lateralis muscle, which is necessary when operating on the patient in a supine position, leads to compromise and traumatization of the muscles attached to the flap. This alters the blood supply to the flap and endangers the ability of the bone flap to heal properly. Thus, MacDonald et al. [3] found a high risk of unintentional trochanteric dislocation of 9%, a need for further surgery of 11%, and only an 89% healing rate of the flap in 45 prosthesis revisions with this approach.

The transfemoral access can be performed from the ventral side, in which case the femur is approached ventrally of the gluteus medius and vastus lateralis muscles, and the flap is then folded dorsally with the musculature lying on top. However, this technique is limited with respect to the length of the flap, so that usually a maximum of only 12 cm is possible. Extension distally entails a high risk of injury to the vessels crossing the flap. Pretterklieber et al. [12] showed in an anatomical study that the perforating vessels coming from the femoral artery could be injured unintentionally and that there is no safe zone 14–36.5 cm from the anterior superior iliac spine to the distal medial side, which would correspond to about 9–30 cm from the greater trochanter.

From all these considerations, the extended posterolateral approach has the advantage of reproducibly achieving all of the above objectives and is therefore the most commonly used approach for transfemoral access and was first described by Heinz Wagner [13–16]. We have modified this technique to improve the ventral osteotomy and to make the healing rate of the flap more reproducible [5, 17]. Warren et al. [18] found that closure of the flap with wires had a significantly better healing rate than suturing the flap as described by Wagner [13–16].

In the following, our technique is described and technical variants of the transfemoral approach are discussed [17] (Figs. 15.12, 15.13, 15.14, 15.15, 15.16, 15.17, 15.18, 15.19, 15.20, 15.21, 15.22, 15.23, and 15.24, Fig. 15.25 for Video 15.1).

The patient is placed in a lateral position. Supports dorsal to the thorax and ventral to the upper pelvis help to stabilize the patient in this position (Fig. 15.12). A vacuum support cushion can also be used. After sterile washing and covering of the surgical site, a posterolateral approach extended distally is performed. Depending on the length of the planned flap, a skin incision approx. 25–40 cm long is first extended to the tuberculum innominatum of the greater trochanter, which can be palpated under the skin, and then extended dorsally at 45° in the same direction as the fibers of the gluteus maximus muscle (Fig. 15.12). The subcutaneous tissue is transected down to the fascia lata, which is also transected in the same direction as the skin incision, and the fibers of the musculus gluteus maximus are bluntly separated (Fig. 15.13). The external rotators are detached close to the insertion point and secured as necessary (Fig. 15.14). The sciatic nerve can be palpated. Since it can be distorted by scarring during revision surgery, only wide, blunt retractors (e.g., box hooks) should be used here. I do not recommend the insertion of pointed Hohmann hooks or even hammering a nail into the ischium, in order not to endanger the ischial nerve. The neocapsule is exposed and opened. At least in the first case of a posterior approach (where the primary implantation was performed via a different approach), the capsule can be opened in a T-shape and cap-

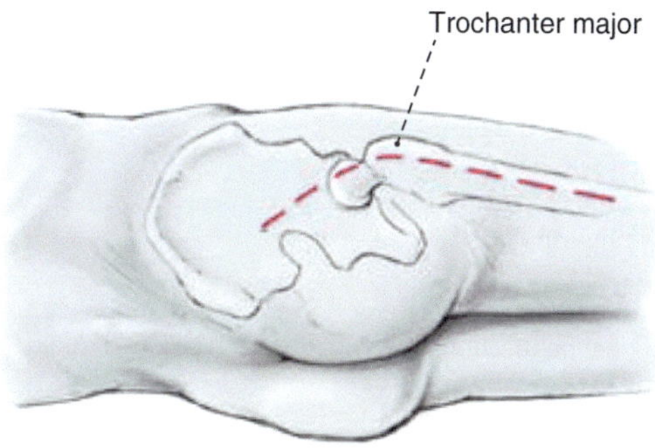

Fig. 15.12 Lateral position. Approx. 30–40 cm long incision; it begins as a posterolateral approach in the direction of the fibers of the gluteus maximus muscle, extends to the greater trochanter, and runs distally approx. 20–30 cm lengthwise along the thigh (with permission of the original publication: Fink B, Grossmann A. Modified transfemoral approach to revision arthroplasty with uncemented modular revision stems. Oper Orthop Traumatol. 2007;19:32–55)

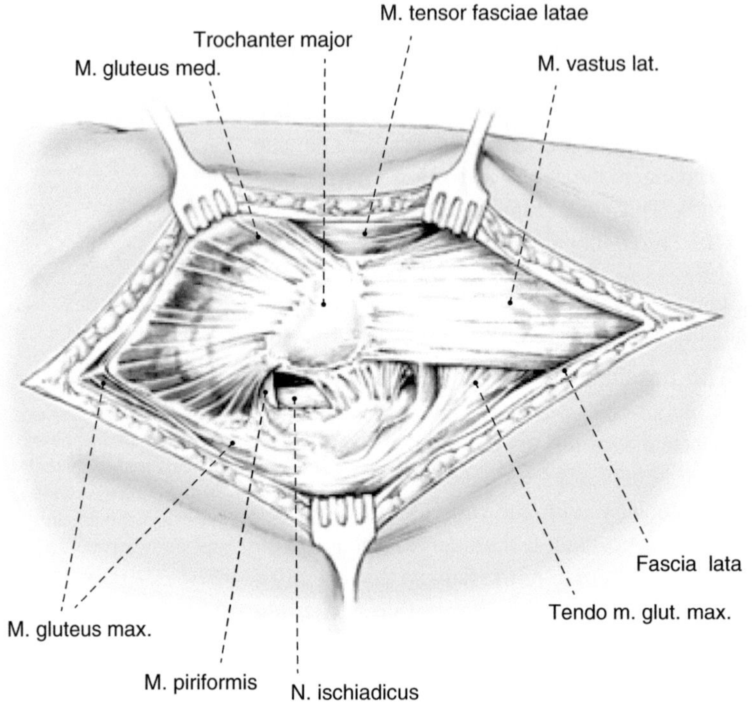

Fig. 15.13 Dissection of the subcutaneous tissue and the fascia lata in the same direction. Blunt separation of the musculus gluteus maximus in fiber direction (with permission of the original publication: Fink B, Grossmann A. Modified transfemoral approach to revision arthroplasty with uncemented modular revision stems. Oper Orthop Traumatol. 2007;19:32–55)

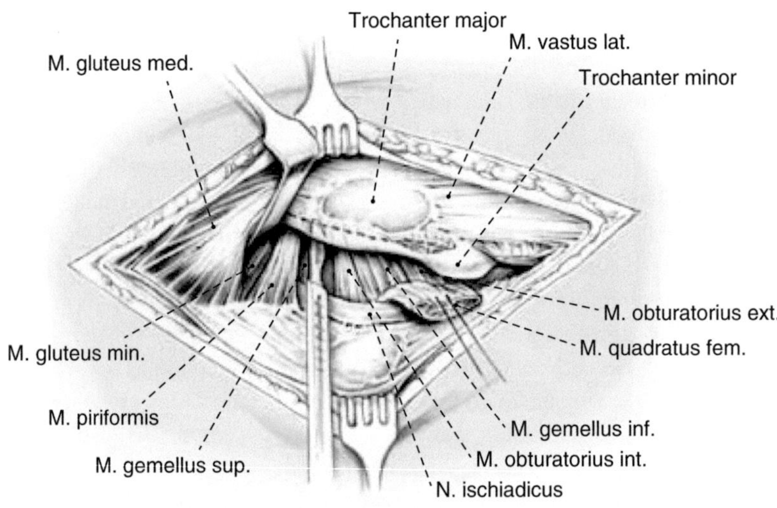

Fig. 15.14 Separation close to the bone and securing the stumps of the external rotators. Identification and protection of the sciatic nerve (with permission of the original publication: Fink B, Grossmann A. Modified transfemoral approach to revision arthroplasty with uncemented modular revision stems. Oper Orthop Traumatol. 2007;19:32–55)

sule flaps prepared (Fig. 15.15). This is also advantageous for revision surgery. After implantation of the new prosthesis, the capsule flaps can then be used as a capsuloplasty to augment the reinsertion of the external rotators. This significantly reduces the risk of dorsal dislocation [19–21]. Goldstein et al. [19], Pellicci et al. [20], and White et al. [21] each showed a significant reduction in the dislocation rate from 3 to 6% without capsuloplasty to less than 1% with capsuloplasty.

The approach is now extended into the intermuscular lateral septum down to the linea aspera of the femur. It is advantageous to do this with an electric knife, since the muscle fibers can be separated more easily from the septum. Proximally, the insertion of the musculus gluteus maximus at the femur is partially incised but only until access to the femur is enabled (Fig. 15.16a, b). If this procedure is carried out carefully and step by step, the branches of the perforating vessels can be located and ligated before they are severed. This reduces blood loss during the operation. Now the end of the flap is prepared. After locating the tip of the greater trochanter, the lower end of the flap is marked using a rule according to the preoperative implant planning. At this point, the lateral half-circumference of the femur is exposed transversely from the vastus lateralis muscle. A 3.2-mm hole is drilled at the lower boundary of the bony flap at each of its dorsal and ventral ends on the femoral circumference, while cooling with Ringer's solution (Fig. 15.16a, b).

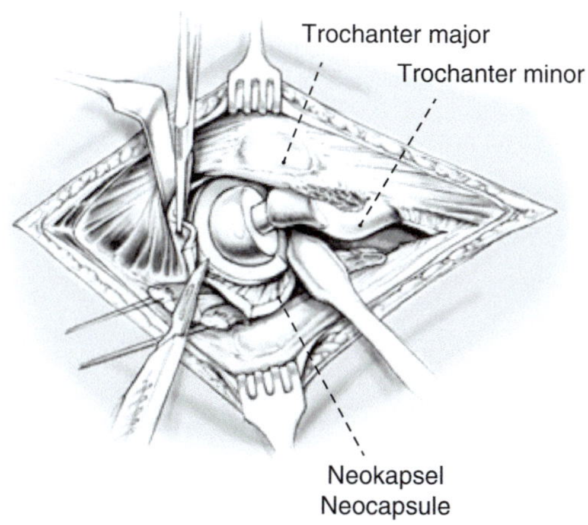

Fig. 15.15 T-shaped opening of the so-called neocapsule and scar tissue to expose the joint (with permission of the original publication: Fink B, Grossmann A. Modified transfemoral approach to revision arthroplasty with uncemented modular revision stems. Oper Orthop Traumatol. 2007;19:32–55)

Next, the ventral proximal osteotomy of the femur is performed (Fig. 15.17a, b). The leg is rotated externally for this. A sterile cushion can be placed under the knee. A small longitudinal incision is made at the ventral vasto-gluteal transition (ventral region of the greater trochanter), opening the interstitium between the musculus gluteus medius and the musculus vastus lateralis. A large osteotomy chisel is inserted here and the ventral proximal osteotomy is executed, whereby the chisel is guided proximally by inclining it slightly in order to completely osteotomize the trochanter region in a proximal direction. It can also be tilted slightly distally to extend the osteotomy a little distally from here.

In the next step, the dorsal osteotomy of the bony flap is carried out with an oscillating saw along the labium externum of the linea aspera while cooling with Ringer's solution (Fig. 15.18a, b). We use a wide saw blade with a thickness of only 0.7 mm to minimize bone loss when creating the bony flap. The osteotomy is initiated at the distal, dorsal drill hole, is advanced from distal to proximal, and ends in a proximal arc to dorsal (Fig. 15.18a). This makes it possible to have the complete greater trochanter with the gluteus medius and minimus muscles attached to the flap.

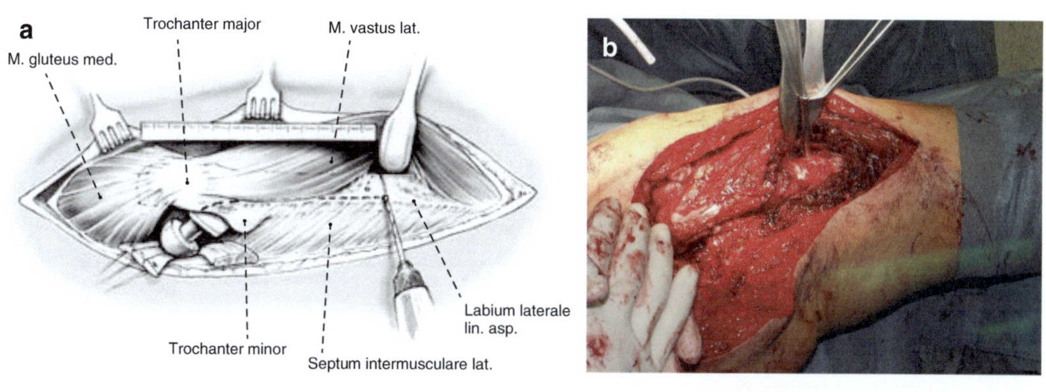

Fig. 15.16 (**a** (drawing) and **b** (photo)) Representation of the femur ventral to the lateral lip of the linea aspera with the lateral intermuscular septum; the perforator vessels are ligated. Representation of the lateral circumference of the femur and drilling of the 3.2-mm-diameter holes at the dorsal and ventral distal ends of the planned bony flap (with permission of the original publication: Fink B, Grossmann A. Modified transfemoral approach to revision arthroplasty with uncemented modular revision stems. Oper Orthop Traumatol. 2007;19:32–55)

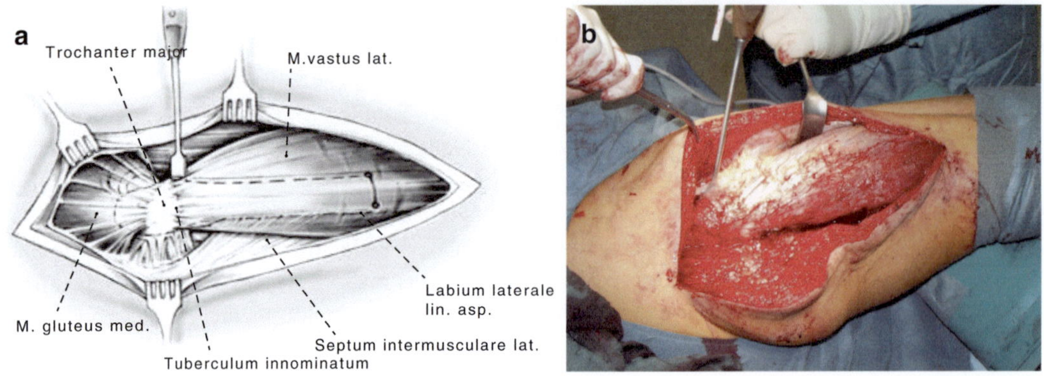

Fig. 15.17 (**a** (drawing) and **b** (photo)) Osteotomy of the femur with a wide osteotomy chisel ventrally proximal at the transition of the vastus lateralis muscle to the gluteus medius muscle with the leg rotated externally (with permission of the original publication: Fink B, Grossmann A. Modified transfemoral approach to revision arthroplasty with uncemented modular revision stems. Oper Orthop Traumatol. 2007;19:32–55)

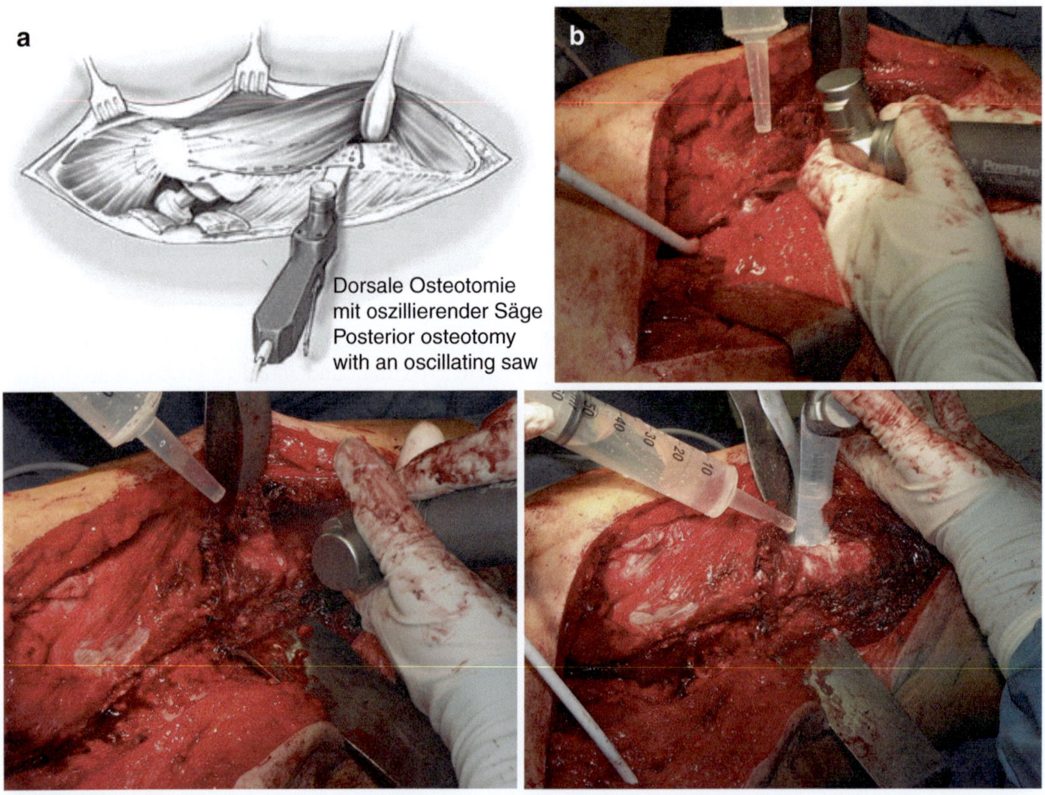

Fig. 15.18–15.20 (**a** (drawing) and **b** (photo)) Dorsal osteotomy ventral to the lateral lip of the linea aspera; transverse osteotomy between the two drill holes with the leg rotated internally; ventral distal osteotomy of approx. 3 cm using an oscillating saw while cooling with sterile Ringer's solution with the leg rotated externally (with permission of the original publication: Fink B, Grossmann A. Modified transfemoral approach to revision arthroplasty with uncemented modular revision stems. Oper Orthop Traumatol. 2007;19:32–55)

In addition, a flap that is too narrow proximally could lead to the distally fixed revision stem that will be inserted later being hindered by contact with the proximal femur bone during its distal anchorage in the isthmus of the femur.

The two distal drill holes are now connected with the oscillating saw under cooling, thus completing the distal transverse osteotomy (Fig. 15.19). The ventral distal osteotomy is then initiated from the distal ventral drill hole with the oscillating saw. Here, just the lead-in for the ventral osteotomy is created with the oscillating saw (again under cooling) (Fig. 15.20). For these steps, it is again recommended to rotate the leg externally by supporting the knee joint with, for example, a sterile pad.

The ventral osteotomy is then completed from the distal side using a narrow osteotomy chisel, which is guided under the vastus lateralis muscle (Fig. 15.21a, b). It is usually sufficient to chisel a few centimeters from distal to proximal. Then, the flap usually breaks automatically as far as the proximal ventral osteotomy created earlier. Now the bony flap is carefully opened from the side using a chisel (Fig. 15.22). During the osteotomy, it is of the utmost importance for the blood supply to the bony flap that the attachment of the vastus lateralis muscle to the flap remains intact.

The old prosthesis and, if necessary, the cement can now be removed completely without difficulty (Fig. 15.23). Direct access to the isthmus of the femur is also possible, so that cement

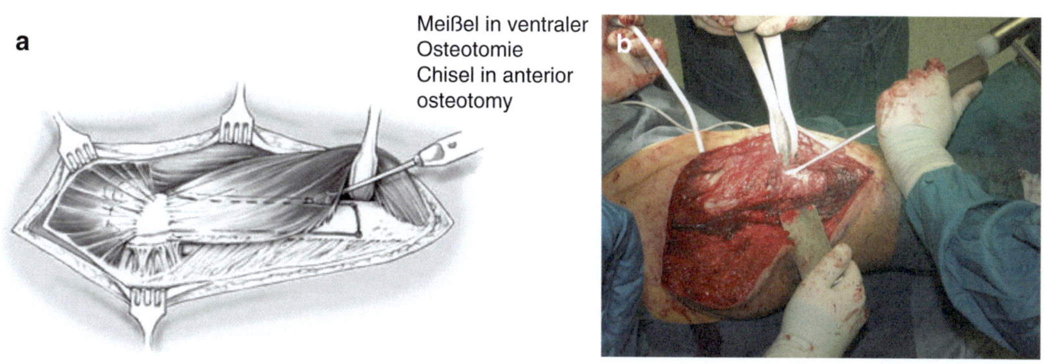

Fig. 15.21 (**a** (drawing) and **b** (photo)) Completion of the ventral osteotomy using a chisel guided from the distal under the vastus lateralis muscle to the proximal side with the leg rotated externally. The attachment of the vastus lateralis muscle to the bony flap remains intact (with permission of the original publication: Fink B, Grossmann A. Modified transfemoral approach to revision arthroplasty with uncemented modular revision stems. Oper Orthop Traumatol. 2007;19:32–55)

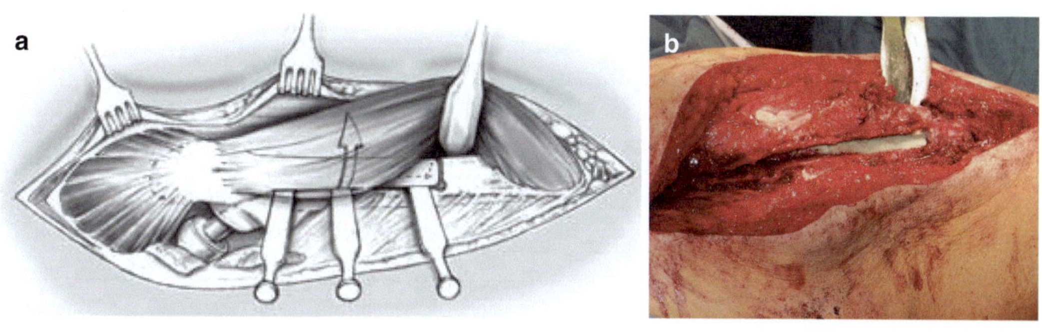

Fig. 15.22 (**a** (drawing) and **b** (photo)) Lifting the osteotomized lateral femoral flap with the vastus lateralis muscle attached medially (with permission of the original publication: Fink B, Grossmann A. Modified transfemoral approach to revision arthroplasty with uncemented modular revision stems. Oper Orthop Traumatol. 2007;19:32–55)

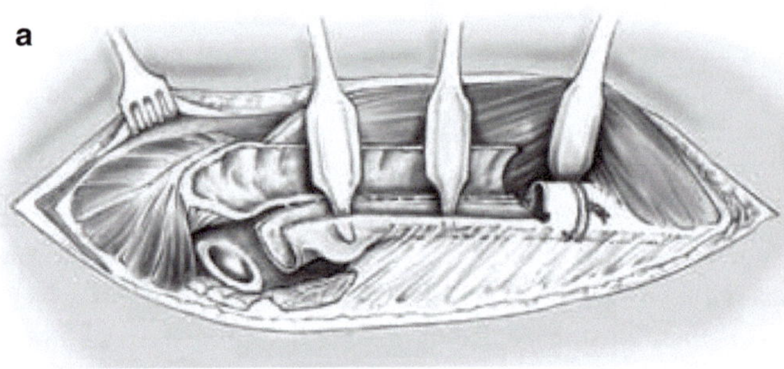

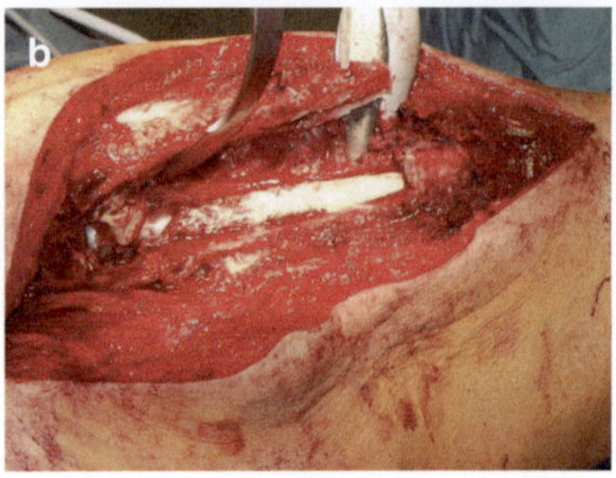

Fig. 15.23 (**a** (drawing) and **b** (photo)) Prosthesis and bone cement are completely removed (with permission of the original publication: Fink B, Grossmann A. Modified transfemoral approach to revision arthroplasty with uncemented modular revision stems. Oper Orthop Traumatol. 2007;19:32–55)

still in the isthmus distal to the flap can be removed directly under visual control (by drilling and chiseling) without risk of perforation.

This access provides a good view of the acetabulum and/or the prosthetic cup, which can now be revised if necessary (Fig. 15.24). Before reaming, milling, or rasping the intact distal femur, we recommend applying a prophylactic double cerclage with a 1.5-mm cerclage wire (passed twice around the femur) or cerclage cable immediately distal to the bony flap. This is intended to prevent the formation of fissures or fractures during reaming, rasping, or when the final implant is inserted, or to prevent the further propagation of a fissure if one occurs. In their series of studies, Miner et al. [22] reported such fissures at a rate of 10.8%.

After implantation of the final stem, the bony flap is closed and usually fixed with two to three double cerclages (1.5-mm cerclage wire) or cerclage cable (Figs. 15.26 and 15.27a, b, Fig. 15.28 for Video 15.2). In a biomechanical study, Wagner et al. [23] demonstrated that double cerclages with a 1.5-mm-thick wire were the most stable of the various cerclage techniques available. Therefore, we prefer to use two double cerclages. One double cerclage is placed at the end of the flap and a second proximal one in the region of the lesser trochanter. The latter can be guided with one turn above and one turn below the lesser trochanter. In a cadaver study, Schab et al. [24] found no difference between 2 and 3 cerclage cables in the closure of the osteotomy with respect to the strength and the axial and rotational displacement of the flap. Zhu et al. [25] came to the same conclusion in a biomechanical study. The cerclage or cable instrumentation should be deployed close to the bone in order to avoid damage to the musculature and vessel nerve structures.

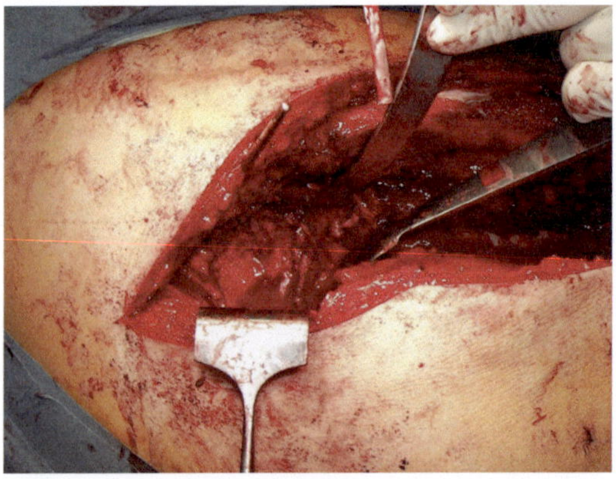

Fig. 15.24 Fit of the prosthetic cup is checked, and an inlay or cup exchange is performed

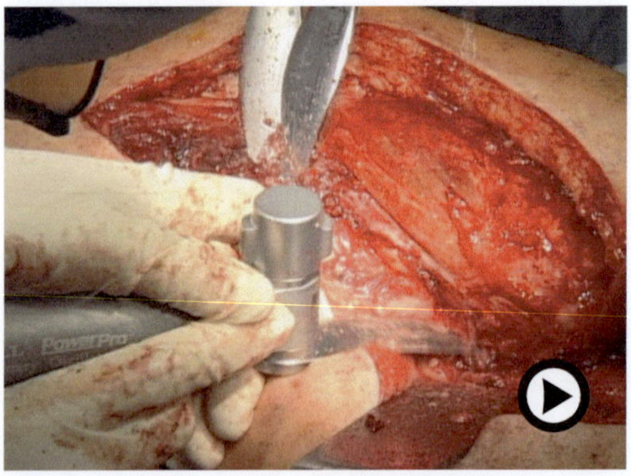

Fig. 15.25 (Video 15.1) Performing the transfemoral approach (with permission of Zimmer Biomet, Winterthur, Switzerland) (▶ https://doi.org/10.1007/000-4pr)

In our experience, cerclage tapes (bands) are less suitable because they do not allow sufficient tension to be applied and because their insertion is more traumatic for the soft tissues. This, together with their large surface area, compromises the blood supply to the femur and the bony flap. The technique of fixing the flap with sutures alone, as described by Heinz Wagner for the original Wagner SL stem (with a CCD angle of 145°), is not recommendable in my opinion. Due to the higher soft tissue tension in modern revision stems with higher offset, there would be a high level of instability of the flap if it were not firmly fixed. Warren et al. [18] were able to show in a comparative study that the healing rate of the flap is significantly higher when the flap is closed with cerclages compared to a suture-only approach. Warren et al. [18] and Wilkes et al. [26] also believe that cerclage-based fixation of the bony flap helps to reduce the risk of stem subsidence in compromised isthmus bone conditions.

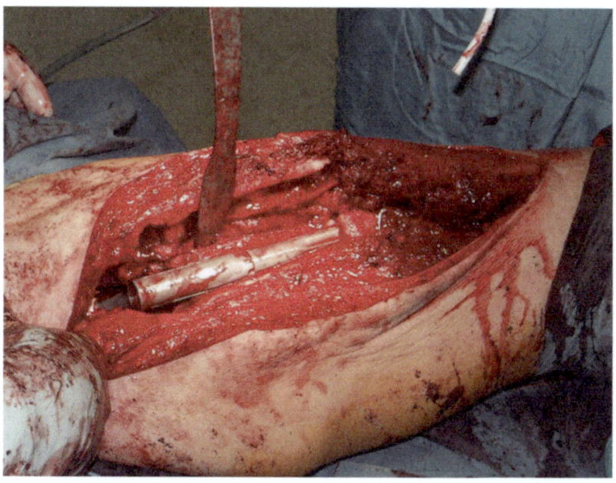

Fig. 15.26 Implantation of the modular revision stem

Although claw plates have shown greater stability in trochanteric fracture fixation, they should only be used in exceptional cases for closure of the bony flap due to the significantly higher incidence of pain in the trochanteric region (17% compared to 3% for cables in a review by Mei et al. [27]).

It is not always possible to close the bony flap with a tight fit, so that sometimes a gap may remain both at the end of the flap (if the flap is proximalized due to gluteal muscle traction) and at the posterior edge of the flap. This can be tolerated, and no attempt should be made to improve the fit by reducing the thickness of the flap internally. Milling debris obtained during preparation of the fixation bed of the new stem can be inserted into these gaps as a bone graft. These gaps will be closed during the first few months after surgery due to the fracture hematoma and the callus formation. To achieve better closure of the osteotomy flap, we use a curved revision stem, since this corresponds to the anatomical profile of the femur and there is not any proximal lateralization of the flap, which can arise from using a straight stem.

After closure of the bony flap, the vastus lateralis muscle is sutured at its insertion point, and then after placement of a Redon drain, the outer rotators are sutured with a capsuloplasty if pos-

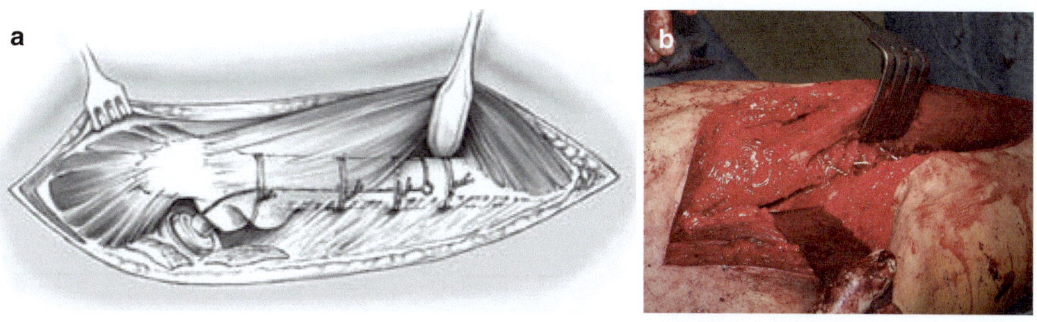

Fig. 15.27 (**a** (drawing) and **b** (photo)) Closure and fixation of the bony with two double cerclages (1.5-mm-thick cerclage wires). Alternatively, cerclage cables can be used (with permission of the original publication: Fink B, Grossmann A. Modified transfemoral approach to revision arthroplasty with uncemented modular revision stems. Oper Orthop Traumatol. 2007;19:32–55)

sible, followed by fascial suturing and further layer-by-layer wound closure. The Redon drain should be connected to a "cell saver" for a typical period of 6 h with low suction (20 mmHg).

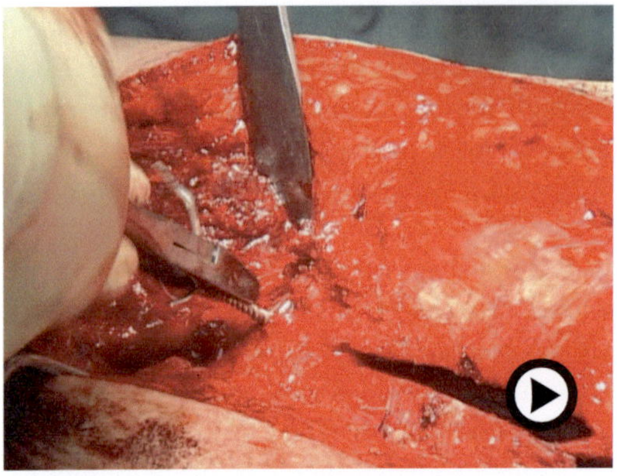

Fig. 15.28 (Video 15.2) Folding back the flap and closing the transfemoral approach with double cerclages (with permission of Zimmer Biomet, Winterthur, Switzerland) (▶ https://doi.org/10.1007/000-4pq)

15.3 Variations

15.3.1 Double Osteotomy

If there is a marked curvature of the femoral axis in the frontal and/or sagittal plane, an additional medial osteotomy is recommended to improve the contact between bone and implant. The medial transverse osteotomy should be above the distal end of the lateral bony flap to provide better stability of the bone fragments. This creates a kind of "zig-zag double osteotomy." The necessity for a double osteotomy becomes apparent firstly during preoperative planning and secondly when there is a considerable distance between the medial femur and the inserted trial stem or the distal reamer or rasp (Fig. 15.29a, b). Prior to implantation of the final distal component, the medial transverse osteotomy is created by drilling and subsequent careful chiseling of the

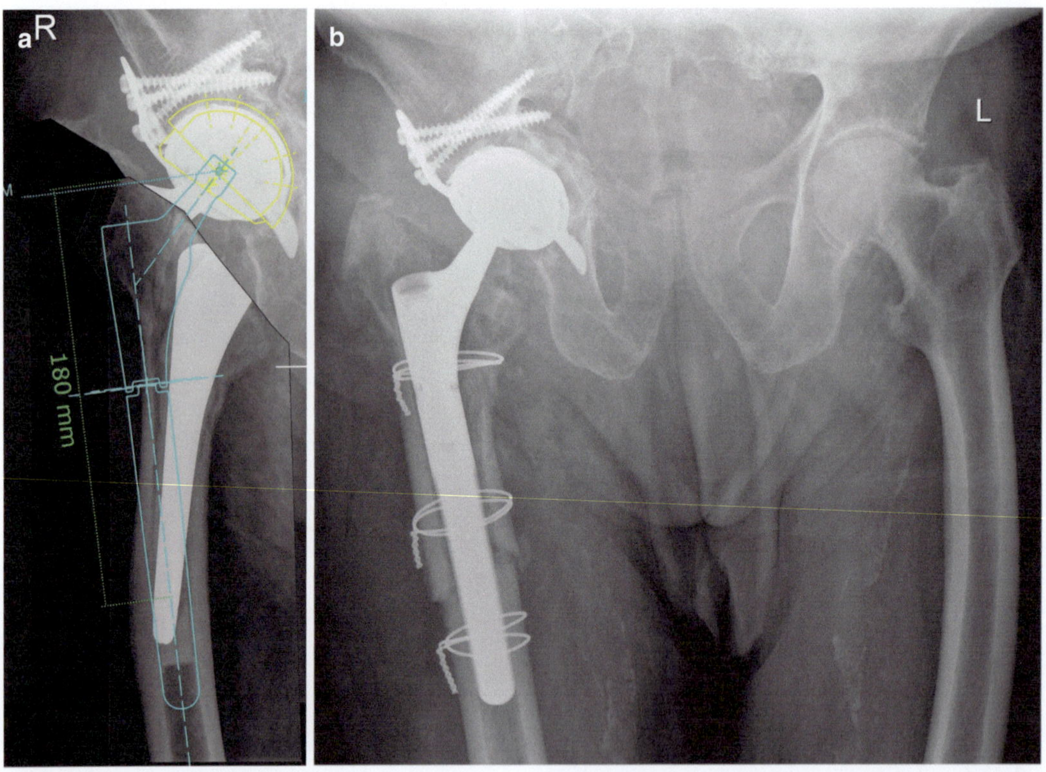

Fig. 15.29 (**a**) Preoperative planning shows a significant axial deviation of the femur, which requires a double osteotomy to avoid unintentional fractures and to improve contact of the prosthesis to the medial femur. (**b**) Completed double osteotomy with contact of the prosthetic stem to the medial bone, also protecting the joint between the modular components (junction)

medial femur. The use of cerclages or cable systems for the closure of the bony flaps additionally increases the stability and contact of the bone fragments with the implant (Fig. 15.30a–c). Secondary displacement of the bone fragments due to muscle traction of the gluteus medius muscle and the iliopsoas muscle is avoided. This promotes bony integration of the prosthetic stem and protects the junction of the modular components from failure due to fatigue that is a recognized mechanical weakness of modular revision stems.

15.3.2 Osteotomy Through the Femur After Prior Removal of the Implanted Stem

The medial osteotomy of the bony flap can also be performed through the femur by lateral sawing after removal of the stem. For this, however, it must be ensured that the stem can be removed without risk of unintentional fracture before the transfemoral access is opened up. This is usually the case with polished cemented stems, which can be removed out of the cement mantle without any problems. Even loosened cementless stems can be removed first, and then, the medial osteotomy can be performed through the femur. In this case, the transfemoral approach and the osteotomy are not intended to facilitate the removal of the inserted stem, but rather to correct any axial deviations of the femur and, if necessary, to remove cement.

15.3.3 Extended Trochanteric Osteotomy

The extended trochanteric osteotomy is basically identical to the transfemoral approach. The difference between the extended trochanteric osteotomy and the transfemoral approach lies in the width and length of the flap. In the case of an extended trochanteric osteotomy, a flap is created in 1/3 of the stem circumference with an average length of 12.6–14.2 cm, depending on the respective study, and widths between 7 and 19 cm [22, 28–34]. The main aim of an extended trochanteric osteotomy is to make it easier to remove the inserted stem. In the transfemoral approach, the

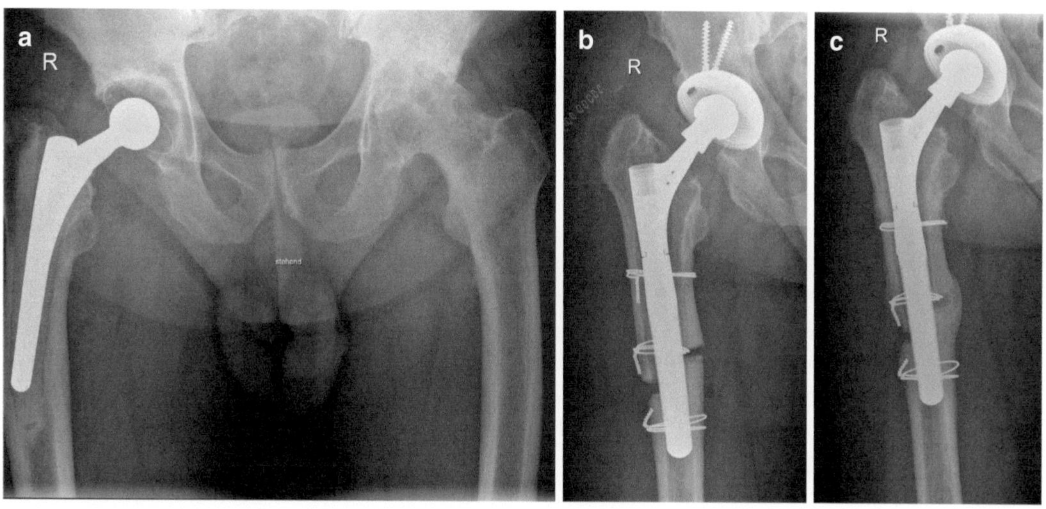

Fig. 15.30 (**a**) Stem loosening with varus deviation of the prosthetic stem and the femur requiring a double osteotomy for axial correction and adaptation of the medial femur to the proximal prosthetic component, also to protect the junction of the modular prosthetic stem. (**b**) Radiograph 7 days after transfemoral prosthesis revision with the modular revision stem Revitan Curved and Allofit-S press-fit cup (Zimmer Biomet, Winterthur, Switzerland) and double osteotomy of the femur. **c:** Radiograph 3 months after surgery showing a bony consolidation of the medial osteotomy

flap is more extensive and its width covers half of the circumference of the stem. Distally, the osteotomy is extended to immediately above the fixation bed of the new prosthesis or to the apex of the deformity [13–16]. In addition to improving access, the transfemoral approach is used for correction osteotomy of proximal femoral axial deviations and, above all, for direct, straight access to the fixation bed of a distally anchored cementless revision stem. In our own study, the length of the flap of the transfemoral approach averaged 17.4 ± 7.8 cm and ranged from 12.3 to 27.8 cm [5]. It is therefore the preferred choice for cementless revision stems with distal diaphyseal fixation.

15.4 Complications

When the bony flap is lifted, osteolysis of the flap area may cause fractures of the flap itself. Since the fragments are connected to the soft tissue of the lateral vastus muscles, only an additional double cerclage is required to hold the fragments together when closing the flap (Fig. 15.31a–c). An intraoperative trochanteric avulsion or fracture can also be stabilized with a transosseous fiber wire cerclage, which is guided through the most cranially located double cerclage (Fig. 15.32a, b). Since the vasto-gluteal sling is retained in the transfemoral approach and the traction forces of the gluteal muscles are neutralized by those of the vastus lateralis muscle, there is no risk of dislocation of the greater trochanter. Postoperative trochanteric avulsions occur rarely and when they occur then below the tubercle innominatum. As a rule, they do not lead to a significant dislocation, are usually stable, and heal with bony remodeling. For this purpose, a prolonged partial weight bearing of 10 kg should be implemented (Fig. 21.2a, b).

The closure of the flap can be difficult, especially with straight revision stems. We generally prefer to close the flap with cerclages or cables. In our opinion, simply suturing the flap by closing the intermuscular septum, as originally described by Wagner and Wagner [16], leads to a less stable closure with the consequent possibility of dislocation of the flap. We also prefer a curved revision stem for transfemoral access because the flap is easier to close.

15.5 Outcomes

In a separate study, 68 hip prosthesis revisions with the Revitan Curved (Zimmer GmbH, Winterthur, Switzerland) implanted via a modified transfemoral approach according to Wagner were followed clinically and radiologically prospectively over 32.3 ± 10.2 months [5]. The average flap length used for transfemoral access was 17.4 ± 7.8 cm and ranged from 12.3 to 27.8 cm. The average distal distance of the osteotomy flap from the resection margin was 6.6 ± 5.9 mm (1–21 mm). In 4 patients, there was a gap below the flap of 26–46 mm because of diaphyseal defects. The intraoperative blood loss was 970 ± 560 mL (420–2100 mL). Intraoperatively, there were 6 cases of a flap fracture due to osteolytic or osteoporotic weakening of the bony flap. The individual flap fragments were stably secured and fixed by double cerclage osteosynthesis. The bony flap underwent complete osseous consolidation in 98.5% of cases, in one case only partial consolidation following a two-stage septic change. Two trochanteric avulsions that occurred postoperatively healed without further intervention under partial weight bearing of 10–20 kg for 8 weeks. The Harris hip score increased continuously from 41.4 ± 14.5 points preoperatively to 85.9 ± 14.6 points 24 months after surgery. These outcomes are comparable to those published in the literature (Tables 15.1 and 15.2).

Good healing rates of the flap between 96% and 100% have also been observed throughout when using the transfemoral approach for the removal of infected prosthetic stems (Table 15.3). To analyze our own results of transfemoral access in two-stage septic replacement with closure of the flap around the interim prosthesis with cerclages and reopening of the bony flap upon reimplantation after 6 weeks, 76 patients were followed up in a study averaging 51.2 ± 23.2 (24–118) months [47]. The post-reimplantation healing rate of the bony flap was 98.7%, the

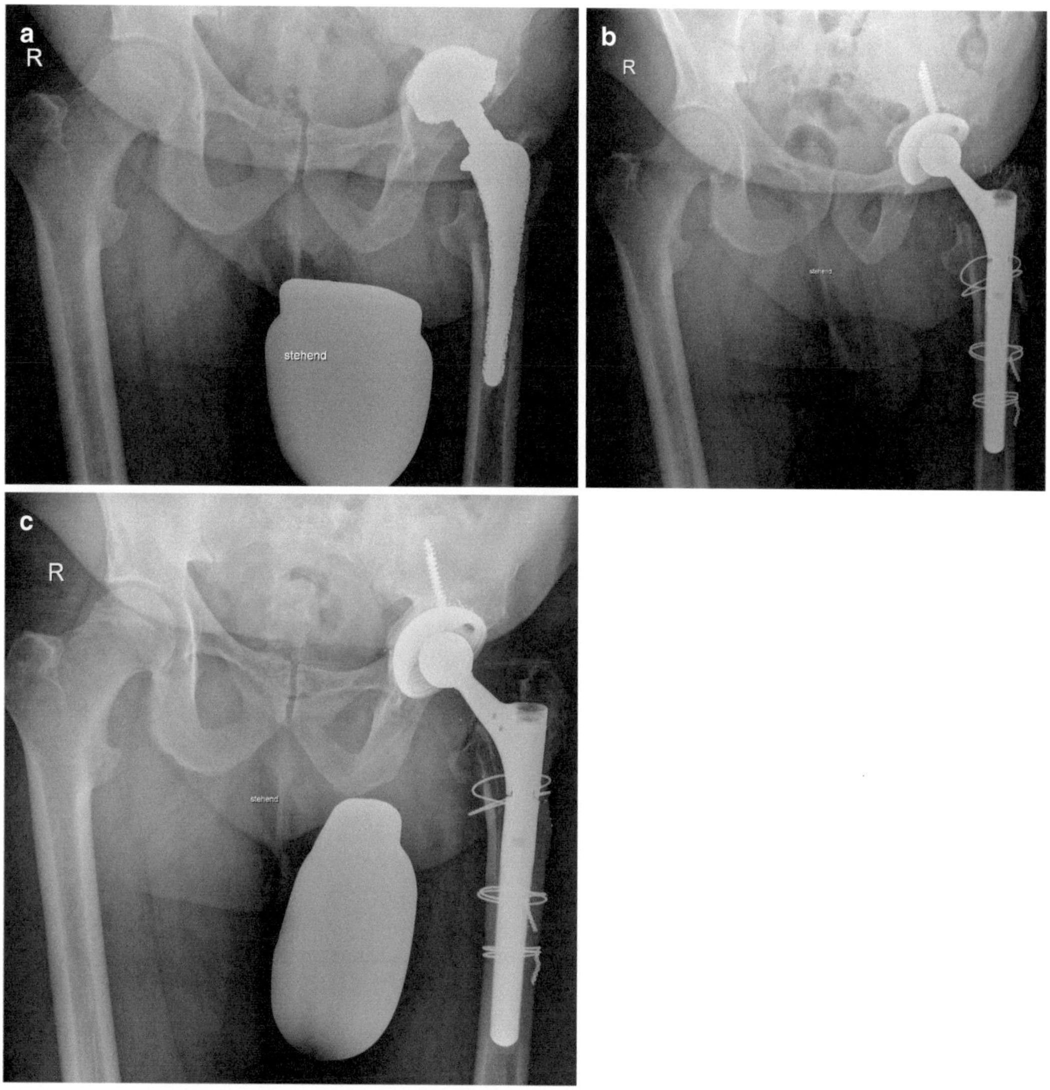

Fig. 15.31 (**a**) Prosthesis loosening of a roughly structured stem and cup (S&G stem, ESKA, Lübeck, Germany) with osteolysis in the trochanteric region. (**b**) Radiograph 7 days after transfemoral prosthesis revision with a modular revision stem Revitan Curved and Allofit-S cup (Zimmer Biomet, Winterthur, Switzerland) with fracture of the bony flap due to osteolysis. The individual segments are fixed with cerclages, and the greater trochanter is secured with a transosseous fiber wire running under the proximal cerclage. (**c**) Radiograph 1 year after surgery shows the bony consolidation of the fractures and osteointegration of the implants

absence of infection was 93.4%, the rate of stem subsidence was 6.6%, and the dislocation rate was 6.6%, with no aseptic loosening of the implants. The Harris hip score was 62.2 ± 12.6 points with the spacer before prosthesis reimplantation and 86.6 ± 15.5 points 2 years after reimplantation. Four fractures of the flap (5.3%) occurred due to osteolysis or osteoporotic bone thinning, but all subsequently healed. Thus, the outcome of the two-stage septic revision with a transfemoral approach can be considered reproducibly good in terms of the healing rate of the flap and freedom from infection. The closure of the flap with cerclage did not have a negative effect on the re-infection rate, despite the introduction of cerclage as foreign material, and the

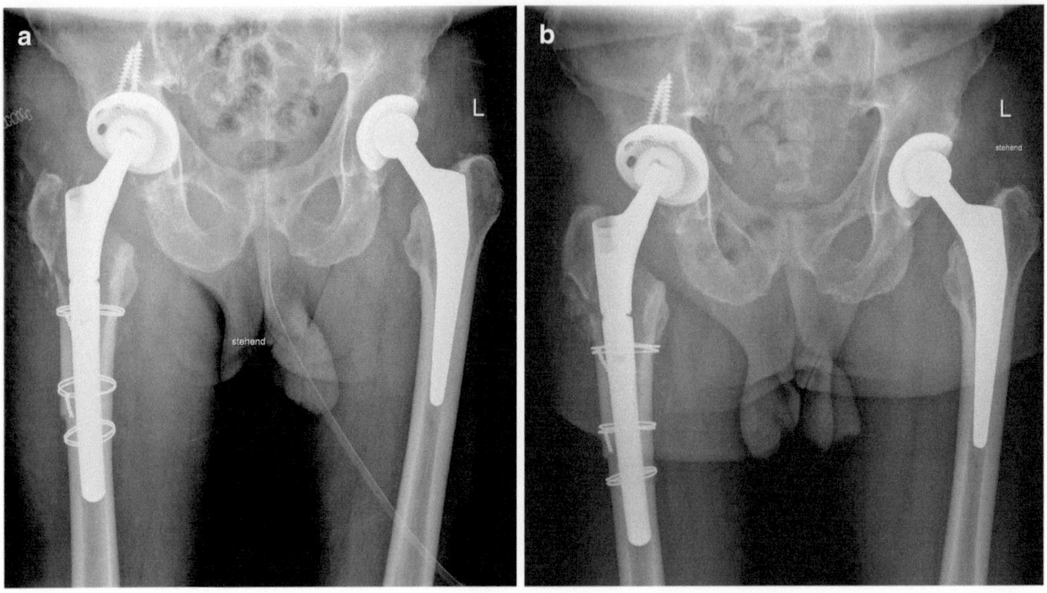

Fig. 15.32 (**a**) Radiograph 7 days postoperatively after transfemoral prosthesis revision on the right side using the modular revision stem Revitan Curved and Allofit-S cup (Zimmer Biomet, Winterthur, Switzerland) with intraoperative trochanteric fracture due to osteolysis. The trochanter was fixed with a transosseous fiber wire passed under the proximal cerclage. An additional proximal autologous bone transplantation was carried out with milled bone. (**b**) Radiograph 3 months after surgery showing almost complete bony consolidation of fractured greater trochanter

Table 15.1 Results of extended trochanteric osteotomy

Author	*n*	Follow-up [years]	Healing of the osteotomy	Flap fracture
Peters [35]	21	3.7	100%	4.4%
Chen [29]	46		97.8%	
Miner [22]	166	3.9	98.7%	2.4%
Huffman [32]	42	1.4	100%	12.0%
Mardones [33]	74	2.0	98.6%	5.4%
Morshed [36]	13 inf.	3.3	100%	23.1%
Levine [39]	17 #	> 2	100%	
Lakstein [37]	105	5.4	99%	5%
Lakstein [38]	53	4.75	98.1%	7.5%
Charity [40]	18	10	100%	

inf. periprosthetic infection, # periprosthetic fracture Vancouver B2 and B3

reopening of the transfemoral access with lifting the flap did not have a negative effect on the healing rate of the flap. However, it is essential for the muscles on the flap to be spared to ensure the blood supply to the bone and, thus, the healing of the flap.

The healing rate of the flaps in the case of transfemoral access or extended trochanteric osteotomy for periprosthetic fractures lies between 91% and 100% in the literature (Table 15.4). In our own study, 22 Vancouver B2 and 10 B3 fractures of 19 cemented and 13 cementless stems were examined [50]. Due to cup loosening, two additional cup exchanges were performed, otherwise the existing cup was left in place or an inlay exchange (23 times) was performed. According to the classification of Paprosky et al. [51], 10 cases had a type 2 defect, 15 cases a type 3A defect, and 7 cases a type 3B defect. The time difference between primary implantation and periprosthetic fracture was 4.9 ± 5.1 (1–20) years.

Table 15.2 Outcomes of transfemoral access with the Wagner SL stem and Revitan Curved [5] and Straight [46]

Author	*n*	Follow-up [years]	Healing of the osteotomy	Flap fracture
Wilkes [26]	24	1.5	83.3%	
Hartwig [41]	23	2.3	95.8%	
Grünig [42]	18	3.9	94.4%	
Isacson [43]	42	2.1	97.6%	
Böhm [44]	60	4.8		60%
Böhm [45]	60	5.4		60%
Warren [18]	17	4–7	70.6%	
Fink [5]	68	2.7	98.5%	8.8%
De Menezes [46]	100	4	95%	

Table 15.3 Outcomes of the transfemoral approach in two-stage septic revision

Author	*N*	Flap technique	Follow-up (mo)	Flap healing (%)	Success rate	Subsidence	Dislocation	Flap fracture	HHS
Morshed [36]	13	No closure + reopening	>24	100%	77%	15.4%	30.8%	23%	
Lim [48]	23	Closure + no reopening	63 (24–123)	100%	96%	4.3%	4.3%	8.7%	81.8 (59–93)
Levine [49]	23	Closure + various reopening options	49.1 (24–82)	96%	87%		8.7%	8.7%	
Fink [47]	76	Closure + reopening	51.2 (24–118)	98.7%	93.4%	6.6%	6.6%	1.3%	86.6 (59–100)

Radiographic examination 6 months after surgery showed fracture healing and bony consolidation of the bone segments and the transfemoral approach in all cases. The average fracture healing time was 14.5 ± 5.2 weeks (8–24 weeks). In accordance with the Engh classification [52] for biological fixation of the stem, bony ingrowth fixation was observed in 28 cases and stable fibrous fixation in 4 cases. The distal fixation zone in the isthmus of the femur in cases with Paprosky 2 and 3A defects where no additional distal locking was required was 4.5 ± 1.1 cm (3.1–6.2 cm). No subsidence of the revision stem or failure of the locking screws was observed during the study period.

Intraoperative blood loss averaged 990 ± 570 mL and ranged from 460 to 2000 mL. The Harris hip score increased continuously after surgery: 3 months postoperatively, it was 59.2 ± 14.6 points, 6 months postoperatively 66.9 ± 14.8 points, 9 months postoperatively 72.1 ± 15.4 points, 12 months postoperatively 75.2 ± 14.9 points, 18 months postoperatively 77.6 ± 15.9 points, and 24 months postoperatively 81.6 ± 16.5 points. One dislocation occurred 6 weeks after the procedure, which was treated conservatively, and one deep vein thrombosis of the leg. In accordance with the classification of Beals and Tower [53], all outcomes of this study were considered excellent.

Ladurner et al. [59] report their results from 43 patients (40 Vancouver B2 and 3 Vancouver B3) who received the same modular revision stem as in our study via a modified transfemoral approach. The transfemoral approach was performed in a supine position, the lateral dorsal osteotomy was performed through the vastus lateralis muscle, and the greater trochanter was split proximally. The idea here was not to involve the posterior capsule and external rotators, as in the posterior approach, in order to reduce the dislocation rate. Comparing the

Table 15.4 Results of the transfemoral approach in Vancouver B2 and B3 periprosthetic fractures

Author	*N* (B2/B3)	Follow-up [mo]	Healing	HHS	Subsidence	Dislocation	Fracture	Infection	Loosening
Sledge [54]	7/0	33	100%	83	28.6%	0%	0%	0%	0%
O'Shea [55]	10/12	33.7	91%	≈75	9.1%	0%	0%	4.5%	0%
Ko [56]	12/0	58.5	100%	≈80	16.6%	0%	8.3%	8.3%	0%
Levine [39]	12/5	44.5	100%	–	17.6%	5.8%	5.8%	5.8%	0%
Mulay [57]	10/12	24	91%	69	77.3%	22.7%	4.5%	4.5%	0%
Fink [50]	22/10	32.2	100%	81.6	0%	3.4%	0%	0%	0%
Drexler [58]	34	57	97%	77		2.9%	2.9%		
Ladurner [59]	40/3	40	97,6%	70	7,5%	5%	0%	5%	2.5%

results of Ladurner et al. [59] with ours [50], similarly high flap and fracture healing rates were found (97.5% in Ladurner et al. and 100% in our study), but the final results in terms of fracture healing and stem stability based on the classification of Beals and Tower [53] were different. 31 of the 40 (77.5%) outcomes followed up by Ladurner et al. [59] could be classified as excellent (prosthetic stem stable and fracture healed without shortening and only minor deformity); in our study, it was 100% [50]. However, the decisive difference is reflected in the functional outcomes, which are significantly worse in the study by Ladurner et al. [59]. While we were able to achieve a Harris hip score of 81.6, Ladurner et al. [59] only achieved a score of 70. In Ladurner et al. [59], only 52.5% of the patients were able to walk without aids and one patient could only be mobilized in a wheelchair. In our study, 2 patients needed a walking stick (93.75% without walking aids). In my opinion, this can be explained by the significantly higher traumatization of the vasto-gluteal sling in the technique used by Ladurner et al. [59]. This also explains the trochanteric escape in 3 cases (7.5%) in Ladurner et al. [59]. The dislocation frequency was not lower in the study by Ladurner et al. [59], at 5%, than in our study at 3.4% [50]. Thus, we believe that the protection of the vasto-gluteal sling and gluteal muscles is more important than the protection of the external rotators and posterior capsule, and therefore, we prefer the technique of transfemoral access via the posterior approach.

In a further evaluation of 120 revision surgeries, in which 42 modular revision prostheses (Revitan Curved, Zimmer Biomet GmbH, Winterthur, Switzerland) were implanted endofemorally and 78 transfemorally (including 21 periprosthetic fractures) were followed up for an average of 34.5 ± 11.6 months, the patients who underwent transfemoral access showed a slower postoperative increase in the Harris hip score and positive Trendelenburg signs for a longer period of time (Figs. 15.33 and 15.34) [60]. However, this was not a randomized study and patients who underwent transfemoral access procedures actually exhibited more severe bone defects and more problematic baseline conditions than patients who received endofemoral implantations. Despite this methodological weakness, this study demonstrated that with transfemoral access patients require a longer rehabilitation period but ultimately achieve similarly good clinical outcomes. The patient should be informed about this preoperatively.

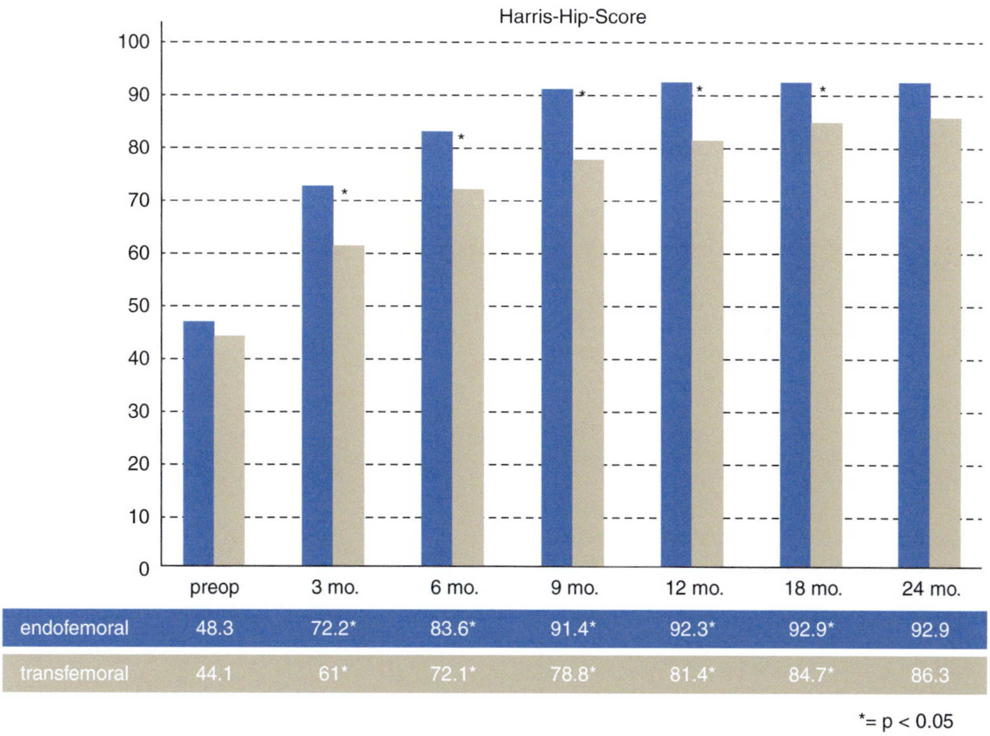

Fig. 15.33 Harris hip score before and during the postoperative follow-up of endofemoral and transfemoral implanted stems

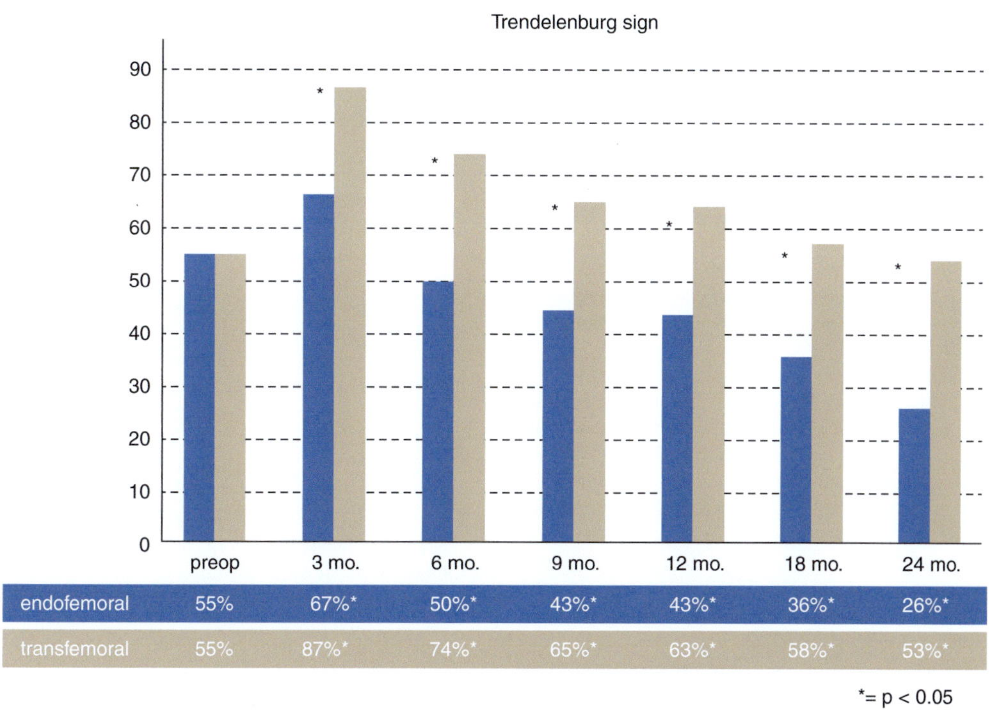

Fig. 15.34 Trendelenburg signs before and during the postoperative follow-up of endofemoral and transfemoral implanted stems

References

1. Lerch M, van Lewinski G, Windhagen H, Thorey F. Revision of total hip arthroplasty: clinical outcome of extended trochanteric osteotomy and intraoperative femoral fracture. Technol Health Care. 2008;16:293–300.
2. Wolf JH. Julius Wolff und sein Gesetz der Transformation der Knochen. Orthopäde. 1995;24:378–86.
3. MacDonald SJ, Cole C, Guerin J, Rorabeck CH, Bourne RB, McCalden RW. Extended trochanteric osteotomy via the direct lateral approach in revision hip arthroplasty. Clin Orthop Relat Res. 2003;(417):210–216.
4. Paprosky WG, Martin EL. Cemented stem failure requires extended trochanteric osteotomy. Orthopedics. 2003;26:28–38.
5. Fink B, Grossmann A, Schubring S, Schulz MS, Fuerst M. A modified transfemoral approach using modular cementless revision stems. Clin Orthop Relat Res. 2007;462:105–14.
6. Fink B. Revision of late periprosthetic infections of total hip endoprostheses: pros and cons of different concepts. Int J Med Sci. 2009;6:287–95.
7. Firestone TP, Hedley EL. Extended proximal femoral osteotomy for severe acetabular protrusion following total hip arthroplasty: a technical note. J Arthroplasty. 1997;12:344–5.
8. Fink B. The transfemoral approach for controlled removal of well-fixed femoral stems in hip revision surgery. J Clin Orthop Trauma. 2020;11:33–7.
9. Meek RM, Garbuz DS, Masri BA, Greidanus NV, Duncan CP. Intraoperative fracture of the femur in revision total hip arthroplasty with a diaphyseal fitting stem. J Bone Joint Surg Am. 2004;86-A:480–5.
10. Park YS, Moon YM, Lim SJ. Revision total hip arthroplasty using a fluted and tapered modular distal fixation stem with and without extended trochanteric osteotomy. J Arthroplasty. 2007;22:993–9.
11. McInnis DP, Horne G, Devane PA. Femoral revision with a fluted, tapered, modular stem. Seventy patients followed for a mean of 3.9 years. J Arthroplasty. 2006;21:372–80.
12. Pretterklieber B, Pablik E, Dorfmeister K, Pretterklieber KL. There are no safe areas for avoiding the perforating arteries along the proximal part of the femur: a word of caution. Clin Anat. 2020;33:507–15.
13. Wagner H. Revisionsprothese für das Hüftgelenk bei schwerem Knochenverlust. Orthopäde. 1987;16:295–300.
14. Wagner H. Revisionsprothese für das Hüftgelenk. Orthopäde. 1989;18:438–53.
15. Wagner H, Wagner M. Femur-Revisionsprothese. Z Orthop. 1993;131:574–7.
16. Wagner H, Wagner M. Hüftprothesenwechsel mit der Femur-Revisionsprothese. Erfahrungen von 10 Jahren. Med Orthop Tech. 1997;117:138–48.
17. Fink B, Grossmann A. Modified transfemoral approach to revision arthroplasty with uncemented modular revision stems. Oper Orthop Traumatol. 2007;19:32–55.
18. Warren PJ, Thompson P, Flechter MDA. Transfemoral implantation of the Wagner SL stem. The abolition of subsidence and enhancement of osteotomy union rate using Dall-Miles cables. Arch Orthop Trauma Surg. 2002;122:557–60.
19. Goldstein WM, Gleason TF, Kopplin M, Branson JJ. Prevalence of dislocation after total hip arthroplasty through a posterolateral approach with partial capsulotomy and capsulorrhaphy. J Bone Joint Surg Am. 2001;83-A Suppl 2(Pt 1):2–7.
20. Pellicci PM, Bostrom M, Poss R. Posterior approach to total hip replacement using enhanced posterior soft tissue repair. Clin Orthop Relat Res. 1998;(355):224–8.
21. White RE Jr, Forness TJ, Allman JK, Junick DW. Effect of posterior capsular repair on early dislocation in primary total hip replacement. Clin Orthop Relat Res. 2001;(393):163–7.
22. Miner TM, Momberger NG, Chong D, Paprosky WL. The extended trochanteric osteotomy in revision hip arthroplasty: a critical review of 166 cases at mean 3-year, 9-month follow-up. J Arthroplasty. 2001;16:188–94.
23. Wagner M, Knorr-Held F, Hohmann D. Measuring stability of wire cerclage in femoral fractures when performing total hip replacement. In vitro study on a standardized bone model. Arch Orthop Trauma Surg. 1996;115:33–7.
24. Schab JH, Camacho J, Kaufman K, Chen Q, Berry DJ, Trousdale RT. Optimal fixation fort he extended trochanteric osteotomy: a pilot study comparing 3 cables ves. 2 cables. J Arthroplasty. 2008;23:534–8.
25. Zhu U, Ding H, Shao H, Zhou Y, Wang G. An in-vitro biomechanical study of different fixation techniques for the extended trochanteric osteotomy in revision THA. J Orthop Surg Res. 2013;8:7.
26. Wilkes RA, Birch J, Pearse MF, Lee M, Atkins RM. The Wagner technique for revision arthroplasty of the hip: a review of 24 cases. J Orthop Rheumatol. 1994;7:196–8.
27. Mei XY, Gong YJ, Safir OA, Gross AE, Kuzyk PR. Fixation options following greater trochanter osteotomies and fractures in total hip arthroplasty: a systemic review. J Bone Joint Surg Rev. 2018;6:e4.
28. Abdel MP, Wyles CC, Viste A, Perry KI, Trousdale RT, Berry DJ. Extended trochanteric osteotomy in revision total hip arthroplasty. Contemporary outcomes of 612 hips. J Bone Joint Surg Am. 2021;103:162–73.
29. Chen WM, McAuley JP, Engh CA Jr, Hopper RH Jr, Engh CA. Extended slide trochanteric osteotomy for revision total hip arthroplasty. J Bone Joint Surg Am. 2000;82-A:1215–9.
30. Della Valle CJ, Berger RA, Rosenberg AG, Jacobs JJ, Sheinkop MB, Paprosky WG. Extended trochanteric osteotomy in complex primary total hip

arthroplasty. A brief note. J Bone Joint Surg Am. 2003;85-A:2385–90.
31. Glassman AH. Exposure for revision: total hip replacement. Clin Orthop Relat Res. 2004;(420):39–47.
32. Huffman GR, Ries MD. Combined vertical and horizontal cable fixation of an extended trochanteric osteotomy site. J Bone Joint Surg Am. 2003;85-A:273–7.
33. Mardones R, Gonzalez C, Cabanela ME, Trousdale RT, Berry DJ. Extended femoral osteotomy for revision of hip arthroplasty: results and complications. J Arthroplasty. 2005;20:79–83.
34. Younger TI, Bradford MS, Magnus RE, Paprosky WG. Extended proximal femoral osteotomy. A new technique for femoral revision arthroplasty. J Arthroplasty. 1995;10:329–38.
35. Peters PC Jr, Head WC, Emerson RH Jr. An extended trochanteric osteotomy for revision total hip replacement. J Bone Joint Surg Br. 1993;75-B:158–9.
36. Morshed S, Huffman R, Ries MD. Extended trochanteric osteotomy for 2-stage revision of infected total hip arthroplasty. J Arthroplasty. 2005;20:294–301.
37. Lakstein D, Kosashvili Y, Backstein D, Safir O, Gross AE. Modified extended trochanteric osteotomy with preservation of posterior structures. Hip Int. 2010;20:102–8.
38. Lakstein D, Kosashvili Y, Backstein D, Safir O, Lee P, Gross AE. The long modified extended sliding trochanteric osteotomy. Int Orthop. 2011;35:13–7.
39. Levine BR, Della Valle CJ, Lewis P, et al. Extended trochanteric osteotomy for the treatment of Vancouver B2/B3 periprosthetic fractures of the femur. J Arthroplasty. 2008;23:527–33.
40. Charity J, Tsiridis E, Gusmao D, Bauze A, Timperley J, Gie G. Extended trochanteric osteotomy followed by cemented impaction allografting in revision hip arthroplasty. J Arthroplasty. 2013;28:154–60.
41. Hartwig C-H, Böhm P, Czech U, Reize P, Küsswetter W. The Wagner revision stem in alloarthroplasty of the hip. Arch Orthop Trauma Surg. 1996;115:5–9.
42. Grünig R, Morscher E, Ochsner PE. Three- to 7-year results with the uncemented SL femoral revision prosthesis. Arch Orthop Trauma Surg. 1997;116:187–97.
43. Isacson J, Stark A, Wallensten R. The Wagner revision prosthesis consistently restores femoral bone structure. Int Orthop. 2000;24:139–42.
44. Böhm P, Bischel O. Femoral revision with the Wagner SL revision stem. Evaluation of one hundred and twenty-nine revisions followed for a mean of 4.8 years. J Bone Joint Surg Am. 2001;83-A:1023–31.
45. Böhm P, Bischel O. The uncemented diaphyseal fixation of femoral revision stems in case of large bone defects—analysis of twelve years experience with the Wagner SL revision stem. Z Orthop. 2001;139:229–39.
46. De Menezes DFA, Le Béguec P, Sieber HP, Goldschild M. Stem and osteotomy length are critical for success of the transfemoral approach and cementless stem revision. Clin Orthop Relat Res. 2012;470:883–8.
47. Fink B, Oremek D. The transfemoral approach for removal of well-fixed femoral stems in two-stage septic hip revision. J Arthroplasty. 2016;31:1065–71.
48. Lim SJ, Moon YW, Park YS. Is extended trochanteric osteotomy safe for use in 2-stage revision of periprosthetic hip infection? J Arthroplasty. 2011;26:1067–71.
49. Levine BR, Della Valle CJ, Hamming M, Sporer SM, Berger RA, Paprosky WG. Use of the extended trochanteric osteotomy in treating prosthetic hip infection. J Arthroplasty. 2009;24:49–55.
50. Fink B, Grossmann A, Singer J. Hip revision arthroplasty in periprosthetic fractures of Vancouver type B2 and B3. J Orthop Trauma. 2012;26:206–11.
51. Paprosky WG, Weeden SH, Bowling JW Jr. Component removal in revision total hip arthroplasty. Clin Orthop Relat Res. 2001;(393):181–193.
52. Engh CA, Glassman AH, Suthers KE. The case of porous-coated hip implants: the femoral side. Clin Orthop Relat Res. 1990;(261):63–81.
53. Beals RK, Tower SS. Periprosthetic fractures of the femur. An analysis of 93 fractures. Clin Orthop Relat Res. 1996;(327):238–246.
54. Sledge JB 3rd, Abiri A. An algorithm for the treatment of Vancouver type B2 periprosthetic proximal femoral fractures. J Arthroplasty. 2002;17:887–92.
55. O'Shea K, Quinlan JF, Kutty S, et al. The use of uncemented extensively porous-coated femoral components in the management of Vancouver B2 and B3 periprosthetic femoral fractures. J Bone Joint Surg Br. 2005;87-B:1617–21.
56. Ko PS, Lam JJ, Tio MK, et al. Distal fixation with Wagner revision stem in treating Vancouver type B2 periprosthetic femur fractures in geriatric patients. J Arthroplasty. 2003;13:446–52.
57. Mulay S, Hassan T, Birtwistle S, et al. Management of types B2 and B3 femoral periprosthetic fractures by a tapered, fluted, and distally fixed stem. J Arthroplasty. 2005;20:751–6.
58. Drexler M, Dwyer T, Chakravertty R, Backstein D, Gross AE, Safir O. The outcome of modified extended trochanteric osteotomy in revision THA for Vancouver B2/B3 periprosthetic fractures of the femur. J Arthroplasty. 2014;29:1598–604.
59. Ladurner A, Zurmühle P, Zdravkovic V, Grob K. Modified extended trochanteric osteotomy for the treatment of Vancouver B2/B3 periprosthetic fractures of the femur. J Arthroplasty. 2017;32:2487–95.
60. Fink B, Grossmann A, Schubring S, Schulz MS, Fuerst M. Short-term results of hip revisions with a curved cementless modular stem in association with the surgical approach. Arch Orthop Trauma Surg. 2009;129:65–73.

16 Technical Implementation of the Stem Implantation of Modular Revision Stems with Distal Fixation

Contents

16.1 **Scratch-Fit Distal Fixation of a Modular Revision Stem** 210

16.2 **Cone-in-Cylinder Distal Fixation of a Modular Revision Stem** 212

16.3 **Cone-in-Cone Distal fixation of a Modular Revision Stem** 212
16.3.1 Basic Sequence of Surgical Steps for a Modular Straight Stem (Arcos) 213
16.3.2 Surgical Procedures with a Tapered Modular Revision Stem (Revitan Curved) 215

16.4 **Comments on Surgical Descriptions or Assembly of Modular Stems** 233

References 235

After the old implant and, if necessary, the cement residues have all been removed, the next step is to prepare the fixation bed for the new prosthetic stem. Depending on the stem system and intended fixation principle (scratch fit with cylinder-in-cylinder fixation, cone-in-cylinder fixation, or cone-in-cone fixation), this is done with cylindrical broaches, flexible medullary reamers, conical broaches, or conical rasps (after prior use of cylindrical medullary reamers). In my opinion, one should always try to get the thickest possible broach, rasp, and then the stem or distal prosthetic component into the fixation bed. This creates the most stable anchorage possible without subsequent subsidence of the stem and avoids implanting long, thin stems, which, especially when straight stems are implanted in the curved femur, carry the risk of unintentional perforation or fracture. For this aim, the preoperative planning is an essential help. However, experience has shown that it is not uncommon to implant a stem or distal component that is one size thicker than specified in the preoperative planning. An awareness of the specific features of each stem system (degree of taper, height of the thickness designation, etc.) helps to select the correct stem thickness.

Supplementary Information The online version contains supplementary material available at [https://doi.org/10.1007/978-3-030-84821-7_16]. The videos can be accessed by scanning the related images with the SN More Media App.

B. Fink, *Femoral Revision Arthroplasty*, https://doi.org/10.1007/978-3-030-84821-7_16

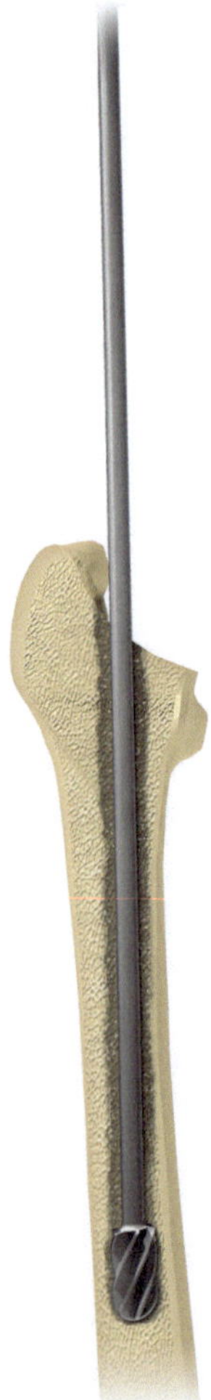

Fig. 16.1 Reaming of the medullary canal distally with a flexible medullary reamer until cortical contact has been established (with permission of ZimmerBiomet, Warsaw, IN, USA)

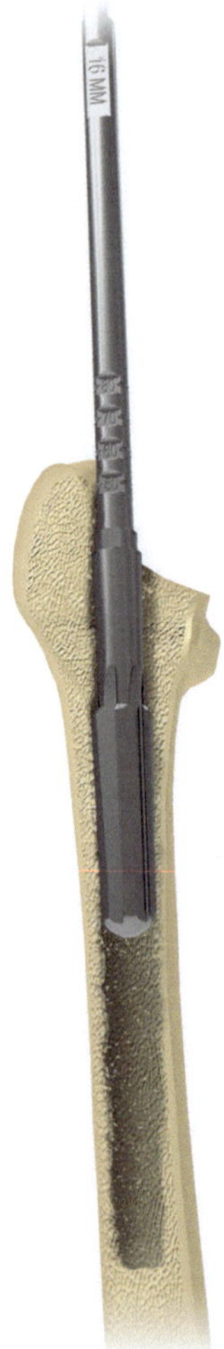

Fig. 16.2 Reaming of the medullary canal with a rigid cylindrical broach until cortical contact has been established (with permission of ZimmerBiomet, Warsaw, IN, USA)

16.1 Scratch-Fit Distal Fixation of a Modular Revision Stem

This principle will be exemplified using this particular version of the Arcos modular revision system (Zimmer Biomet, Warsaw, IN, USA). First, the distal femoral canal is reamed with a flexible medullary reamer to create a sound cortical contact (Fig. 16.1), followed by a rigid cylindrical broach (Fig. 16.2). Other systems use a rigid broach directly. A trial distal component can be used to check whether there are still any obstacles that could prevent the distal seating of the components (Fig. 16.3). This is followed by implantation of the final distal components (Fig. 16.4). For stem systems that are implanted by means of scratch fit (cylinder-in-cylinder fixation), a distal prosthesis component 0.5 mm–1 mm thicker than the last intramedullary reamer is selected, depending on the manufacturer's recommendation [1, 2]. A guide is inserted on the implanted final distal component to create the extra room

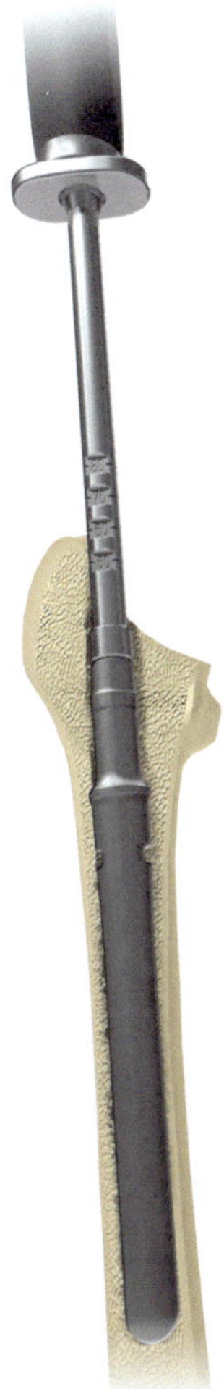

Fig. 16.3 Insertion of the trial component (with permission of ZimmerBiomet, Warsaw, IN, USA)

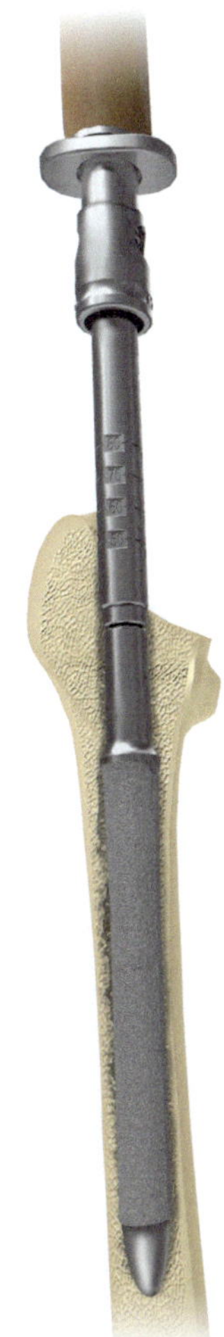

Fig. 16.4 Implantation of the final distal component

required for the proximal component with proximal reamers, if this is necessary (Fig. 16.5). With the trial proximal component in place, a trial reduction can be performed (Fig. 16.6). This is used to check whether the leg length, range of motion, antetorsion, offset, and stability can be recreated or achieved as desired. If necessary, a reduction with another proximal component is made. Once the tests have been completed satisfactorily, the proximal components are mounted in situ on the final distal components (Fig. 16.7).

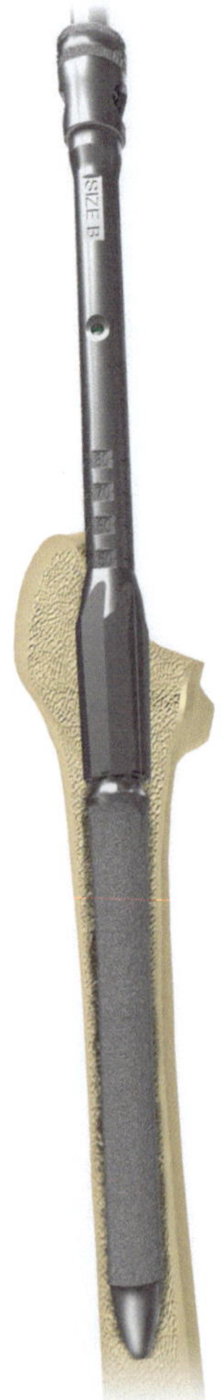

Fig. 16.5 Creating room for the proximal component with a proximal reamer utilizing a guide mounted on the distal component

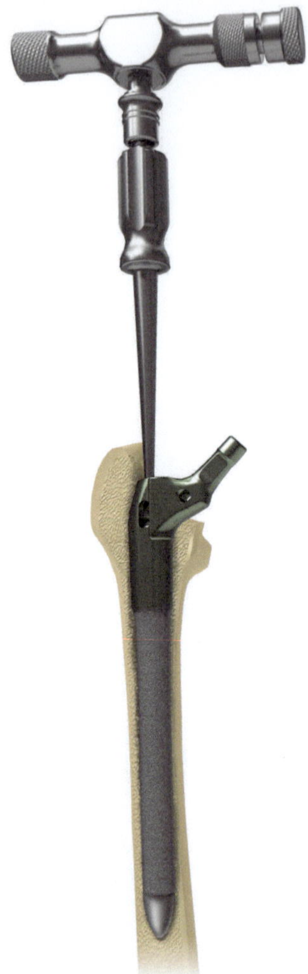

Fig. 16.6 Insertion of the trial proximal component

16.2 Cone-in-Cylinder Distal Fixation of a Modular Revision Stem

In some curved, distally tapered revision stems, preparation of the fixation bed is performed exclusively using a cylindrical flexible medullary reamer (e.g., MRP stem, Peter Brehm, Weisendorf, Germany). This then creates a cone-in-cylinder fixation. Depending on the manufacturer and cortical thickness, a distal component that is nominally 2–3 mm thicker than the last used thickness of the medullary reamer is implanted [3, 4]. The reason for this is the difference between the actual thickness of the stem at the distal start of the tapered section and the quoted nominal diameter (Table 8.1).

16.3 Cone-in-Cone Distal fixation of a Modular Revision Stem

The distal revision systems with dual conical fixation have their own characteristics that depend on the taper of the stem (the angle of the tapered portion of the distal stem). The basic

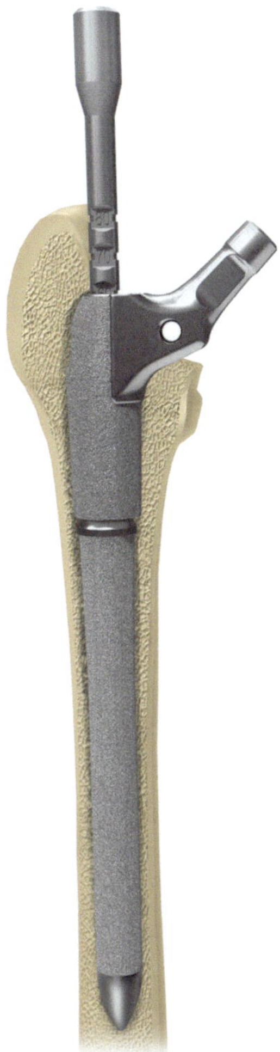

Fig. 16.7 In situ assembly of the proximal and the final components

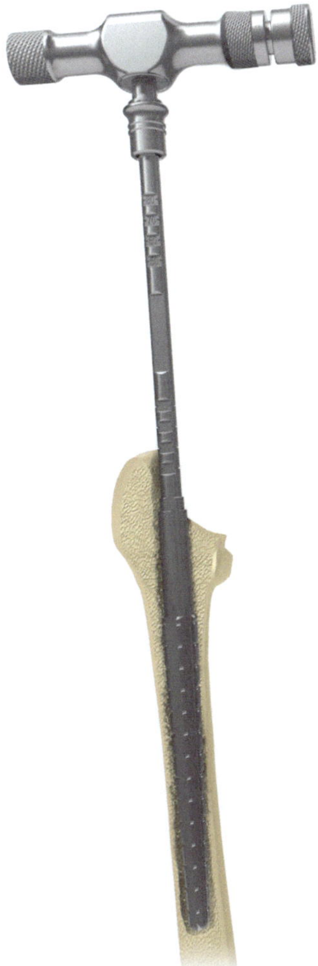

Fig. 16.8 Reaming of the medullary canal distally with a conical broach to create a conical fixation bed

principles of the surgical procedure will first be described using the example of a modular straight stem system (Arcos, Zimmer Biomet, Warsaw, IN, USA). This will be followed by a more detailed description of the surgery involved in the implantation of a modular Revitan Curved revision stem (ZimmerBiomet GmbH, Winterthur, Switzerland).

16.3.1 Basic Sequence of Surgical Steps for a Modular Straight Stem (Arcos)

First, the distal femoral canal is reamed with a conical reamer (broach) until a conical bed has been cut into the cortex (Fig. 16.8). A trial distal

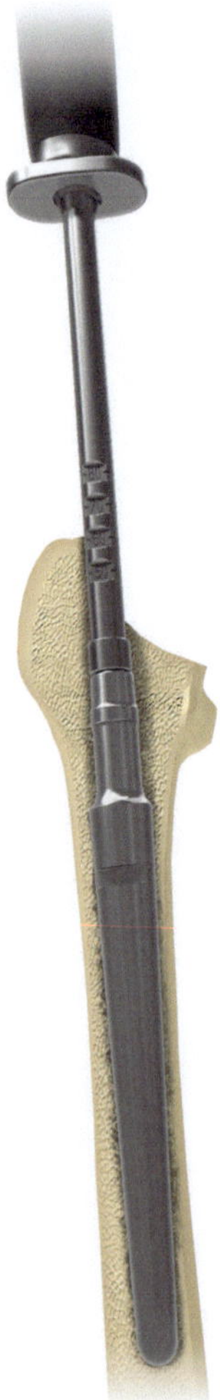

Fig. 16.9 Insertion of the trial distal component

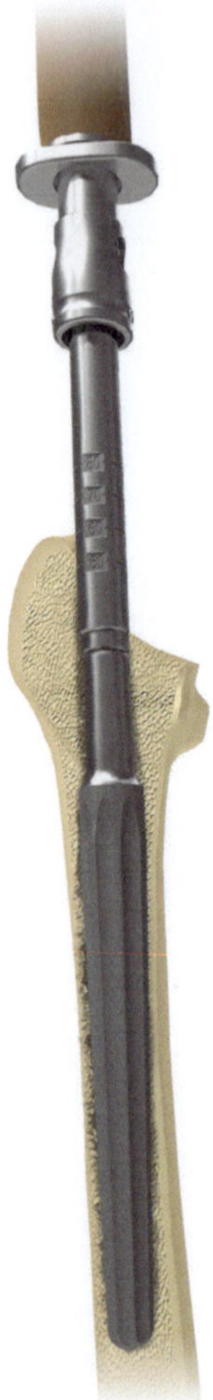

Fig. 16.10 Implantation of the final distal component

component can be used in some systems to check whether there are still obstacles preventing distal fixation of the component (Fig. 16.9). This is followed by implantation of the final distal component (Fig. 16.10). Here, the nominal diameter and length of the distal component correspond to that of the last broach used. If necessary, the room required for the proximal component is then created with proximal reamers using a guide mounted on the implanted final distal component (Fig. 16.11). With the trial proximal component than in place, a trial reduction can be performed

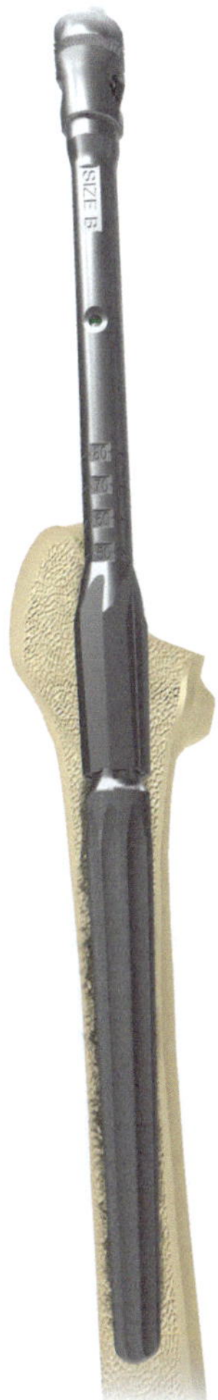

Fig. 16.11 Creating room for the proximal component with a proximal reamer utilizing a guide mounted on the distal component

(Fig. 16.12). This is used to check whether the range of motion, stability, and anatomical reconstruction is as desired. If necessary, the alignment or the components are changed again. After satisfactory testing, the proximal components are mounted in situ onto the final distal components (Fig. 16.13).

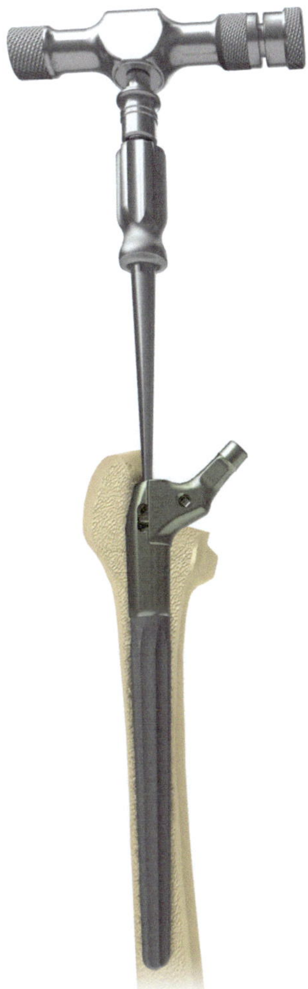

Fig. 16.12 Insertion of the trial proximal component

16.3.2 Surgical Procedures with a Tapered Modular Revision Stem (Revitan Curved)

16.3.2.1 Transfemoral Implantation

Prior to preparation of the fixation bed in the isthmus of the femur, a prophylactic double cerclage

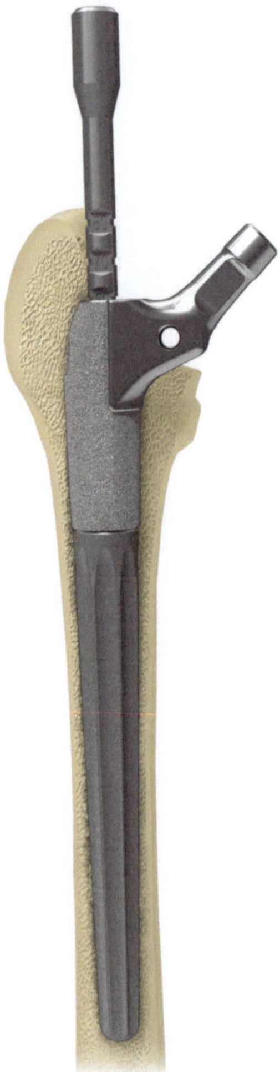

Fig. 16.13 In situ assembly of the final proximal and distal components

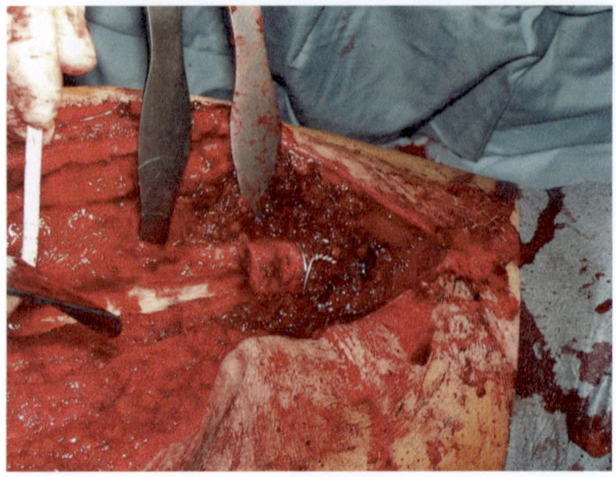

Fig. 16.14 Placement of a prophylactic double cerclage below the flap of the transfemoral access at the proximal end of the still intact isthmus of the femur

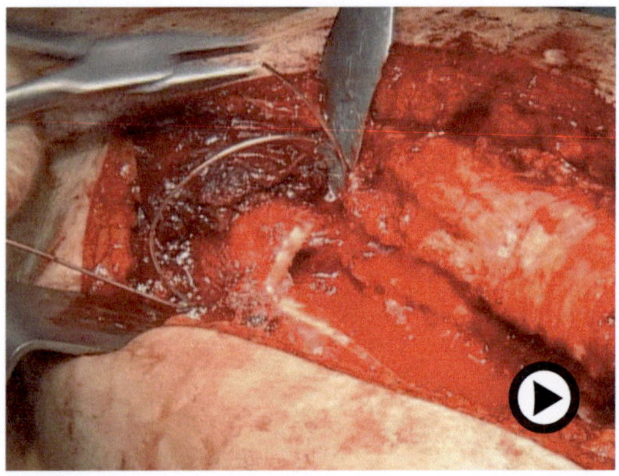

Fig. 16.15 (Video 16.1) Applying a prophylactic double cerclage below the flap of the transfemoral approach at the commencement of the intact isthmus (with permission of Zimmer Biomet, Winterthur, Switzerland). Placement of a prophylactic double cerclage below the flap of the transfemoral approach at the beginning of the intact isthmus (▶ https://doi.org/10.1007/000-4pz)

or cable is placed just below the opened flap at the beginning of the intact femoral shaft. This is to prevent the extension of any fissure that may have developed during preparation of the fixation bed with conical broaches or rasps, or during impaction of the stem. We do this with a 1.5 mm cerclage wire passed around twice. Alternatively, cerclage cable (e.g., Cable Ready system, Zimmer Biomet, Warsaw, IN., USA) can be used (Figs. 16.14 and 16.15 for Video 16.1).

It has been shown that, for transfemoral implantation of the 2° tapered Revitan Curved modular revision stem (Zimmer Biomet, Winterthur, Switzerland), the distal component should have a nominal diameter that is 4 mm greater than the diameter of the last cylindrical intramedullary reamer that had formed firm cortical contact in the isthmus of the femur (Fig. 16.16). The reference point for defining the nominal diameters of this system, which is 11 cm above the tip, dictates this difference. The taper of 2° results in a decrease in diameter distally such that a true cone-in-cone fixation zone of 3–5 cm occurs at the tip of the 140-mm-long distal component with nominal diameter + 4. Specifically, the diameter at the distal onset of the tapered portion of the distal component is

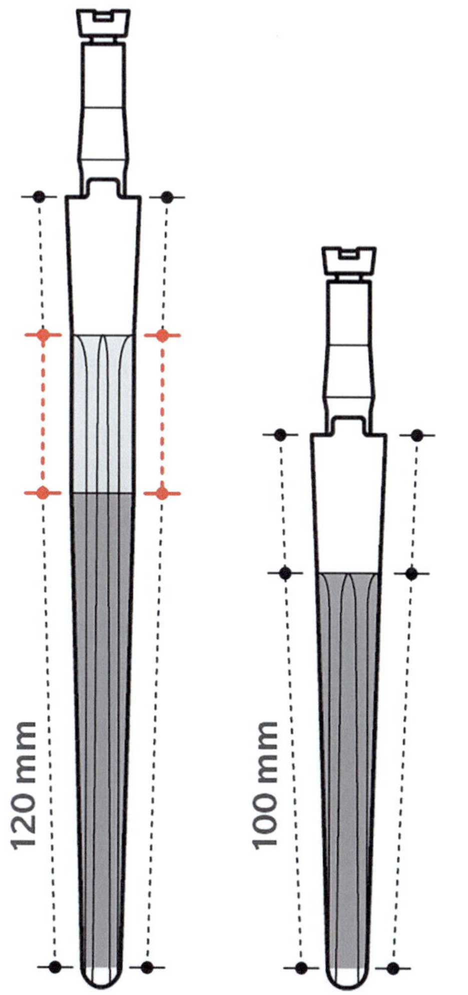

Fig. 16.16 Visualization of the tapered area of the 200 mm long (left) and 140 mm long (right) distal component of the Revitan system (with permission of Zimmer Biomet, Winterthur, Switzerland)

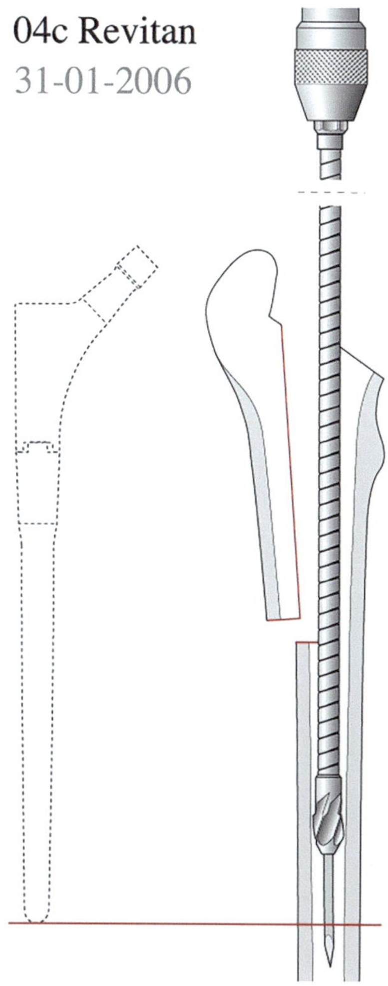

Fig. 16.17 Reaming the distal fixation zone in the isthmus of the femur with a flexible medullary reamer until a firm cortical contact is achieved. This creates an initially cylindrical fixation bed (with permission of Zimmer Biomet, Winterthur, Switzerland)

3.8 mm less than the quoted nominal diameter. Thus, with this stem system, the preparation is done in such a way that a sound cortical contact is created with the cylindrical medullary reamer and then the conical fixation bed is gradually created with a series of conical distal rasps with increasing diameters (Figs. 16.17 and 16.18). Here, the appropriate fixation bed is created at the tip of the conical rasp starting with a rasp of the same diameter as the last intramedullary reamer and finishing with a rasp that is 4 mm larger. Rotational movements should be used to confirm the robust rotational stability of the inserted rasp (Fig. 16.19 for Video 16.2). Care must be taken to ensure that the antecurvature of the rasp corresponds to that of the femur. The position of the patella is helpful for orientation. If the difference between the last cylindrical medullary reamer and the conical rasp diameter (and thus the distal prosthetic component) is then chosen to be 3 mm, the cone-in-cone fixation zone of the same length will be located somewhat higher than at the tip of the distal component (Fig. 16.20). Thus, when the distal component is fixed in this way, it extends

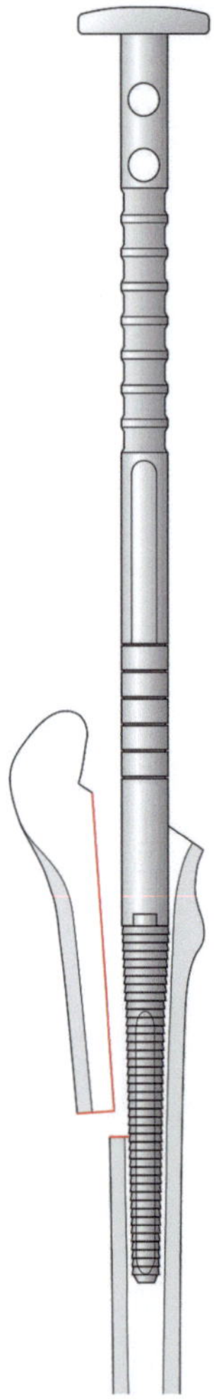

Fig. 16.18 Creation of the conical fixation bed in the isthmus of the femur with conical rasps, whereby a nominally 4 mm larger rasp than the last medullary reamer achieves a fixation bed of 3–4 cm in the isthmus (with permission of Zimmer Biomet, Winterthur, Switzerland)

slightly further into the femur. A similar principle can be applied to the MRP stem (Peter Brehm, Weisendorf, Germany) for the first three lengths of the distal component, since here the difference between the nominal diameter and the diameter at the distal start of the tapered section is 4 mm. However, the fixation bed is not prepared conically for the curved components of the MRP system, instead it is cylindrical and created with intramedullary reamers alone.

Theoretically, this principle can also be applied to the tapered straight stems and distal

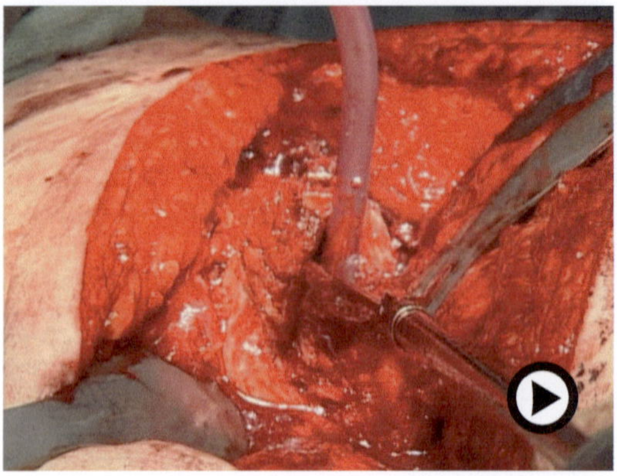

Fig. 16.19 (Video 16.2) Preparation of the fixation bed with initially a cylindrical medullary reamer and then creation of a conical fixation bed by using increasing sizes of conical rasps (with permission of Zimmer Biomet, Winterthur, Switzerland) (► https://doi.org/10.1007/000-4pt)

components. If one knows the difference between the nominal diameter of the distal component or straight stem and the diameter at the distal start of the tapered section (Table 8.1), one could prepare the fixation bed with a cylindrical medullary reamer, and then, after preparing the conical fixation bed with the conical broach, implant (for 2-degree tapered stems) a stem with a diameter that reflects this difference. This procedure would result in a cone-in-cone fixation zone at the tip of the stem of 3–5 cm for a 2-degree conical stem, and slightly shorter for stems with a greater taper. However, for highly tapered stems (e.g., ZMR stem with 3.5° taper), the fixation zone cannot start at the distal tip of the stem. Rather, it starts well above the tip (Figs. 7.2 and 7.16a–c). In this case, one would implant a stem with a nominal diameter that is not greater by the entire amount of the difference between the nominal diameter and the actual diameter at the distal start of the tapered section. For example, in the case of the ZMR stem, this difference is approximately 6 mm (Table 8.1). But here a stem only 4 or 5 mm thicker than the diameter of the last medullary reamer would be implanted (after preparation of the fixation bed with the broaches). Nevertheless, this surgical technique helps to achieve a firm fixation using short stems and thus avoids the use of unnecessarily long stems.

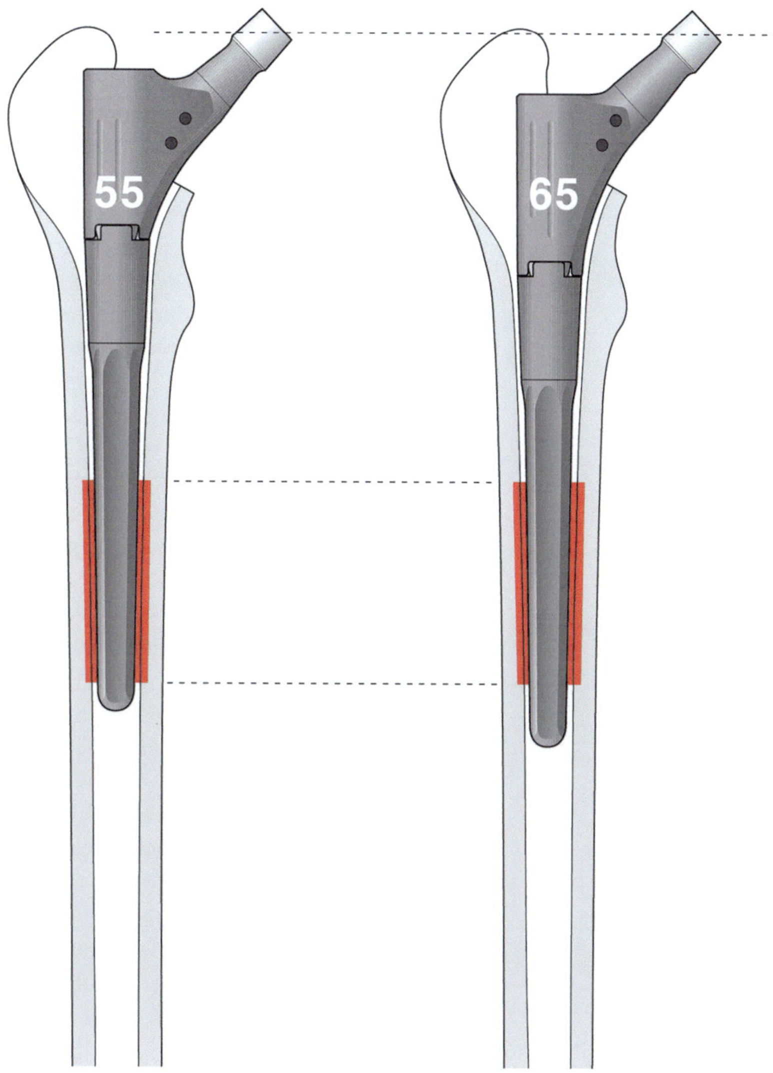

Fig. 16.20 Depiction of the fixation area for the distal component with a + 4 mm difference between the last medullary reamer thickness and the selected diameter of the distal component (left) and a + 3 mm difference (right) with a more proximal fixation zone for the stem (with permission of Zimmer Biomet, Winterthur, Switzerland)

After preparation of the distal fixation bed with the conical reamers or rasps, the expected length of the proximal component or the total length of the stem (in the case of monoblock stems) can be read from the conical reamer or distal rasp component last inserted into the prepared fixation bed. The tip of the greater trochanter serves as the reference point here (Fig. 16.18). In the transfemoral procedure, the bony flap, which is folded away ventrally with the greater trochanter, is folded back for better legibility. If the shortest proximal component length is used, it is now important to ensure that a reduction with the final components at a later stage will be successful. A trial reduction with trial components can be carried out for this purpose. With the Revitan Curved system, the proximal rasp component is placed on the distal rasp component and the trial reduction is carried out. If the trial reduction is not successful because the prosthesis combination is too long, the stem system must be moved lower. If the cortical bone is supportive enough, the conical reamers or the cylindrical medullary reamers can be used to ream one size further and the entire procedure repeated with the trial prosthesis components or rasp components that are thus positioned somewhat lower (Fig. 16.20). If further reaming is not possible

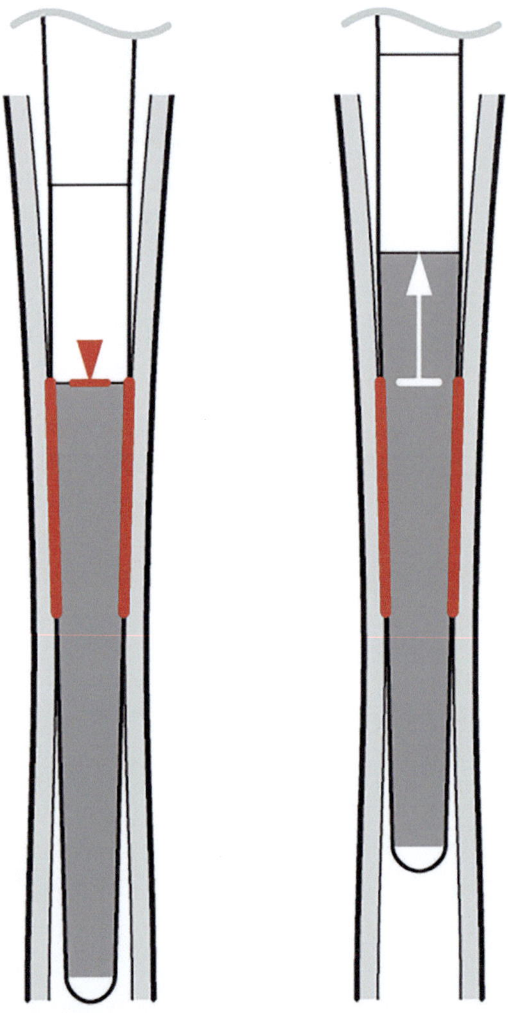

Fig. 16.21 Change from a thicker distal component (right) to a thinner one (left) with lowering of the junction (with permission of Zimmer Biomet, Winterthur, Switzerland)

because of the quality of the cortical bone, the next thinner stem (or trial stem or rasp) is selected, resulting in a conical fixation zone that is further down. The latter alternative results in a longer combination of stem components (Fig. 16.21).

If the readout of the length of the proximal component at the greater trochanter shows that the longest component ought to be selected, then if the isthmus of the femur is intact, it is important to check whether it is possible to select the next larger size of distal component, which would further proximalize the construct and thus shorten the stem combination (Fig. 16.22). Thus, the next larger size of conical reamer or rasp is selected and so will exhibit a more proximal fixation zone; again, this can be read off the scale at the greater trochanter. This latter procedure is performed for three reasons. First, if the isthmus is intact, it is very rarely necessary to use a combination with the longest proximal component. Second, this procedure will result in an overall shorter prosthesis combination with less risk of perforation or fracture. Thirdly, if the final component is fixed slightly deeper than the trial component, conical reamer, or rasp, it is still possible to restore the correct leg length because there is a greater range of proximal component lengths available to the surgeon. If the longest proximal component is chosen and this stem combination then sits slightly deeper in the femur than the trial component, only extra-long modular head sleeve systems with all their disadvantages in terms of corrosion and fretting would still be available to correct for leg length [5, 6].

If the seat of the conical broach or rasp is in the optimal zone between the second-shortest and second-longest proximal components, either a trial prosthesis can be used (in some cases, this can be modular as with the Wagner SL stem (Zimmer Biomet GmbH, Winterthur, Switzerland) for trial reduction as described or the final distal components can be implanted directly) (Figs. 16.23, 16.24, and 16.25 for Video 16.3).

The distal component or the monoblock stem should be impacted with measured hammer blows. Vigorous hammering increases the risk of fissures appearing at the site of fixation. The decisive factor for seating the stem correctly is not the applied force, but the momentum acting on the stem. For this reason, I recommend using only blows from the wrist with a 600-g hammer.

After implantation of the final distal component, the length of the trial proximal component can again be read from the implantation guide at the greater trochanter. The tip of the folded-back bony flap at the greater trochanter is again used as a reference for this purpose. The trial proximal

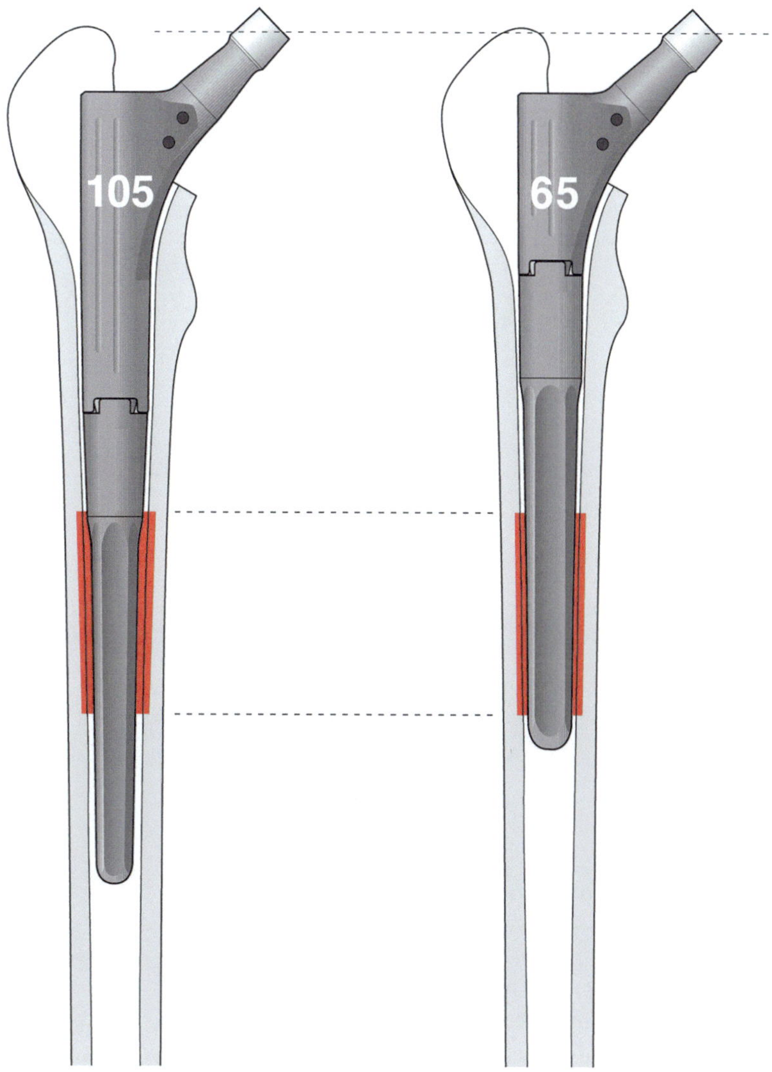

Fig. 16.22 Change from a thinner distal component (left) to a thicker one (right) with proximalization of the junction and shortening of the proximal component (with permission of Zimmer Biomet, Winterthur, Switzerland)

component is now placed on the final distal component, and a trial reduction is performed with a trial head (Figs. 16.26 and 16.27 for Video 16.4). The leg length and antetorsional adjustment of the proximal component are then checked for impingement-free movement and stability. After satisfactory testing and any correction of the length or position of the proximal component and retesting, the selected proximal implant is fitted in situ to the distal component with the appropriate torque wrenches (Figs. 16.28 and 16.29 for Video 16.5). A trial reduction can be performed again and the locking screw can then be inserted with the torque wrench. After another trial reduction with the trial head, the selected final prosthesis head is attached. Then, in the case of a transfemoral approach, the flap is closed by means of double cerclages or cables followed by stepwise wound closure (Figs. 16.30a–c, 16.31a–c, and 16.32 for Video 16.6).

16.3.2.2 Endofemoral Implantation

An endofemoral approach will result in a cone-in-cone fixation of the Revitan Curved by means of a three-surface fixation (see Chap. 7) (Fig. 16.33a–c). Here, the difference between the last cylindrical medullary reamer and the distal conical rasp component finalizing the fixation

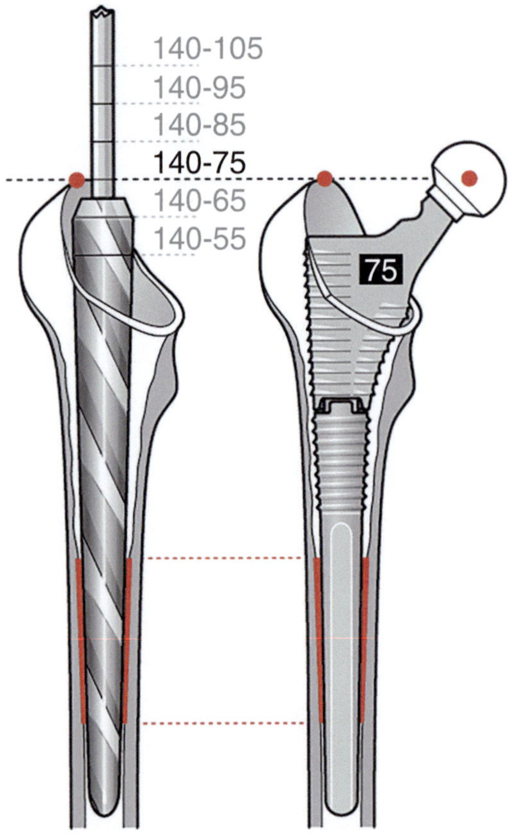

Fig. 16.23 Insertion of a trial prosthesis with the Revitan Straight (with permission of Zimmer Biomet, Winterthur, Switzerland)

bed will never be 4 mm. Depending on the radius of the antecurvature of the femur and the thickness of the femoral cortical bone, the difference required to create a solid fixation with the distal component in the diaphysis of the femur is 2 or 3 mm. Mumme et al. [3] and Wimmer et al. [4] reported similar data for the implantation of an MRP stem (Peter Brehm, Weisendorf, Germany), where a nominally 2–3 mm thicker distal component was inserted into the fixation bed prepared with cylindrical intramedullary reamers (cone-in-cylinder fixation).

After the medullary canal has been reamed with the flexible medullary reamer, the length of the expected proximal component can be read from the rasp application guide at the level of the greater trochanter (Figs. 16.34a, b and 16.35 for Video 16.7). If the surgeon decides to choose the shortest length and wishes to be sure that a reduc-

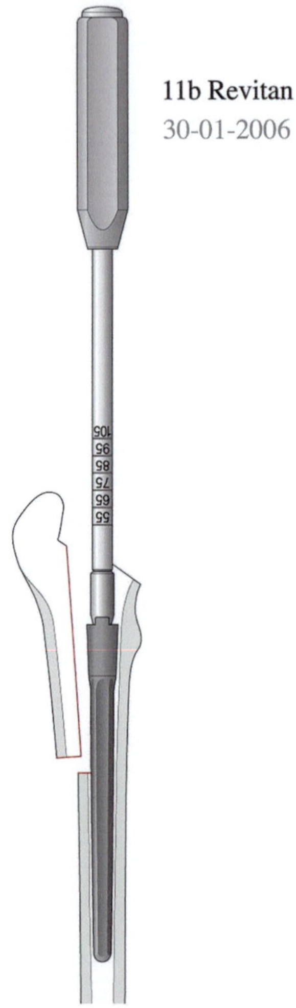

Fig. 16.24 Implantation of the final distal components of the Revitan Curved according to the selected final rasp thickness (with permission of Zimmer Biomet, Winterthur, Switzerland)

tion is still possible with the Revitan Curved stem then, with the distal rasp component still inserted, a trial can be carried out by attaching the shortest proximal rasp component to the distal one. However, during the endofemoral procedure it must be ensured that there is sufficient room for the proximal rasp component in the trochanter region and that there is no risk of an unintentional fracture of the trochanter (Fig. 16.36). If there is insufficient room available for the proximal rasp or proximal trial component, this must be created by careful manual preparation with chisels and prosthesis-specific reamers. In my opinion, it is

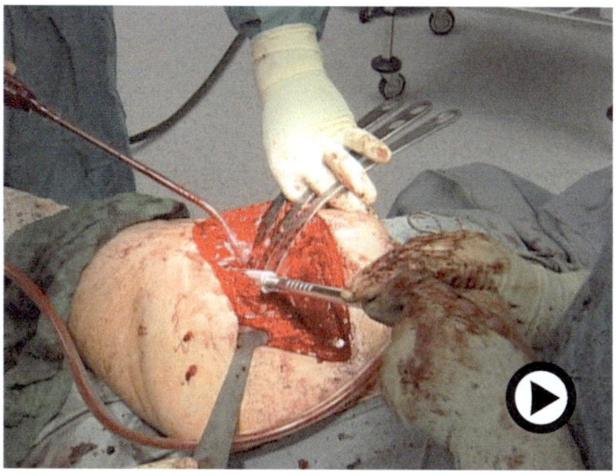

Fig. 16.25 (Video 16.3) Implantation of the final distal component (with permission of Zimmer Biomet, Winterthur, Switzerland) (▶ https://doi.org/10.1007/000-4pv)

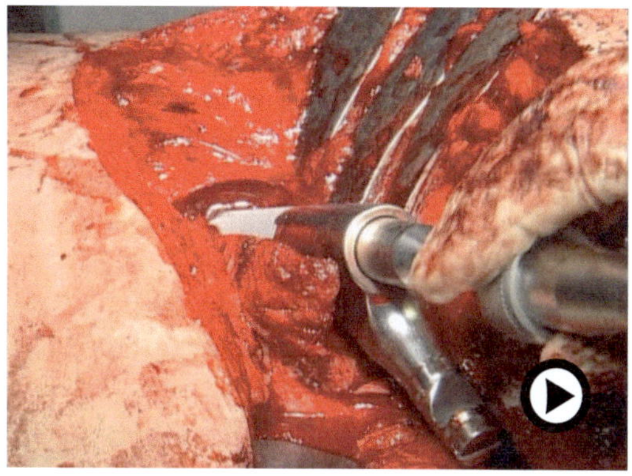

Fig. 16.27 (Video 16.4) Trial reduction with trial proximal component (with permission of Zimmer Biomet, Winterthur, Switzerland). Repositioning with a trial proximal component for testing (▶ https://doi.org/10.1007/000-4pw)

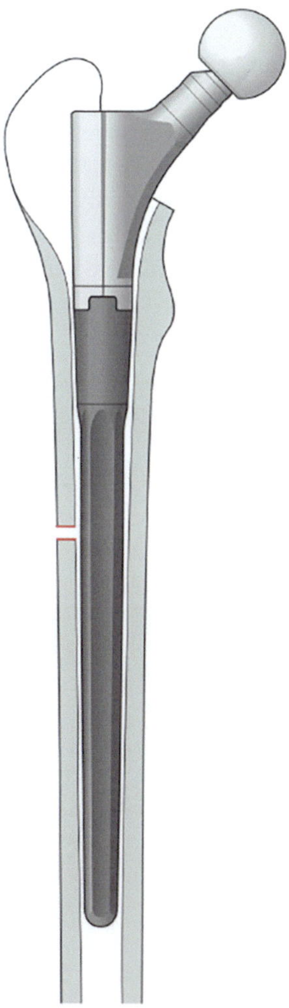

Fig. 16.26 Trial reduction with the trial proximal component and trial head on the final distal component (with permission of Zimmer Biomet, Winterthur, Switzerland)

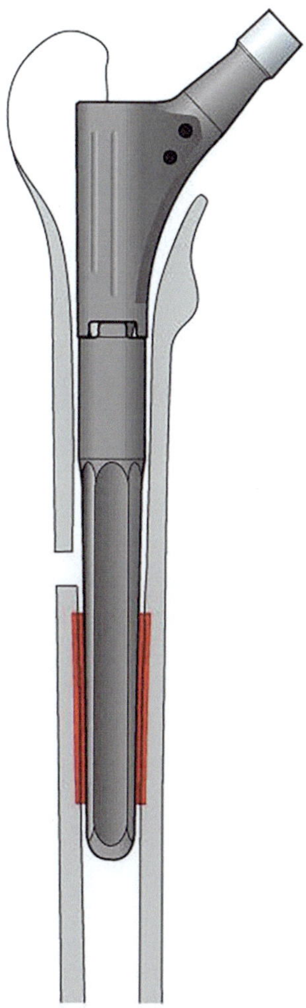

Fig. 16.28 In situ mounted final components (with permission of Zimmer Biomet, Winterthur, Switzerland)

not advisable to use the proximal rasp component as such, as this exerts unnecessary pressure on the trochanter region and could result in unintentional trochanter fractures. We therefore do not use the proximal rasp components, or at most the shortest one, to test the reduction capability with such a combination of components.

In the endofemoral procedure, the final distal components or the monoblock stem should also be impacted with measured hammer blows to avoid fissures or even fractures (Fig. 16.37). Here, too, I recommend using a 600-g hammer and a wrist action to give the stem the appropriate momentum to set it in place (Fig. 16.38 for Video 16.8).

After implantation of the final distal components, the length of the trial proximal component can again be read from the implantation guide at the greater trochanter (Fig. 16.37). It must now be ensured that there is sufficient room for the proximal trial component and that there is no unnecessary pressure on the greater trochanter with an accompanying risk of fracture. For this reason, we choose purely cylindrical proximal components for distally fixed stems and never conical ones. The stem already has a solid distal fixation, and there is no need for any fixation with the proximal component. Therefore, cylindrical components are sufficient to realize the correct adjustment of leg length, antetorsion, and offset through the proximal component. The use of conical proximal components only increases the risk of trochanteric fracture. Usually, a chisel, or a hollow reamer placed on the distal component, is used to carefully remove bone in the greater tro-

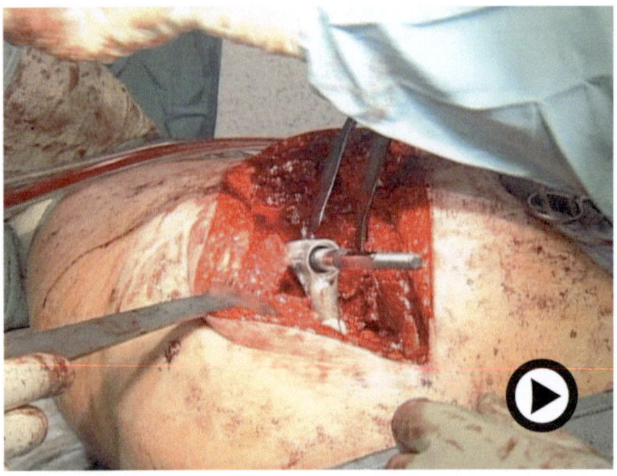

Fig. 16.29 (Video 16.5) In situ assembly of the final proximal component and the final distal component (with permission of Zimmer Biomet, Winterthur, Switzerland) (▶ https://doi.org/10.1007/000-4px)

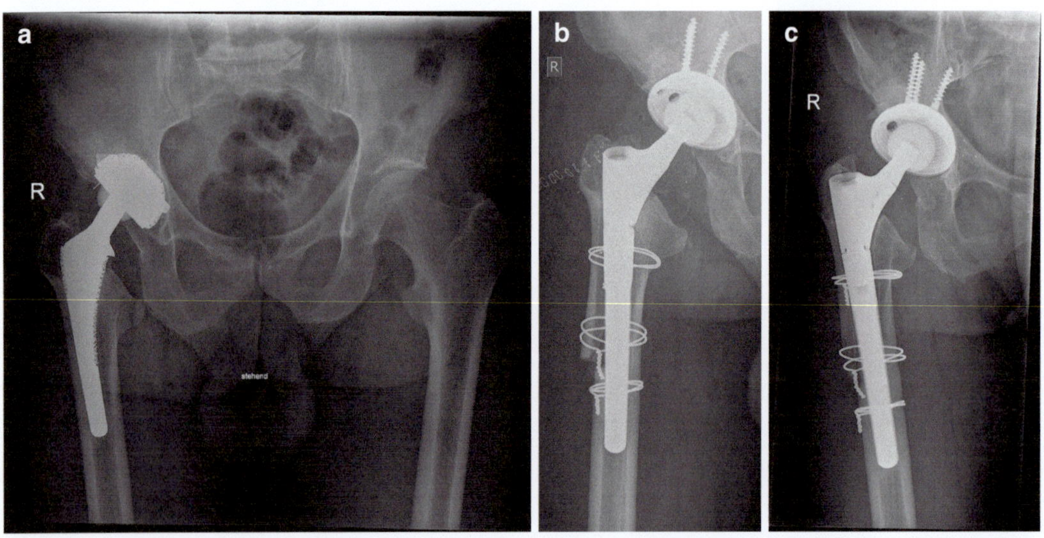

Fig. 16.30 (**a**) Loosened cementless hip prosthesis with coarse surface structure on the right (ESKA, Lübeck, Germany). (**b**) Transfemoral revision to modular revision stem Revitan Curved and Allofit-S cup (Zimmer Biomet, Winterthur, Switzerland). Because of a favorable cortical thickness, a short distal fixation zone can be achieved with a difference of 4 mm between the diameter of the last intramedullary reamer and that of the stem. (**c**) Radiograph 12 months postoperatively with unchanged position of the implants

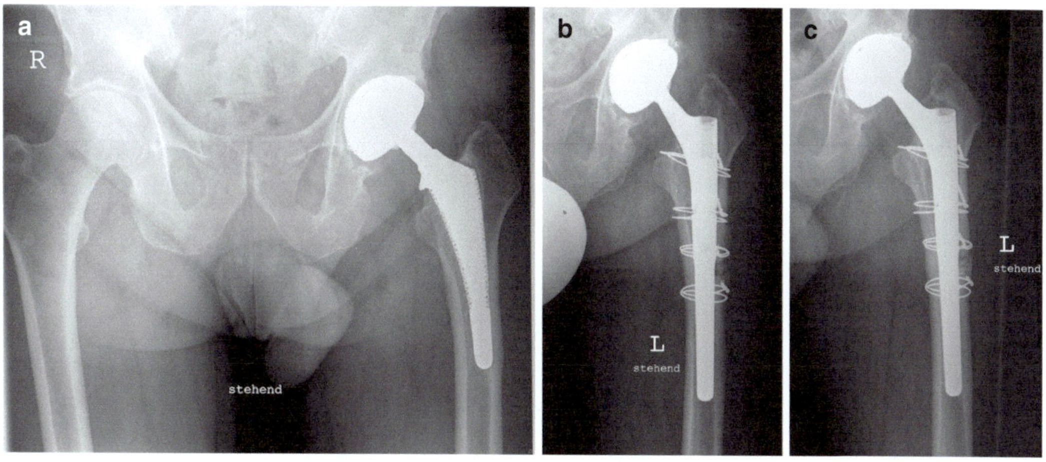

Fig. 16.31 (**a**) Loosened cementless hip prosthesis with coarse surface texturing on the left (ESKA, Lübeck, Germany). (**b**) Transfemoral stem revision to modular revision stem Revitan Curved (Zimmer Biomet, Winterthur, Switzerland). Because of the chosen difference of 3 mm between the last intramedullary reamer diameter and the last nominal diameter of the distal rasp and/or distal prosthesis component, the distal component penetrates deeper into the femur. (**c**) Radiograph 12 months postoperatively with unchanged position of the implants

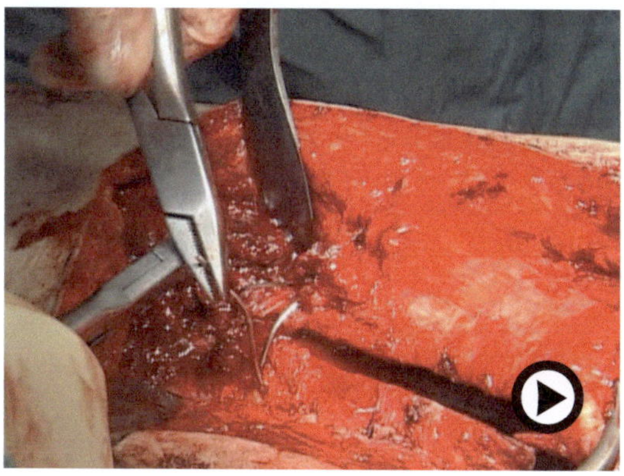

Fig. 16.32 (Video 16.6) Closure of the transfemoral access with double cerclages (▶ https://doi.org/10.1007/000-4py)

chanter area by hand so that the proximal trial component can be matched with the final distal component in situ without exerting pressure on the greater trochanter (Figs. 16.39 and 16.40 for Video 16.9). This bone, which has to be removed from the greater trochanter with the hollow reamer, is the section of bone that prevents correct distal placement of the stem due to premature proximal contact if the modular components are assembled on the operating table. Subsidence of the stem will then occur later when the patient is mobilized and weight is applied to the joint. Therefore, I would never recommend performing a tabletop assembly of the modular components, but always an in situ assembly.

A trial reduction is now carried out with the trial proximal component assembled in situ with the final distal component (Fig. 16.41 for Video 16.10). Leg length, range of motion, impingement-free motion, and dislocation risk are checked. If necessary, the trial proximal component is again modified in length, offset, or position with respect to antetorsion. After a satisfactory trial reduction, the trial proximal component is removed and the final proximal component is combined with the final distal component in situ using the appropriate specialized instruments (torque wrench) (Figs. 16.42 and 16.43 for Video 16.11). Afterward, trial reduction and testing for mobility as well as stability are performed again with the corresponding trial heads, followed by implantation of the selected final head component (Fig. 16.44).

16.3.2.3 Distal Locking

A special situation exists in the case of a deficient femoral isthmus (Paprosky type IIIB and IV) that is no longer suitable for normal distal fixation

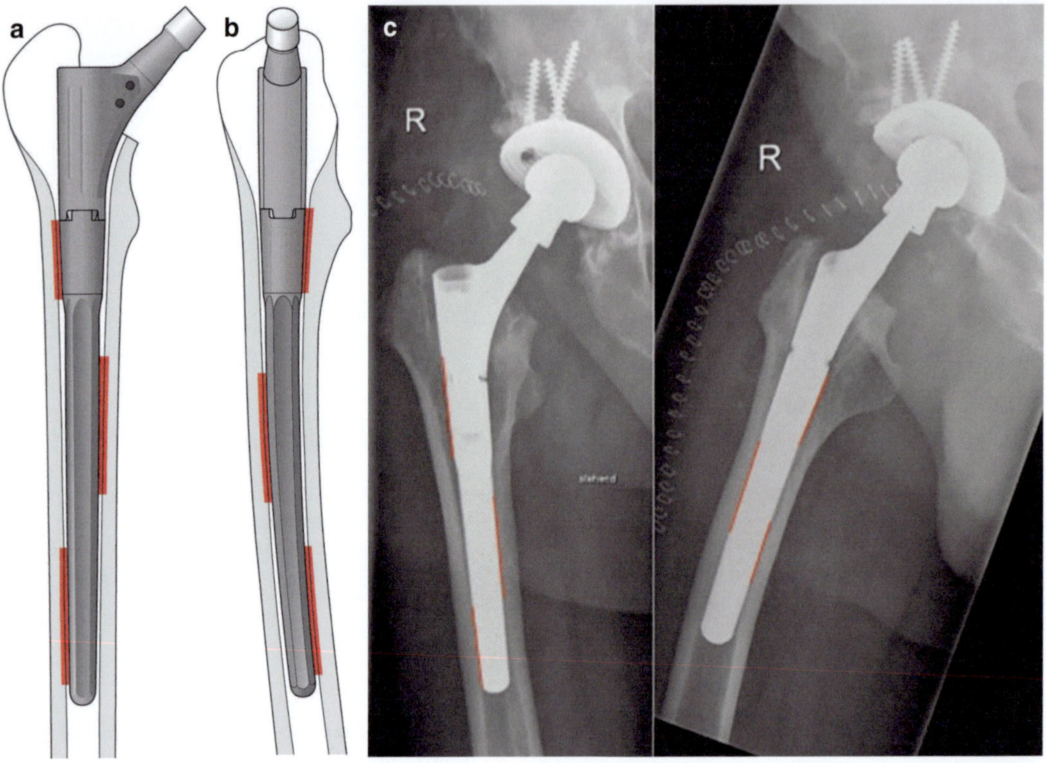

Fig. 16.33 Three-surface fixation of an endofemorally implanted Revitan Curved (with permission of Zimmer Biomet, Winterthur, Switzerland). (**a**) Anterior–posterior view, (**b**) Lateral view. (**c**) Three-surface fixation of the Revitan Curved shown on the radiograph. The surfaces of the stem responsible for fixation are highlighted in red

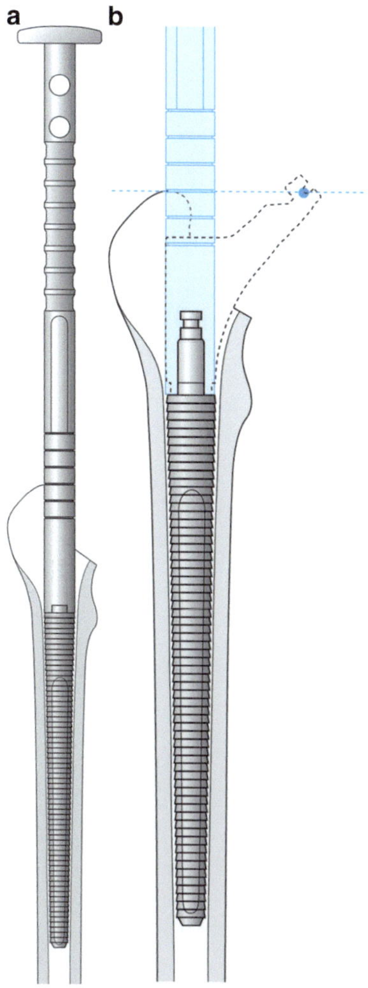

Fig. 16.34 (**a**) Creating the conical distal fixation bed with the conical rasp component. The expected length of the proximal component can be read from the guiding device at the level of the greater trochanter (with permission of Zimmer Biomet, Winterthur, Switzerland). (**b**) Expected length of the proximal component according to the readout on the insertion guide of the distal rasp component (with permission of Zimmer Biomet, Winterthur, Switzerland)

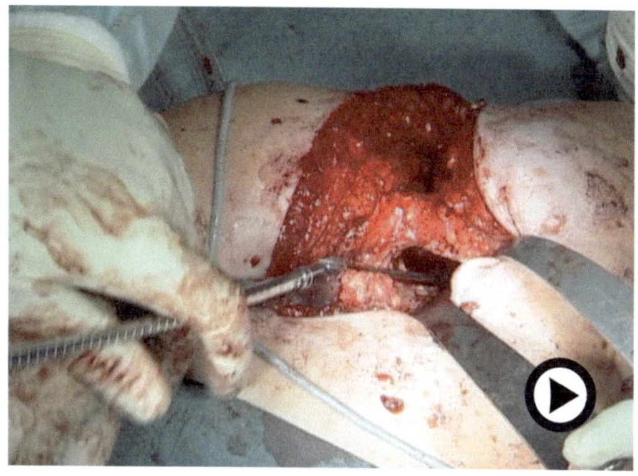

Fig. 16.35 (Video 16.7) Preparation of the fixation bed by first using cylindrical medullary reamers followed by conical rasps (with permission of Zimmer Biomet, Winterthur, Switzerland) (▶ https://doi.org/10.1007/000-4ps)

(using any fixation principle) [1]. In this case, some revision stem systems offer the possibility of additional fixation by means of distal locking screws. It is important here, as already discussed in Chap. 7, that the fixation is not based purely on the locking screws, but rather that a (depending on the stem) cone-in-cone or cone-in-cylinder fixation that cannot meet the respective minimum fixation distance is given temporary support by the locking screws. I recommend performing this only with the transfemoral approach (extended trochanteric osteotomy). In the first place, the short distal fixation of the distal component can be managed better in this way. Secondly, the femoral bone is fragile in these cases, so the risk of fracture during an endofemoral approach is very high. The transfemoral approach addresses this risk. Finally, the osteotomy in the transfemoral approach results in an almost intentional fracture-related callus formation, which leads to bone on-growth and osteointegration of the proximal stem

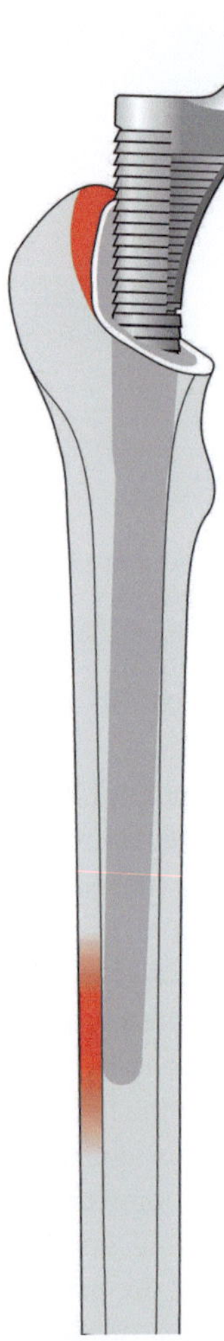

Fig. 16.36 Proximal rasp component makes contact with the greater trochanter. The proximal area of the trochanter shown in red must be carefully removed beforehand to ensure that the proximal rasp component can be positioned without undue pressure (with permission of Zimmer Biomet, Winterthur, Switzerland)

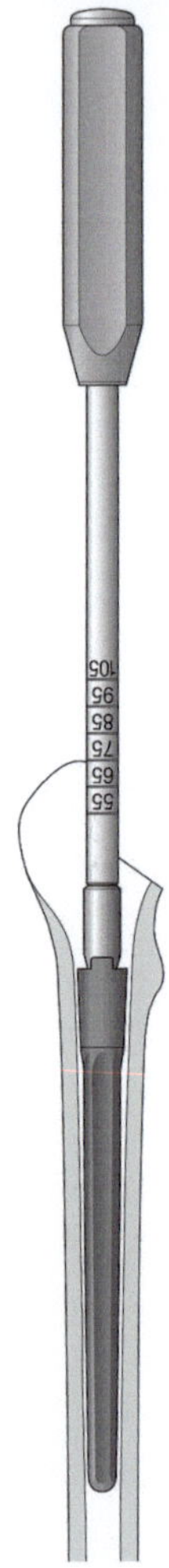

Fig. 16.37 Implantation of the final distal component with the installation instruments. The expected length of the proximal component can be read off at the level of the greater trochanter (with permission of Zimmer Biomet, Winterthur, Switzerland)

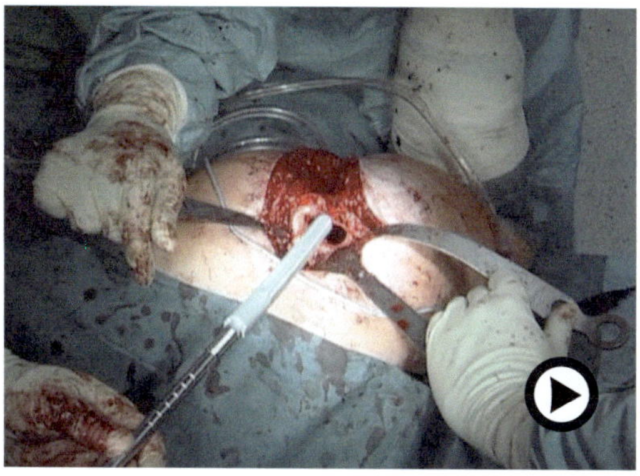

Fig. 16.38 (Video 16.8) Implantation of the final distal components (with permission of Zimmer Biomet, Winterthur, Switzerland) (▶ https://doi.org/10.1007/000-4q0)

region. This ultimately ensures the stability of the stem and eliminates the need for locking screw function once osteointegration has occurred.

Here, the fixation bed of the distal component is prepared as usual for the stem system used. Preoperative planning will show that the minimum fixation distance for the stem and the fixation principle in the isthmus of the stem cannot be attained because of the bone defects or an existing fracture. In the case of cone-in-cylinder fixation, the selected oversize of the stem should be only 0.5 mm larger than the last intramedullary reamer in order to avoid the risk of periprosthetic fractures. For this purpose, attention must be paid to the respective nominal stem-specific diameter of the distal component. In the case of cone-in-cone fixation with distal locking (Revitan Curved), a difference between the cylindrical medullary reamer and the final stem thickness of

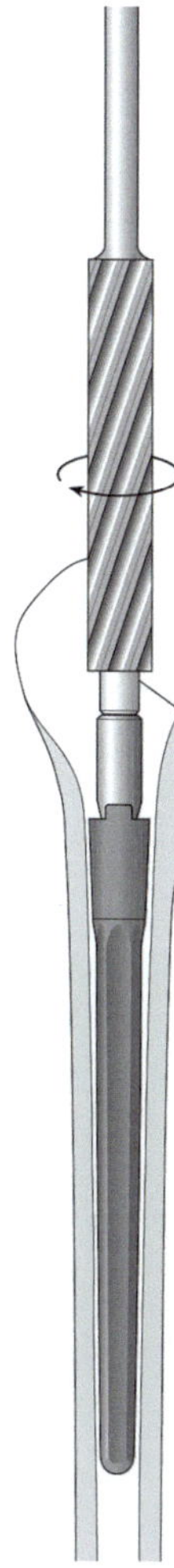

Fig. 16.39 Removal of bone in the region of the greater trochanter using a hollow reamer so that the cylindrical trial component and later the final components can be positioned on the greater trochanter without pressure (with permission of Zimmer Biomet, Winterthur, Switzerland)

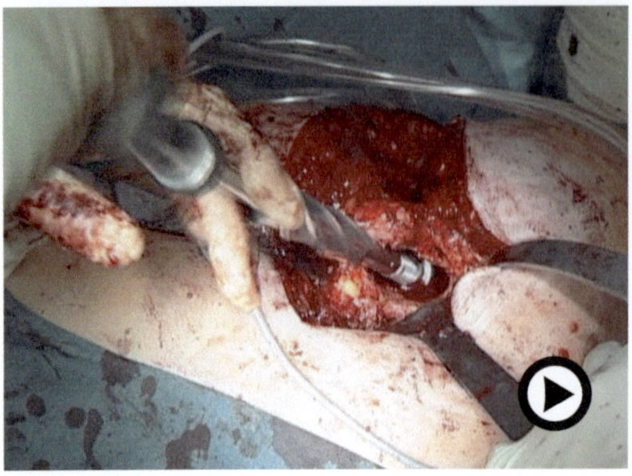

Fig. 16.40 (Video 16.9) Creation of room for the cylindrical trial proximal component and then the final components using cylindrical hollow reamers (with permission of Zimmer Biomet, Winterthur, Switzerland) (▶ https://doi.org/10.1007/000-4q1)

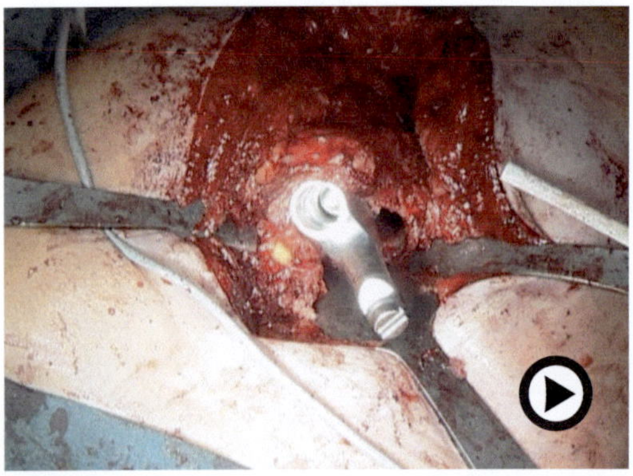

Fig. 16.41 (Video 16.10) Attaching the trial proximal component and trial reduction (with permission of Zimmer Biomet, Winterthur, Switzerland) (▶ https://doi.org/10.1007/000-4q2)

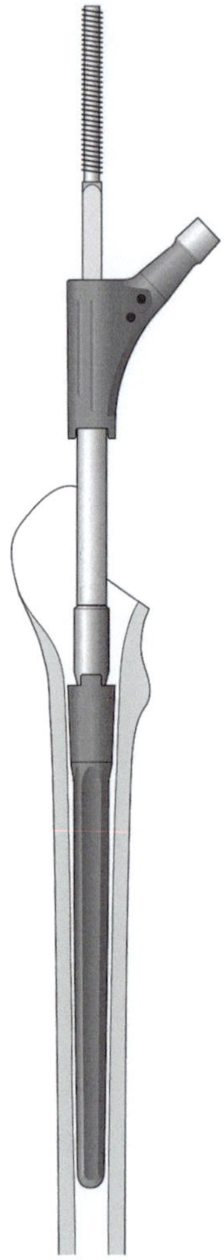

Fig. 16.42 Attaching the trial proximal component in situ to the final distal component. This combination is then used to perform a trial reduction with a trial head (with permission of Zimmer Biomet, Winterthur, Switzerland)

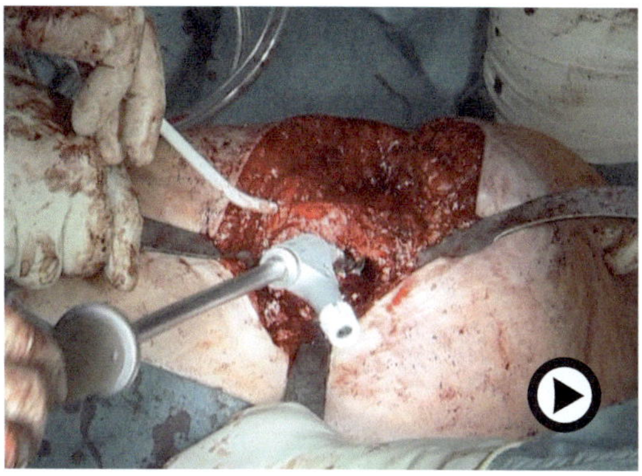

Fig. 16.43 (Video 16.11) In situ assembly of the proximal and final distal components (with permission of Zimmer Biomet, Winterthur, Switzerland) (▶ https://doi.org/10.1007/000-4q3)

only 1 or 2 mm is selected so that an appropriately well-positioned fixation zone is created for the stem in the residual isthmus and so that the distal locking screws can be placed distally to this (Fig. 16.45a, b).

The corresponding targeting guide for the placement of the distal locking screws is now attached to the implanted distal component, which, after careful impacting, has come to rest in the short fixation zone (Figs. 16.46 and 16.47 for Video 16.12). Subsequently, the corresponding locking screws are placed through the targeting guide (Figs. 16.48 and 16.49). The distal component of the stem should not be implanted with the targeting guide attached (as is the case

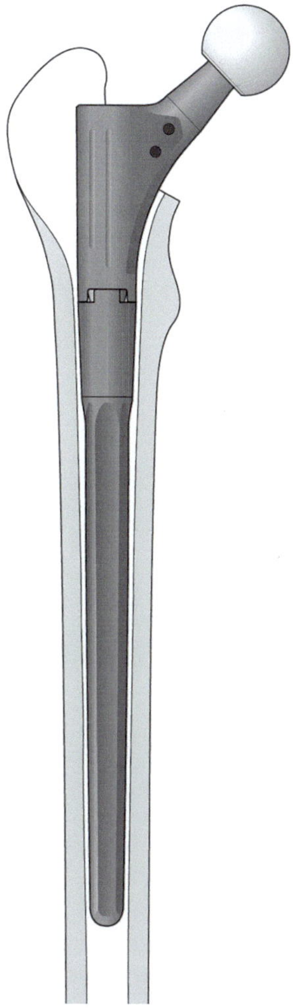

Fig. 16.44 In situ assembled final components (with permission of Zimmer Biomet, Winterthur, Switzerland)

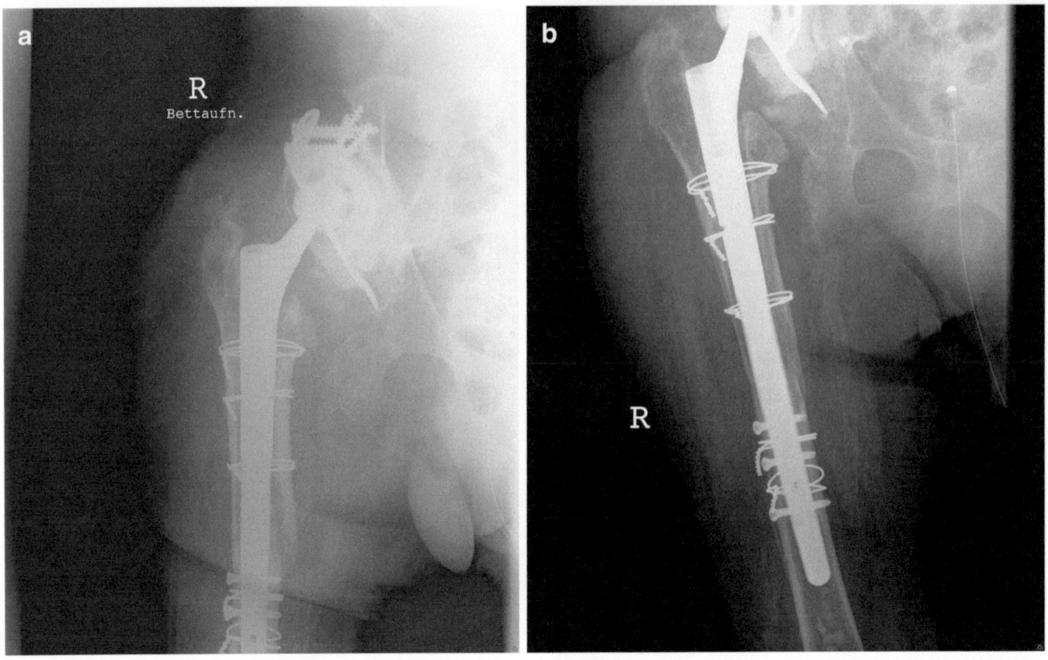

Fig. 16.45 (**a**) Postoperative radiograph after transfemoral stem revision because of a periprosthetic fracture with progression into the isthmus of the right femur. Due to this Vancouver B3 fracture with fractured isthmus, additional distal locking was carried out distal to the fracture and isthmus. (**b**) Radiograph 12 months postoperatively with unchanged position of the implants and consolidated periprosthetic fracture and osteotomy from the transfemoral approach

with an intramedullary nail), as this may cause deformation of the targeting guide during impaction and the corresponding screw holes will be misaligned. Some systems do not have a screw targeting guide (e.g., Prevision stem, Aesculap, Tuttlingen, Germany, or MUTARS RS, implantcast, Buxtehude, Germany). Here, distal locking must be performed using a fluoroscope. After distal locking of the distal component, the trial proximal component is fitted and a trial reduction is performed as described above.

After in situ assembly of the final proximal component, trial reduction with the trial head, and subsequent change to the selected final head, the transfemoral access is closed with double cerclages (double 1.5 cerclage wire) or cable systems and the wound is closed (Fig. 16.45a, b).

The following points should generally be checked before assembling the final prosthesis and its subsequent implantation:

(a) Is there perforation or infraction of the femur?

This can be checked with a probe. If necessary, one should check by means of fluoroscopy in 2 planes to be on the safe side.

(b) Is the selected prosthesis stem not too small? Otherwise, there is a risk of later subsidence. This can also be checked by fluoroscopy.

(c) Has premature three-point fixation occurred, e.g., due to the curvature of the proximal femur? In this case, using the distal fixation technique, there is no circular surface fixation of the stem in the isthmus and there is a risk of subsidence (Fig. 16.50). In addition, the three-point fixation at the tip of the prosthesis can lead to "stress cracks," which can become the starting point for a subsequent femur fracture. The fixation zones can be checked with the aid of the fluoroscope.

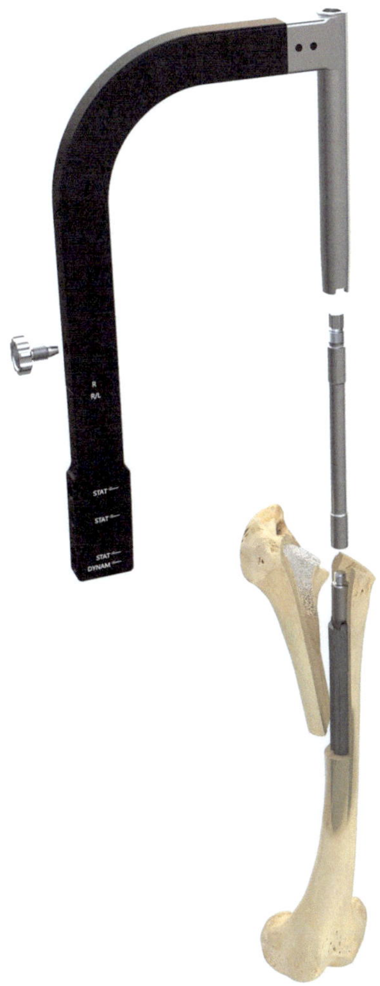

Fig. 16.46 Placement of the targeting guide on the transfemorally implanted distal component (with permission of Zimmer Biomet, Winterthur, Switzerland)

(d) Has the distal component been inserted with the correct rotation? Otherwise, in the case of a curved variant this can lead to the same complications as described under (c). In addition, depending on the stem, antetorsion may no longer be correctly adjusted and dislocation may result. This results in:

(e) Can the antetorsion of the proximal component be adjusted correctly or are there limitations because of incorrect positioning of the distal component that could promote hip dislocation? (Fig. 16.51).

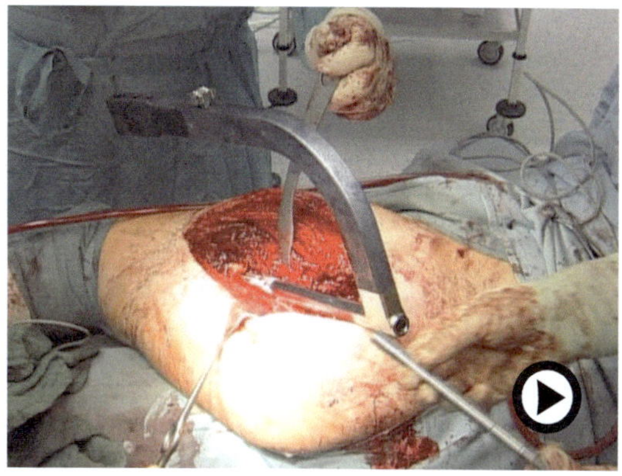

Fig. 16.47 (Video 16.12) Attachment of the targeting guide for distal locking (with permission of Zimmer Biomet, Winterthur, Switzerland). Positioning the alignment guide for distal locking (▶ https://doi.org/10.1007/000-4q4)

16.4 Comments on Surgical Descriptions or Assembly of Modular Stems

Some surgical descriptions describe other implantation techniques, such as tabletop assembly or use of proximal rasp systems. I cannot recommend either of these. Tabletop assembly, as mentioned above, turns a modular system into a nonmodular system, with all the resulting disadvantages of the need to achieve multiple surgical goals simultaneously in one surgical step (reliable implant fixation, correct leg length, anteversion, and offset). The advantage of in situ assembly is to take advantage of the modular design of the prosthesis and to perform the two tasks of revision surgery (implant fixation and restoration of leg length, offset, and antetorsion) in a stepwise manner, independently of each other. First, a reliable distal fixation is established with the distal component and, in the second step, the correct leg length and antetorsion and, if necessary, offset are adjusted with the proximal component.

Because of the force required, the use of proximal rasps carries a higher risk of unintentional fracture in the region of the greater trochanter compared to the careful use of manual hollow

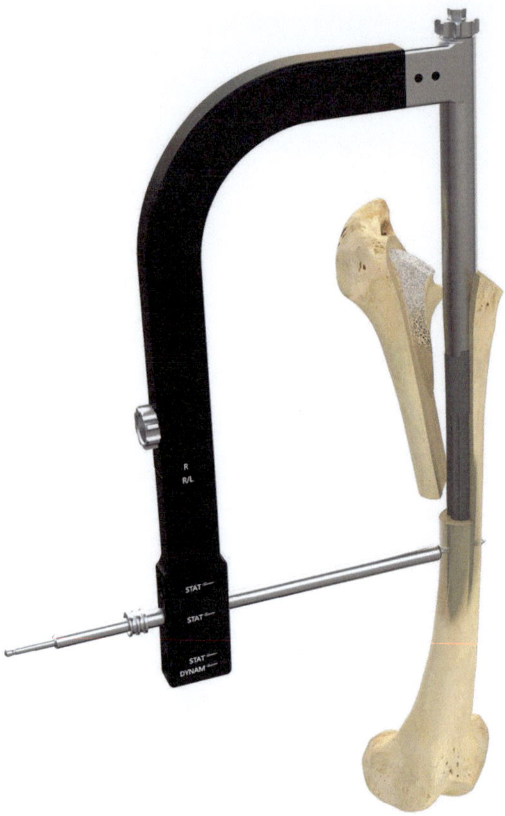

Fig. 16.48 Drilling the holes for the locking screws through the targeting guide. (With permission of Zimmer Biomet, Winterthur, Switzerland)

reamers. The same risk exists for monoblock prostheses, which, if inserted immediately after distal preparation, also pose an increased risk of fracture of the greater trochanter if adequate room has not previously been created for the

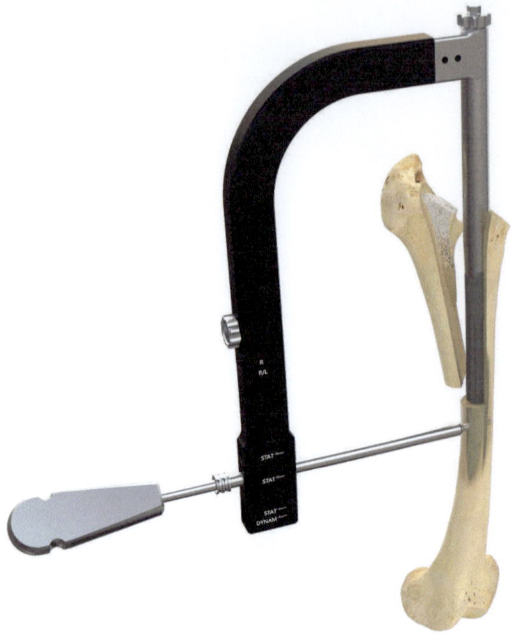

Fig. 16.49 Insertion of the distal locking screws. (With permission of Zimmer Biomet, Winterthur, Switzerland)

proximal portion by hollow reaming. This bone, which has to be removed from the greater trochanter with the hollow reamer, is the bone that prevents the distal placement of the stem due to the premature proximal contact when the modular components are assembled on the operating table. Subsidence of the stem will then occur later during weight bearing. Therefore, again, I recommend never performing a tabletop assembly of the modular components, but always an in situ assembly.

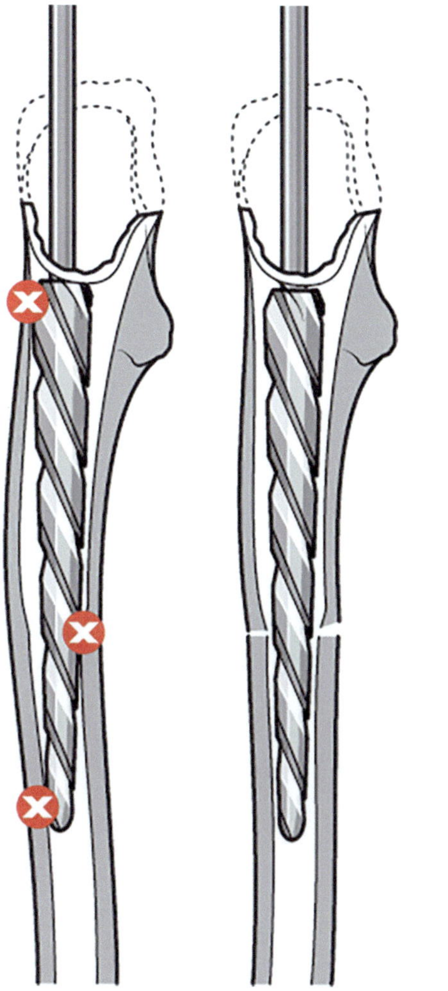

Fig. 16.50 Impending three-point fixation of a stem converted to distal surface fixation in the form of a cone-in-cone fixation by a transfemoral approach and/or a double osteotomy. (With permission of Zimmer Biomet, Winterthur, Switzerland)

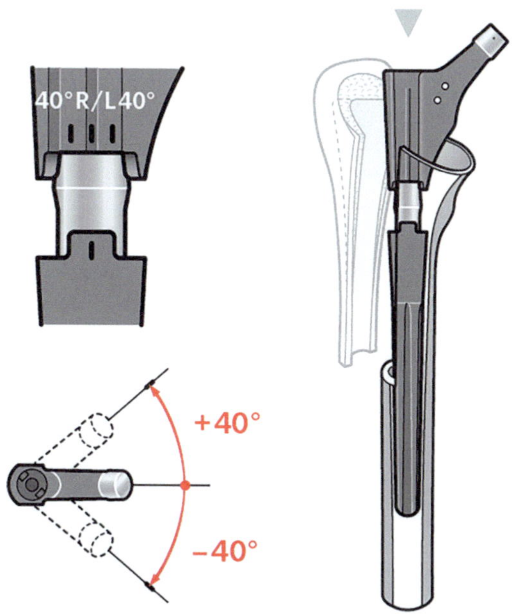

Fig. 16.51 Adjustment range of the proximal component with regard to antetorsion of the Revitan modular revision stem (Zimmer Biomet, Winterthur, Switzerland). (With permission of Zimmer Biomet, Winterthur, Switzerland)

References

1. Paprosky WG, Greidanus NV, Antoniou J. Minimum 10-year-results of extensively porous-coated stems in revision hip arthroplasty. Clin Orthop. 1999;369:230–42.
2. Weeden SH, Paprosky WG. Minimal 11-year follow-up of extensively porous-coated stems in femoral revision total hip arthroplasty. J Arthroplasty. 2002;17Suppl:134–7.
3. Mumme T, Müller-Rath R, Andereya S, Wirtz DC. Zementfreier Femurschaftwechsel in der Moularen Revisions Prothese MRP-Titan-Revisionsschaft. Oper Orthop Traumatol. 2007;19:56–77.
4. Wimmer MD, Randau TM, Deml MC, Ascherl R, Nöth U, Forst R, Gravius N, Wirtz D, Gravius S. Impaction grafting in femur in cementless modular revision total hip arthroplasty: a descriptive outcome analysis of 243 cases with the MRP-titan revision implant. BMC Musculoskelet Disord. 2013;14:19.
5. Lanting B, Naudie DD, McCalden RW. Clinical impact of trunnion wear after total hip arthroplasty. JBJS Rev. 2016;4:e3.
6. MacDonald DW, Chen AF, Lee GC, Klein GR, Mont MA, Kurtz SM, Taper Corrosion Writing Committee, Cates HE, Kraay MJ, Rimnac CM. Fretting and corrosion damage in taper adapter sleeves for ceramic heads: a retrieval study. J Arthroplasty. 2017;32:2887–91.

Necessary Length of the Revision Stems

17

Content

References 244

The required length of a revision stem depends on several factors, namely

1. The bone defect: In simple terms, the larger the defect, the greater the length of the stem required. While Paprosky I defects can be treated with standard stems and Paprosky II defects with lengthened standard stems or proximal fixation revision stems with a slightly greater length than standard stems, the distal fixation stems for Paprosky IIIA defects must extend at least into the isthmus, where they are then fixed (Fig. 17.1a, b). For Paprosky IIIB and IV defects, the stems must extend beyond the isthmus of the femur, with either additional fixation below the isthmus by locking (e.g., Revitan Curved, MPR stem) or by cementing (Link MP stem) (Fig. 17.2a, b), or by profiting from their greater taper to provide a short fixation zone in the isthmus above the level of the tip of the stem (e.g., ZMR stem) (Fig. 17.3a, b).
2. The type of fixation principle used: As already explained in Chap. 7 different fixation principles result in different minimum fixation zones. In the case of cylinder-in-cylinder fixation of an extensively porous-coated stem, this is 4 cm. Cone-in-cone fixation of a 2-degree tapered stem requires at least 3 cm, and in the case of a 3.5-degree tapered stem, if the bone in the fixation zone is sound, the length of the zone can be reduced to 2 cm (see Chaps. 7 and 8). In the case of the 2-degree tapered stem, this fixation zone may be located at the tip of the stem or distal component (Figs. 17.1a, b, 17.3a, and 17.4b, c). But in the case of the 3.5-degree tapered stem, the greater taper means that it can only be located above the tip (Fig. 17.3b). Thus, if the revision stems have a greater taper, and all else is equal, this automatically leads to an implantation of a longer stem.
3. The taper of the revision stem used: As already mentioned, in the case of a 2-degree tapered stem, the stem can be anchored at the tip in the isthmus of the femur. Thus, the revision stem can be short. The greater the taper of the stem, the further proximal the region where the stem cuts into the cortex of the isthmus to create the cone-in-cone fixation (Figs. 7.2 and 7.11a, b). As a result, with increasing taper the stem automatically becomes longer and the fixation zone in the isthmus remains the same.

B. Fink, *Femoral Revision Arthroplasty*, https://doi.org/10.1007/978-3-030-84821-7_17

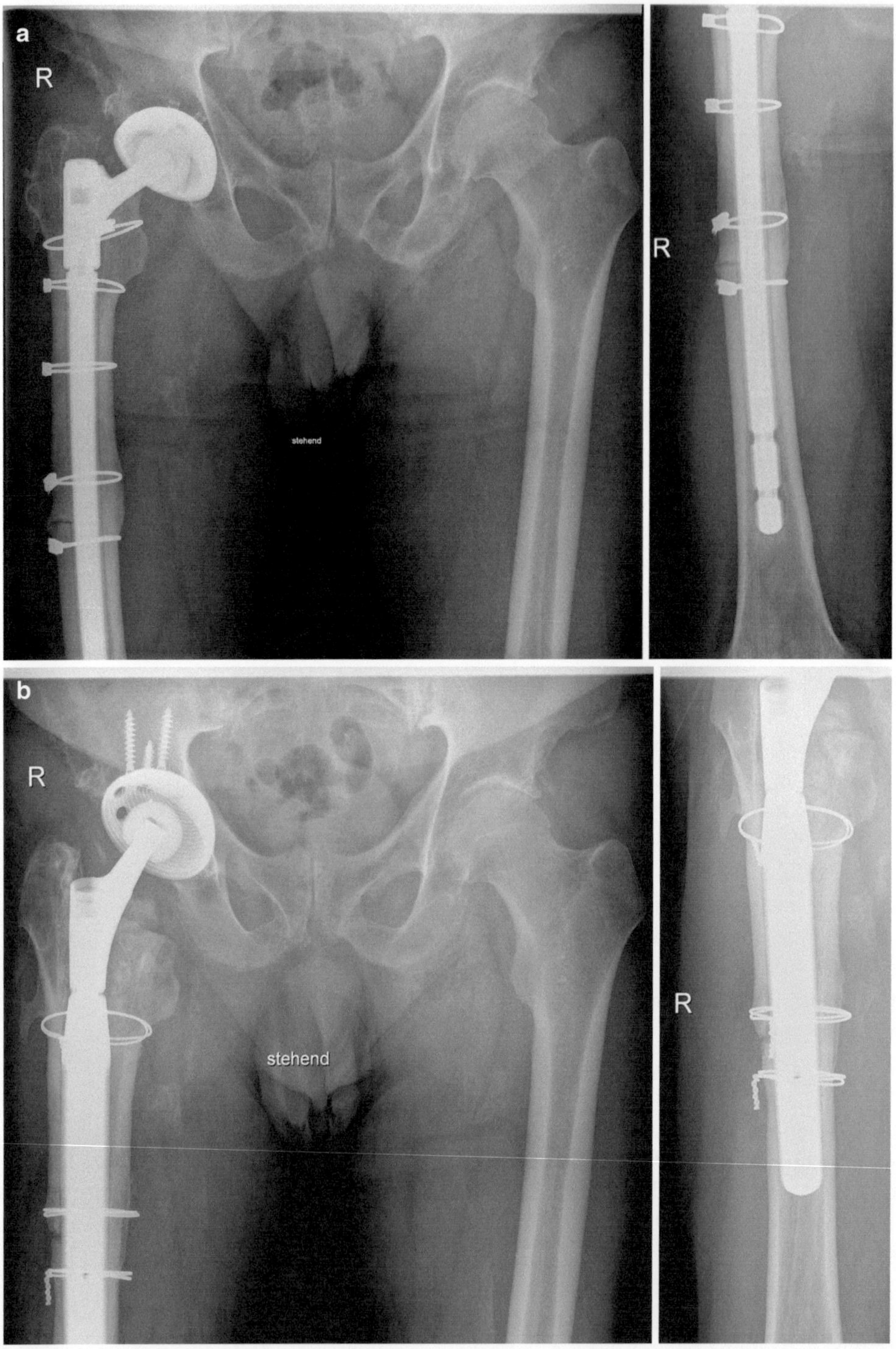

Fig. 17.1 (**a**) A loose modular revision stem that is too thin and too long after extramural transfemoral implantation 6 months previously. The patient complained of pain in the thigh during weight-bearing and rotational movements. (**a1**) Pelvic overview radiograph. (**a2**) A.p. radiograph of the distal femur. Radiolucency can be seen around the stem. (**b**) Radiographs 6 months after transfemoral prosthesis revision to a shorter and thicker modular revision stem Revitan Curved, and a press-fit cup Allofit-S following intraoperative observation of movement of the cup (Zimmer Biomet, Winterthur, Switzerland). Osteointegration of the implants is evident. (**b1**) Pelvic overview radiograph. (**b2**) A.p. radiograph of the thigh

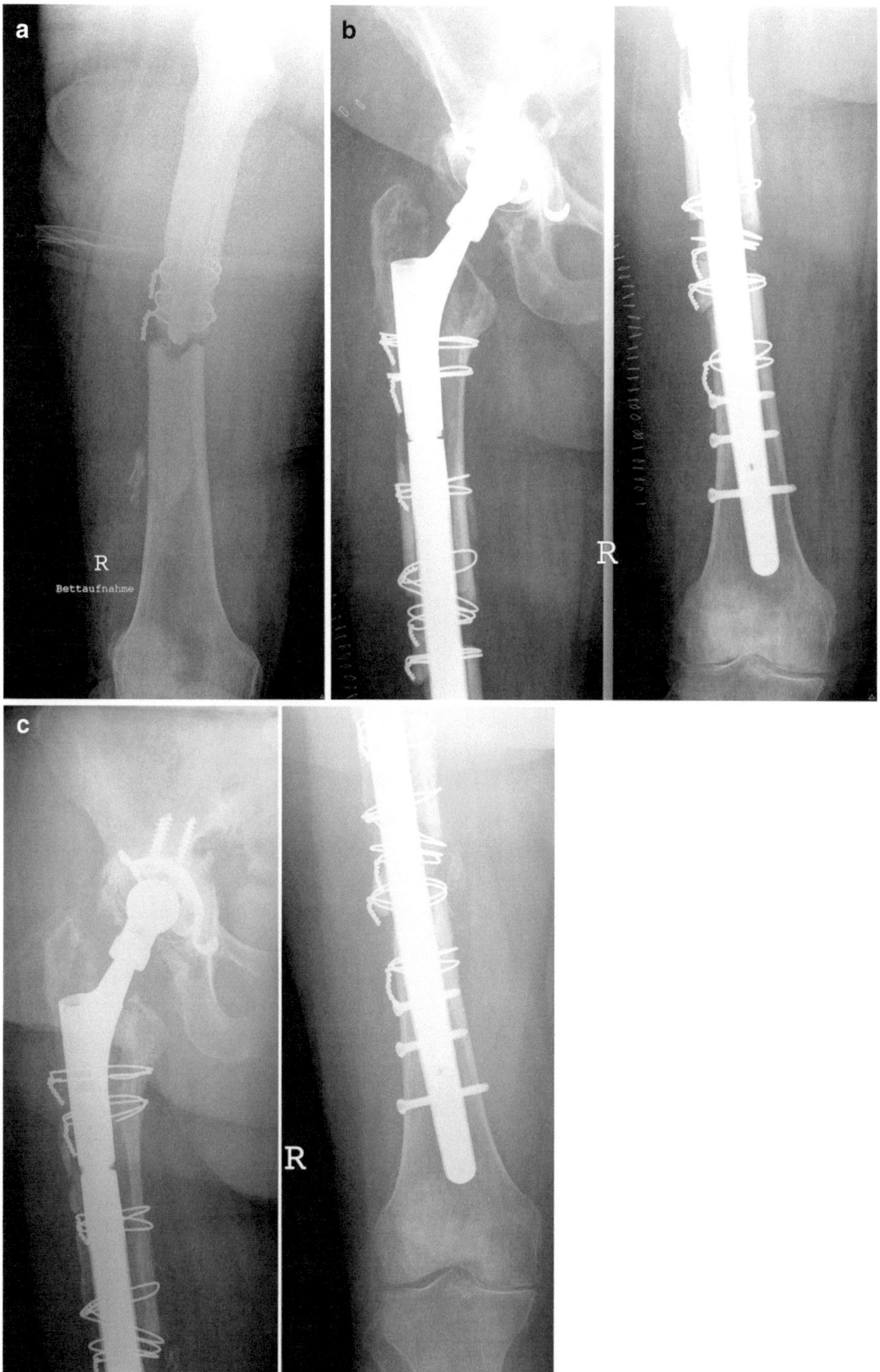

Fig. 17.2 (**a**) Periprosthetic fracture after extramural stem revision with a cemented revision prosthesis and a window at the level of the stem tip and a long distal, firmly seated cement plug. (**b**) Radiograph 7 days following transfemoral stem revision to a modular revision stem Revitan Curved (Zimmer Biomet, Winterthur, Switzerland) with distal locking because of the short region of intact isthmus (<3 cm) (Paprosky type IIIB defect). (**c**) Radiograph 6 months after surgery with consolidation of the osteotomy flap and bone regeneration proximally and medially

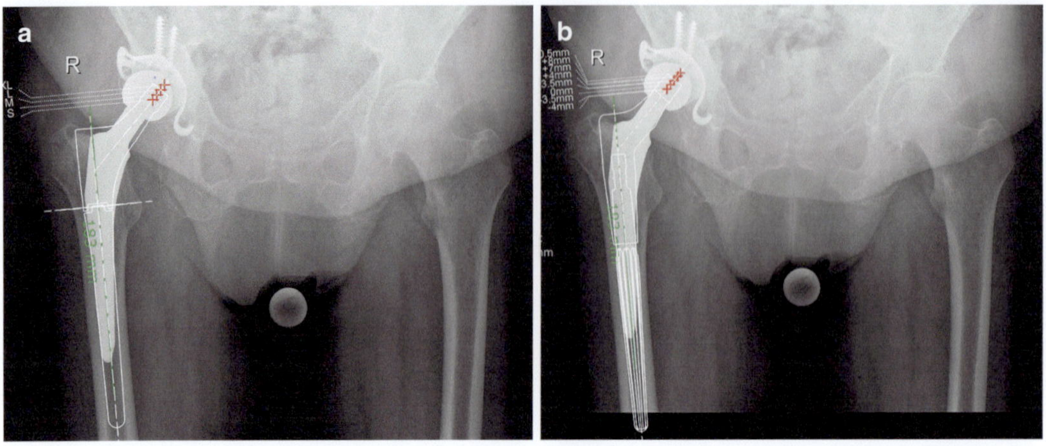

Fig. 17.3 (**a**) Planning the stem revision with 2-degree tapered modular revision stem Revitan Curved (Zimmer Biomet, Winterthur, Switzerland). (**b**) Planning the stem revision with 3.5-degree tapered modular revision stem ZMR (Zimmer Biomet, Warsaw, IN, USA). Because of the greater taper, the fixation zone is above the tip of the stem, which means that the combined stem length is greater than the Revitan stem

4. The thickness and quality of the remaining cortical bone in the fixation zone: The thinner the cortical bone, the higher the risk of fracture and the less aggressive the preparation of the conical fixation bed by the surgeon. In this case, the only way to achieve sufficient fixation is by means of an extended region of contact of the prosthetic stem with the bone, which leads to longer revision stems (see Chap. 7) (Figs. 17.4a–c and 17.5a, b).

In general, the revision stem should be as short as possible. This guideline is based on the following reasoning:

1. In the case of an intact isthmus, fixation can be achieved at the tip of the stem (with a 2-degree tapered stem) (Figs. 17.1b and 17.4b, c). This avoids traversing the isthmus of the femur with the revision stem, thus reducing the risk of unintentional periprosthetic fractures. Especially, when using straight revision stems, implantation beyond the isthmus in the curved femur can lead to ventral contact of the stem with the cortex, thus increasing the risk of periprosthetic fracture. Periprosthetic fractures associated with long, straight revision prostheses have been described in two-digit percentages in some reports (Tables 6.5, 6.8, and 6.9 in Chap. 6). In contrast, no periprosthetic fractures were observed in two of our own studies with consistent use of the shortest distal component (140 mm) and an intact isthmus [1, 2].
2. In the event of a further revision becoming necessary (e.g., because of a periprosthetic infection), the use of short revision stems has the advantage that they can be revised more easily than long, osseointegrated revision stems. Equally, in the event of a transfemoral access than being necessary, there is an opportunity to remove the revision stem without completely exposing the isthmus. This has the advantage that when the new stem is implanted using a two-stage procedure, there is still an adequate fixation zone in the isthmus.
3. Concurrent implantation of a stemmed knee endoprosthesis does not result in only a short stretch of metal-free bone between the ends of the two implants. This reduces the risk of interprosthetic fracture (type D in the united classification system [3]).
4. If the isthmus is intact, shorter distal components of 2° tapered modular distal fixation revision stems can usually be implanted. This

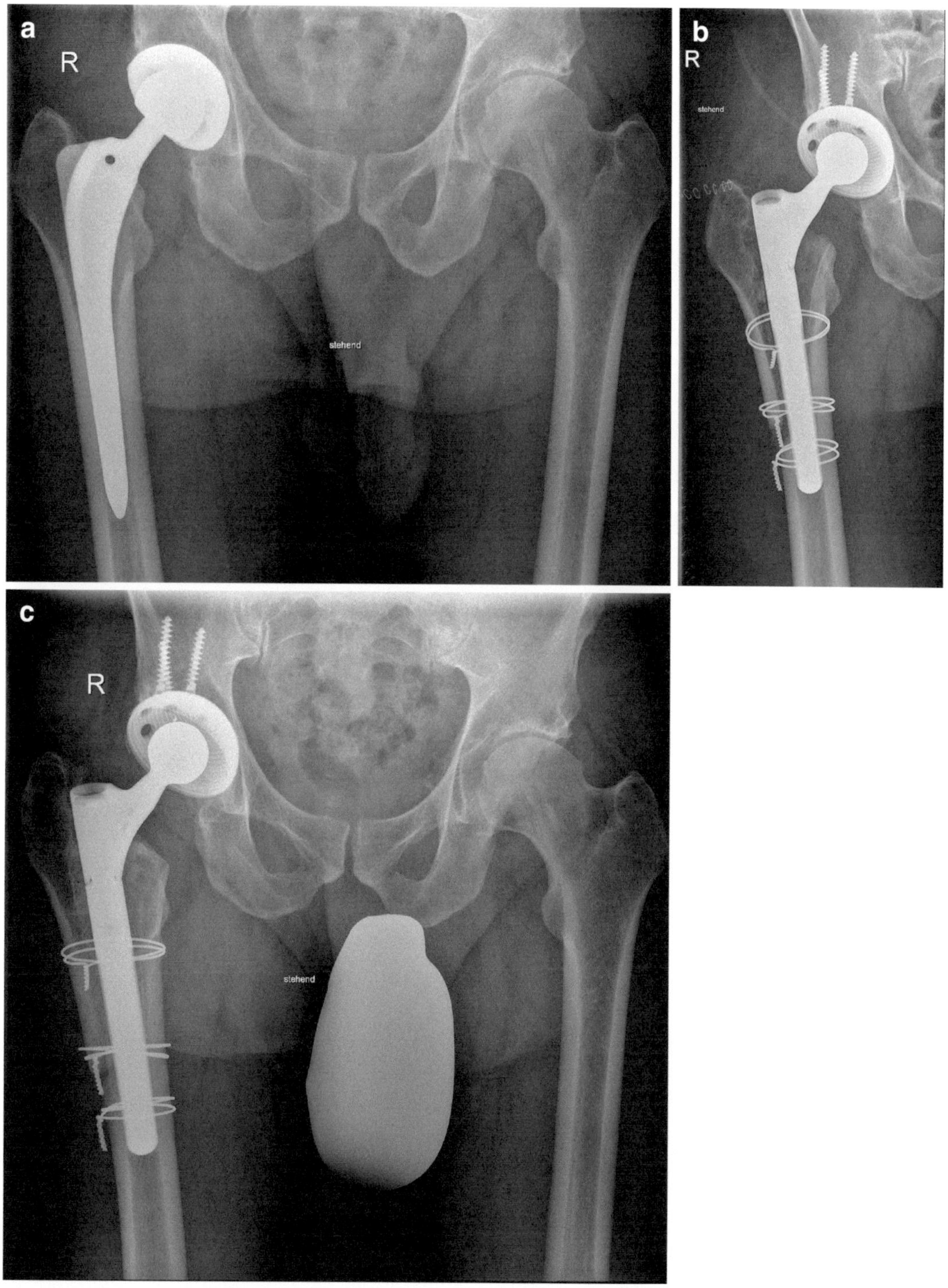

Fig. 17.4 (**a**) Preoperative radiograph of a cementless, firmly fixed prosthesis with periprosthetic late-stage infection. A two-stage septic revision was performed using a transfemoral approach at each stage. (**b**) Radiograph 10 days after transfemoral reimplantation of a modular revision stem Revitan Curved and a cementless press-fit cup Allofit-S (Zimmer Biomet, Winterthur, Switzerland). Because of the thick cortical bone, a shortened fixation zone can be achieved in the isthmus of the femur at the level of the tip of the stem. (**c**) Radiograph 2 years after surgery. Unchanged position of the implants and consolidation of the osteotomy

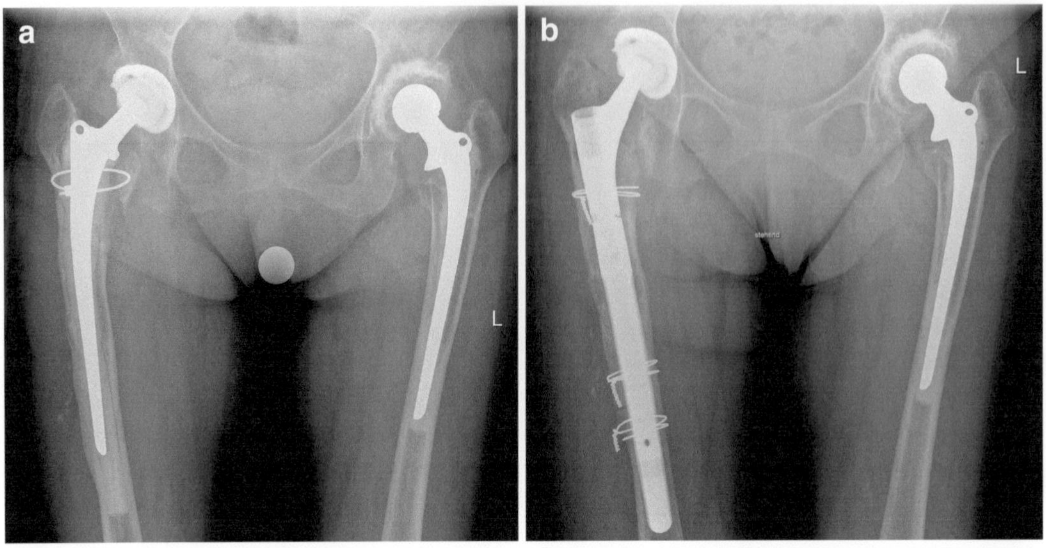

Fig. 17.5 (**a**) Loosened long cemented revision stem with relatively thin cortical bone in the isthmus of the femur in Paprosky type IIIA bone defect. (**b**) Radiograph 3 months after transfemoral revision to a modular revision stem Revitan Curved (Zimmer Biomet, Winterthur, Switzerland). The fixation zone in the distal isthmus is longer than in the previous example because the thinner cortex requires a longer stem to be implanted in the isthmus (Fig. 12.4a–c)

results in the mechanically weakest point of the modular revision endoprosthesis, the junction, being located further distally in the femur and thus gaining medial bone support. This localization with medial support of the junction prevents the rare, but nevertheless possible, fracture of the junction [4].

In an analysis of 202 Revitan Curved prostheses (Zimmer Biomet, Winterthur, Switzerland) implanted in an intact isthmus (58 Paprosky type II and 146 type IIIA defects) (62 endofemoral and 140 transfemoral including 38 Vancouver B2 periprosthetic fractures), 96.8% of endofemoral and 97.8% of transfemoral implanted stems utilized the shortest distal component of 140 mm [2, 5, 6]. Figure 17.6 shows the distribution of stem lengths used in this study [2].

Within the mean follow-up period of 7.44 ± 2.09 years (3–13 years), 3.3% (2 patients) of the endofemorally implanted stems and 2.1% (2 patients) of the transfemorally implanted stems showed a nonprogressive stem subsidence of more than 5 mm. The fixation lengths of the two endofemorally implanted stems (the sum of the two distal fixation lengths in the radiograph) were 5.2 and 6 cm, and that of the transfemorally implanted stems 3 cm in both cases. Loosening was not seen in any of the 202 cases in the study [2].

Thus, we were able to show that in the case of an intact isthmus, i.e., defect types of Paprosky II and IIIA, shorter stem combinations with the short distal component of 140 mm length (when using the Revitan system (ZimmerBiomet, Winterthur, Switzerland)) can regularly be used and that reproducibly good results can be achieved with respect to the incidence of aseptic loosening, subsidence of the stem, and periprosthetic fracture. The use of longer stems does not result in a longer fixation zone in cone-in-cone fixation, but rather in a fixation zone of the same length as shorter stems, but higher up, above the tip of the stem (Fig. 17.7). The subsidence rate of 2.5% and aseptic loosening rate of 0% in that study are in the range of the best outcomes in publications on modular revision stems, where usually significantly longer tapered revision stems were used [7–12]. This corresponds to the observations of de Menezes et al. [13], who were able to show with 100 straight Revitan stems

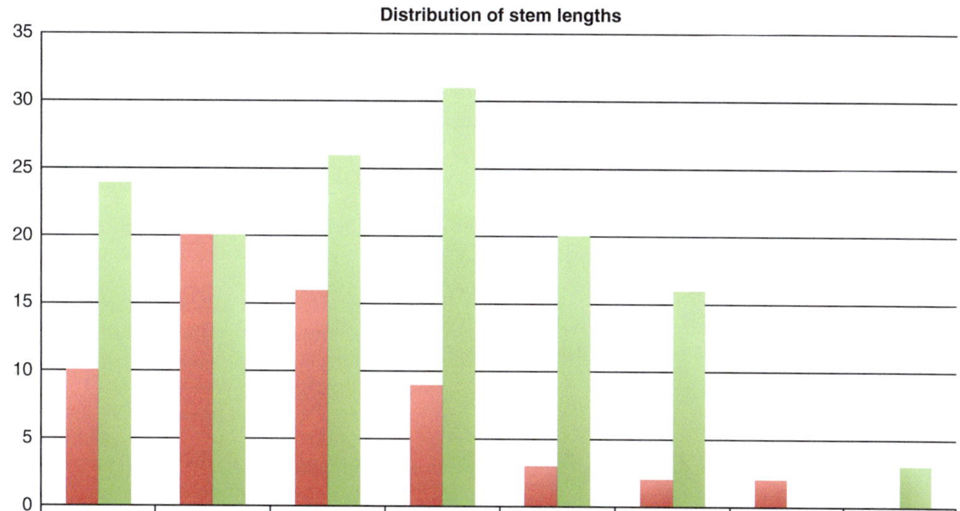

	195	205	215	225	235	245	255	265
endofemoral	10	20	16	9	3	2	2	
transfemoral	24	20	26	31	20	16		3

Fig. 17.6 Distribution of stem lengths used in a study of 202 implanted Revitan Curved prostheses

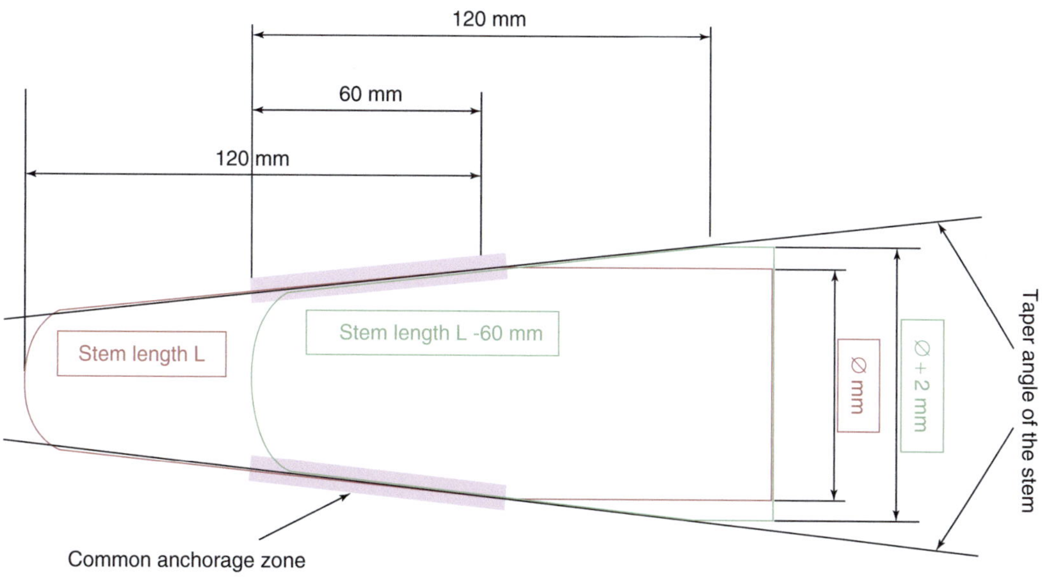

Fig. 17.7 Fixation zone of a shorter stem compared to that of a longer one

implanted via a transfemoral approach that the subsidence rate was significantly lower with short stems with fixation at the tip of the prosthetic stem than with longer stems. Thus, the use of short revision stems resulted in at least similarly low rates of subsidence and loosening as compared to long revision stems. Conversely, the use of long revision stems offers no advantages but only disadvantages (high risk of unintentional periprosthetic fractures).

However, if the isthmus of the femur no longer has a sufficiently long intact fixation zone for the planned revision stem (Paprosky type IIIB and IV defects), distal locking may be used as an additional fixation method for some stems (e.g., Revitan Curved, Zimmer Biomet, Winterthur, Switzerland; MRP stem, Peter Brehm, Weisendorf, Germany; Prevision stem, Aesculap, Tuttlingen, Germany). This distal locking is located below the isthmus of the femur. Therefore, long revision stems with the longer distal components must be used for Paprosky type IIIB and IV defects. Here, the weaker the cortex below the isthmus, the longer the stem has to be in order to ensure a sufficiently long intramedullary seating of the stem (Fig. 17.2b, c).

References

1. Fink B, Urbansky K, Schuster P. Mid term results with the curved modular tapered, fluted titanium Revitan stem in revision hip replacement. Bone Joint J. 2014;96-B(7):889–95.
2. Fink B, Buntenbroich U, Oremek D. Fixation of a modular curved revision stem with a taper of two degrees in the femur. Arch Orthop Trauma Surg. 2019;139:127–33.
3. Duncan CP, Haddad FS. The unified classification system (UCS): improving our understanding of periprosthetic fractures. Bone Joint J. 2014;96-B:713–6.
4. Fink B. What can the surgeon do to reduce the risk of junction breakage of modular revision stems. Arthroplasty Today. 2018;31:306–9.
5. Paprosky WG, Lawrence J, Cameron H. Femoral defect classification. Clin Appl Orthop Rev. 1990;19(Suppl):9–15.
6. Paprosky WG, Greidanus NV, Antoniou J. Minimum 10-year results of extensively porous-coated stems in revision hip arthroplasty. Clin Orthop Relat Res. 1999;369:230–42.
7. Artiaco S, Boggio F, Titolo P, Zoccola K, Bianchi R, Bellomo F. Clinical experience in femoral revision with the modular Profemur R stem. Hip Int. 2011;21:39–42.
8. Köster G, Wald TA, Willert HG. Five- to 10-year results using a noncemented modular revision stem without bone grafting. J Arthroplast. 2008;23:964–70.
9. Kwong LM, Miller AJ, Lubinus P. A modular distal fixation option for proximal bone loss in revision total hip arthroplasty. A 2- to 6-year follow-up study. J Arthroplast. 2003;18:94–7.
10. Pattyn C, Mulliez A, Verdonk R, Audenaert E. Revision hip arthroplasty using a cementless modular tapered stem. Int Orthop. 2012;36:35–41.
11. Wirtz DC, Heller KD, Holzwarth U, Siebert C, Pitto RP, Zeiler G, Blencke BA, Forst R. A modular femoral implant for uncemented stem revision in THR. Int Orthop. 2000;24:134–8.
12. van Houwelingen AP, Duncan CP, Masri BA, Greidanus NV, Garbuz DS. High survival of modular tapered stems for proximal femoral bone defects at 5 to 10 years follow-up. Clin Orthop Relat Res. 2013;471:454–62.
13. De Menezes DFA, Le Béguec P, Sieber H-P, Goldschild M. Stem and osteotomy length are critical for success of the transfemoral approach and cementless stem revision. Clin Orthop Relat Res. 2012;470:883–8.

Stem Revision in Periprosthetic Fractures

18

Contents

18.1 **Principles of Stem Revision in Periprosthetic Fractures** 246
18.2 **Treatment of Vancouver Type B2 Fractures (UCS Type IV.3-B2)** 250
18.3 **Treatment of Vancouver Type B3 Fractures (USC Type IV.3-B3)** 251
18.4 **Surgical Techniques of Revision Prostheses in Periprosthetic Fractures** 251
18.5 **Failed Osteosynthesis of Vancouver B1 Fractures (UCS Type IV.3-B1)** 254
References 257

Periprosthetic fractures of the femur are a relatively rare but difficult to treat complication of total hip arthroplasty. Numerous classifications for periprosthetic fractures can be found in the literature. The so-called Vancouver classification originally presented by Duncan et al. [1] has become generally accepted and has been integrated into and extended by the UCS (unified classification system) of periprosthetic fractures [2].

The goals of treatment of periprosthetic fractures are early fracture healing, preservation or reconstruction of the bone, restoration of correct bone alignment and length, stable prosthetic fixation, early mobilization, and restoration of leg function that should be equal to or better than that prior to the fracture [3–6]. The gluteal musculature in particular is of decisive importance for function, so that the protection of this musculature and the vasto-gluteal sling is beneficial and the preservation of the trochanter major is essential.

In the case of a periprosthetic fracture, it is necessary to exchange the prosthesis if it is loosened (Vancouver type B2 and B3 fractures) or if the implants are also fractured (Fig. 18.1) [1, 2, 4–9]. According to the study by Bethea et al. [10], 75% of postoperative periprosthetic fractures involved loosened prosthetic stems, and in the Swedish Prosthesis Registry, 555 (53%) of 1049 periprosthetic femoral fractures were of type B2 and 43 (4.1%) of type B3 [11]. According to Lindahl et al. [12], 51–66% of patients with a periprosthetic fracture exhibited a loose stem. According to Duncan and colleagues [1], 82% of type B fractures in their study had loosened implants, while Abdel et al. [13] and Lindahl et al. [11] reported in more than 70% Vancouver type B2 and B3 fractures (75% reported by Lindahl [11]).

B. Fink, *Femoral Revision Arthroplasty*, https://doi.org/10.1007/978-3-030-84821-7_18

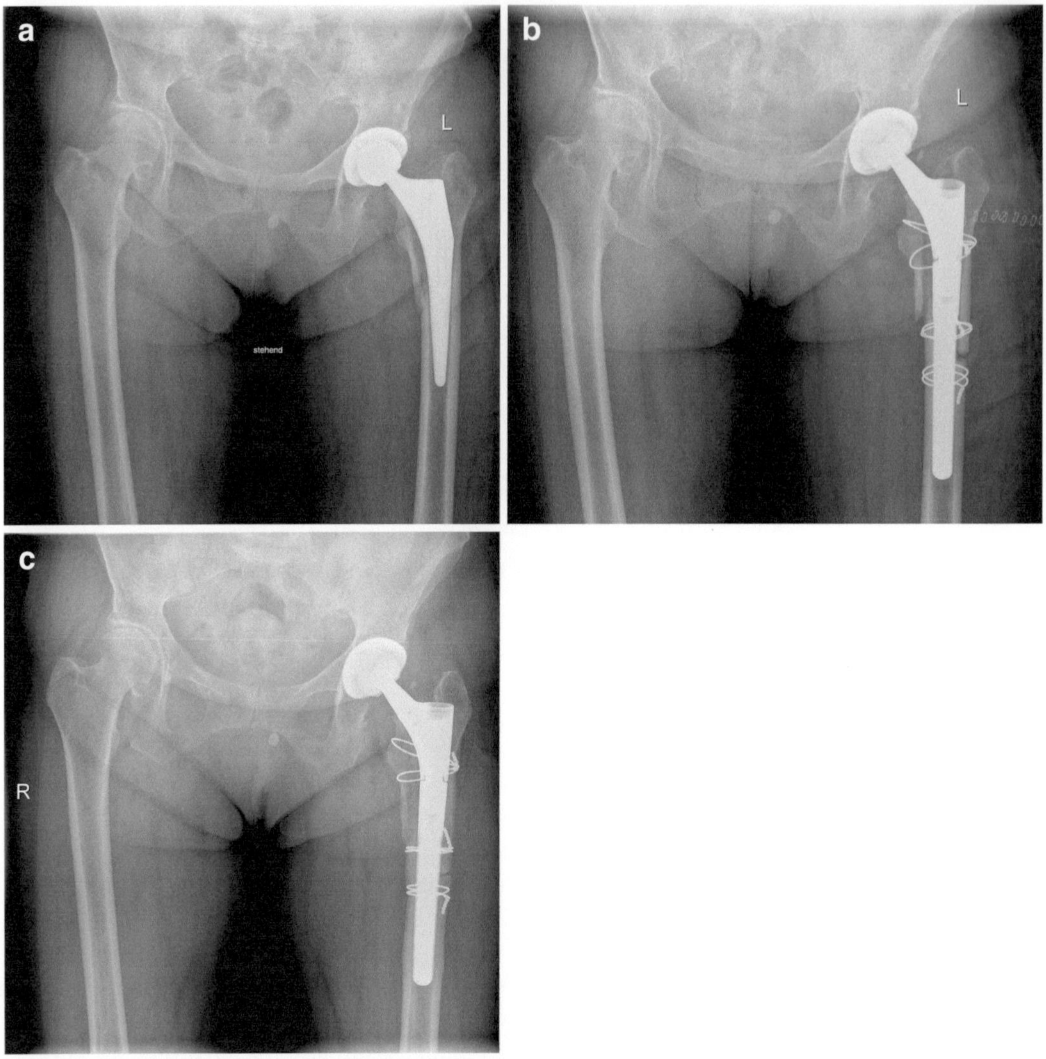

Fig. 18.1 (**a**) Periprosthetic Vancouver type B2 fracture with subsided cementless stem. (**b**) Radiograph 7 days after transfemoral stem revision with a modular revision stem Revitan Curved (Zimmer Biomet, Winterthur, Switzerland). (**c**) Radiograph 6 months after surgery showing complete consolidation of the fracture and osteo-integration of the stem

18.1 Principles of Stem Revision in Periprosthetic Fractures

In principle, prosthesis revision can be performed with either cemented or cementless stems. Although, as Beals et al. [3] have shown, cemented stems can be used, they have the disadvantage that intrusion of cement into the fracture gap can impede healing of the fracture (Fig. 18.2). Moreover, the interdigitation of the cement and thereby the quality of cementation are reduced in cases of periprosthetic fractures (Fig. 18.2). For example, Beals et al. [3] found nonunion in 31% of revisions with cemented stems, renewed fractures in 15%, and persistent bone defects in a further 15%, whereas revision with cementless stems showed renewed fractures in only 7%. Springer et al. [14] observed that only 60% of 42 patients with type B2 and B3 fractures treated with a cemented long stem had a stable implant

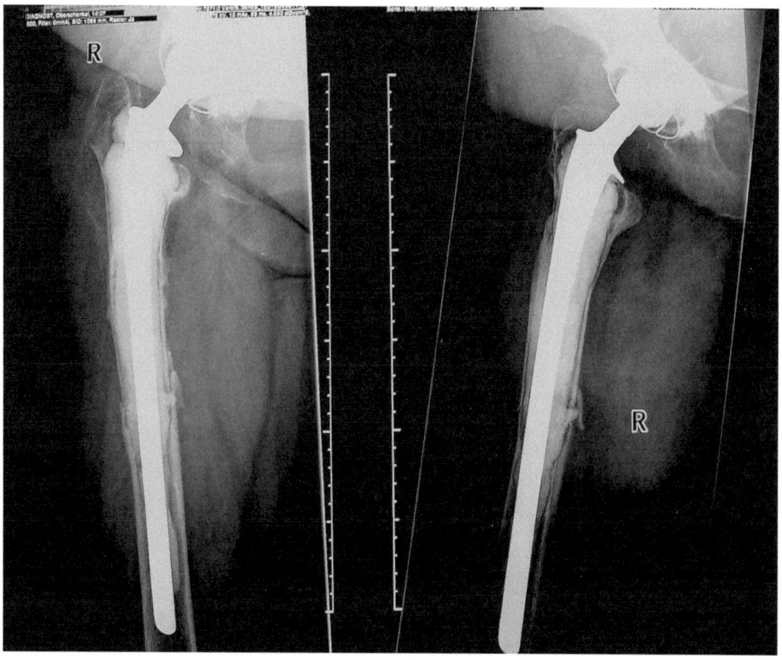

Fig. 18.2 Radiograph 6 months after stem revision ex domo with a long cemented revision stem in a case of a Vancouver type B2 periprosthetic fracture with cement leakage in the fracture area

with a healed fracture after an average of 68 months. Six patients underwent revision due to loosening, nonunion, or dislocation and two patients due to infection. 18% of the unrevised stems showed radiographic evidence of loosening. Therefore, an exchange with cemented stems is recommended only in exceptional cases in elderly patients and/or osteoporotic bones that make cementless fixation impossible [3, 15–17].

Thus, cementless stem revision is the standard procedure for Vancouver B2 and B3 fractures. Cementless implants are classified into those that achieve primary anchorage in the proximal femur and those with distal fixation. The disadvantage of the first mentioned prosthesis types in periprosthetic fractures is that their fixation zone is in the unstable fracture region. In these cases, movement between the proximal fracture fragments and the prosthesis may hinder the bony incorporation of the implant [18]. Therefore, the use of these stems in isolation in periprosthetic fractures does not yield reproducibly good results [19]. To improve proximal stability, these prosthesis types are usually combined with a strut graft in cases of periprosthetic fracture. Nevertheless, Incavo et al. [18] reported 50% stem loosening in normally healed periprosthetic fractures. Other authors, however, did not observe these problems [20, 21]. Overall, however, the case numbers in all the studies mentioned are small (fewer than 10 cases each) so reliable conclusions cannot therefore be drawn (Table 18.1).

Cementless prostheses with distal fixation have the advantage that the prosthesis anchorage is achieved distally to the fracture area, thus bridging the fracture with the fixation zone. The fracture fragments are bound with cerclages around the distally fixed prosthesis and thereby get an osteosynthesis. This technique appears to be a reliable way of achieving good outcomes, as shown by the studies published to date (Fig. 18.1a–c).

The new implant must provide a sufficiently long bridge across the entire fracture. Earlier data indicated that the fracture should be bridged with at least twice the stem diameter [1, 7–9]. As a general rule, the length of the required bridge will depend on the type of fixation of the distal stem and the quality of the bone below the fracture. A cylindrical stem implanted with scratch-fit fixation requires a minimum fixation distance of 4 cm [22]. Since the fixation distance could be at the tip of the stem, the fracture zone must be bridged by a stem long enough to ensure a

Table 18.1 Outcomes of prosthesis revisions for periprosthetic fractures

Author	*N*	Vancouver type	Follow-up	Healing rate	Loosening	Complications
Wang [21]	6 PC + SG	B2, B3	6 months	100%	0%	0%
Sledge III [20]	7 PC + SG	B2	33 months	100%	0%	0%
Incavo [18]	8 PC + SG	B2	49 months	100%	50%	12.5% #
	5 EPC	B2	49 months	100%	0%	0%

AG allograft, *PC* + *SG* proximal coated with strut grafts, proximal fixation, *EPC* extensively porous-coated, distal fixation, # fracture

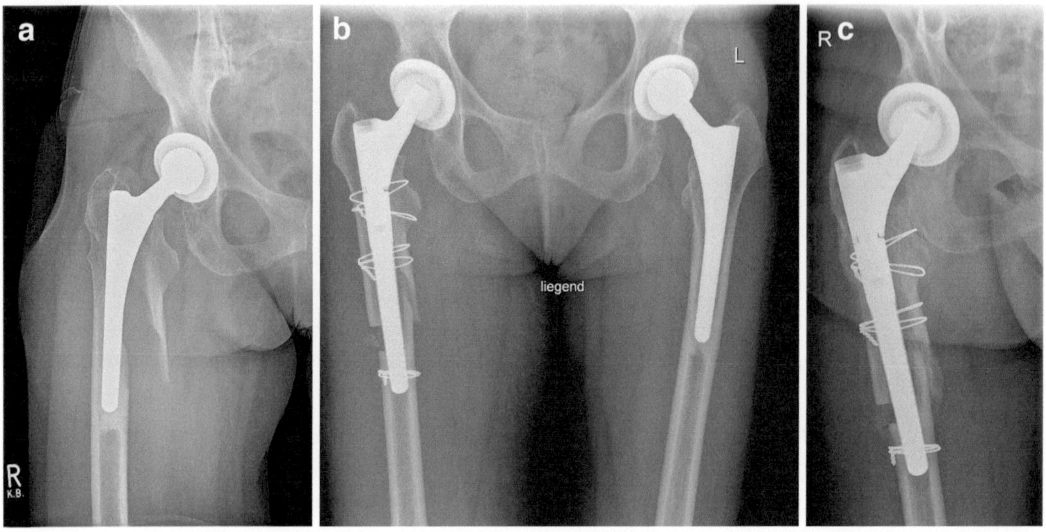

Fig. 18.3 (**a**) Periprosthetic Vancouver type B2 fracture of a cementless stem with an unstable fixation detected intraoperatively. (**b**) Postoperative radiograph after transfemoral prosthesis revision with the modular revision stem Revitan Curved (Zimmer Biomet, Winterthur, Switzerland). The fixation zone at the tip of the stem in the isthmus of the femur is only 3 cm. Due to the sound cortical bone, this short cone-in-cone fixation is sufficient for adequate stability. (**c**) Radiograph 6 months after surgery shows complete bony consolidation of the fracture and osteointegration of the stem

minimum fixation distance of 4 cm in the isthmus. A minimum fixation distance of 3 cm is required when using a 2-degree tapered stem with distal cone-in-cone fixation [23]. This can also be at the tip of the stem, so that the same principle applies as mentioned above, but with a distance of 3 cm instead of 4 cm (Fig. 18.3a–c). If a tapered stem with a greater taper angle is used and the isthmus of the femur has a sound cortex, the fixation zone can be as little as 2 cm according to the studies of Tangsataporn et al. [24]. However, the taper angle of these stems means that the fixation zone is not at the tip but above the tip, so the position of the fixation zone together with the more distal portion of the stem determines the minimum bridging length of the fracture with such a stem. The general prerequisite for a shorter bridging length is sufficient stability of the bone below the fracture (Fig. 18.3a–c). If this is not the case, the fracture must be bridged with a longer stem. This longer stem is then thinner than the abovementioned configurations, but is fixed in the same place in the femur as the shorter, thicker prosthetic stems. Particularly in Vancouver B3 fractures, involving a thin cortical bone that corresponds to a Paprosky type IV bone defect, a long revision stem with additional distal interlocking must be implanted, since a sufficient cone-in-cone fixation in the isthmus can no longer be achieved (Fig. 18.4a–c).

Another treatment option is the so-called distal locking. Here, the fracture area is bridged with

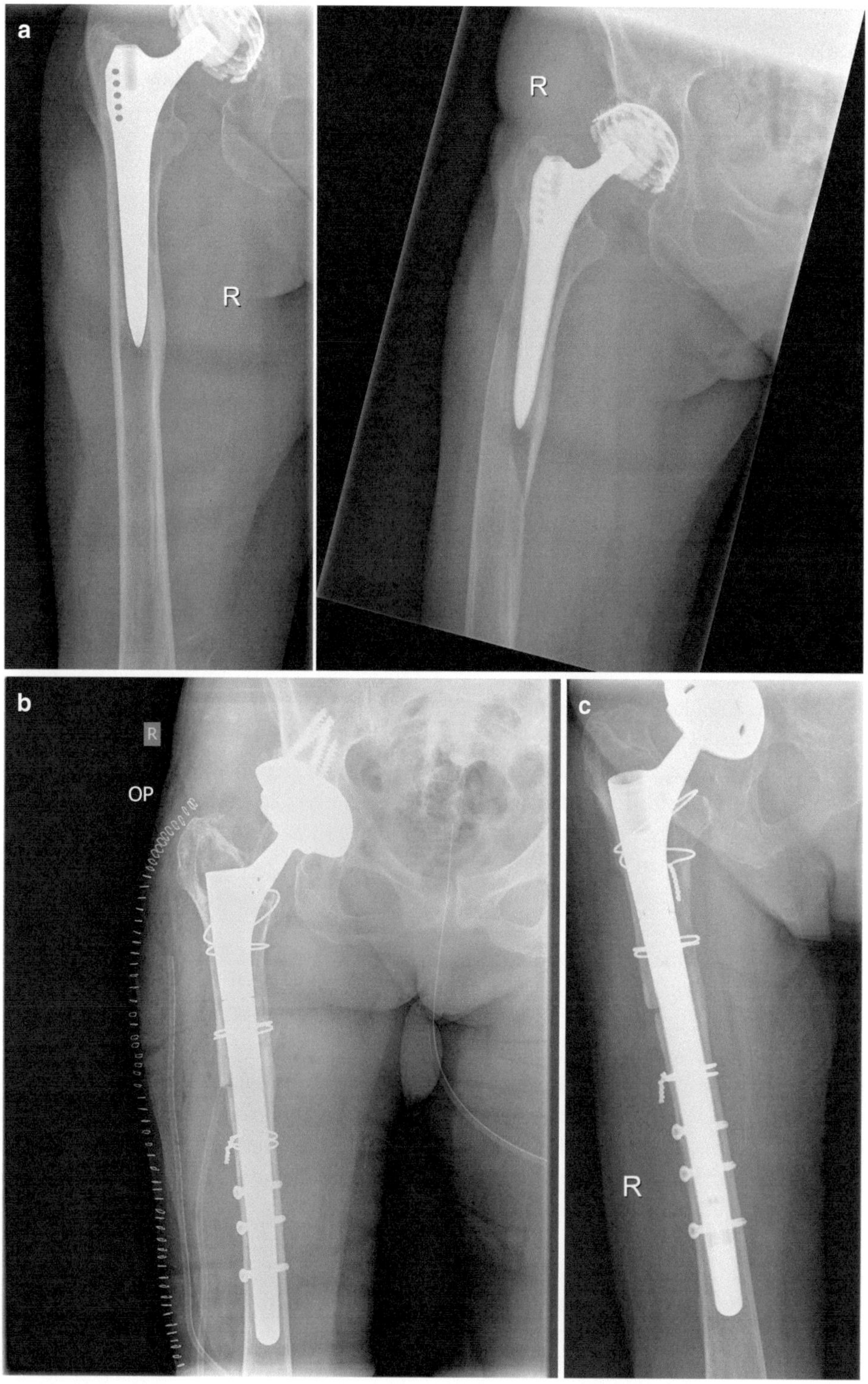

Fig. 18.4 (**a**) Radiographs a.p. (**a1**) and lateral (**a2**) of a periprosthetic Vancouver type B3 fracture with loosened cementless Alloclassic stem and loosened Alloclassic screw cup. (**b**) Postoperative radiograph after transfemoral prosthesis revision with a modular revision stem Revitan Curved with distal locking below the inadequate isthmus and TMT cup with augmentation (Zimmer Biomet, Warsaw, IN, USA). (**c**) Radiograph 12 months after surgery showing a consolidated fracture

a prosthetic stem, which is locked distally to the fracture like an intramedullary nail on a regular base. Once the fracture has healed, the locking screws are removed (6–9 months postoperative) and the following subsidence of the prosthesis (because these cylindrical stems do not get distal press-fit fixation) is expected to result in proximal fixation of the stem. Eingartner et al. [25] reported a 100% fracture healing rate and no prosthesis loosening in 12 periprosthetic fractures of the Vancouver type B2 with a follow-up of 2 years. It seems to me that this procedure would not be completely under the control of the surgeon, and it would be difficult to achieve reproducibly high-quality outcomes. In a later study, in 41 periprosthetic fractures (2 Vancouver type A, 14 B1, 8 B2, and 13 Vancouver B3 fractures) with the then mildly tapered revision stem Bicontact Revision (Aesculap, Tuttlingen, Germany) (0.6 degrees of taper) and additional locking, Eingarnter et al. [26] reported failure in over 12% (5 cases).

This procedure should not be confused with distal locking in cases of a type B3 fracture where an intact isthmus region equivalent to the required fixation length is not available for sufficient cone-in-cone fixation. In this case, the short cone-in-cone fixation (e.g., Revitan Curved, Zimmer Biomet GmbH, Winterthur, Switzerland) or cone-in-cylinder fixation (e.g., MRP stem, Peter Brehm, Weisendorf, Germany) can be improved by additional distal interlocking. These stems are then elongated because of the additional distal interlocking, and the bridging of the fracture with these stems is correspondingly more extensive.

Another option for treating periprosthetic Vancouver B3 fractures is the allograft prosthesis composite (APC). Here, a conventional prosthesis is cemented into the allograft and the remaining proximal bone fragments are fixed with cerclages around the allograft [27, 28]. An APC may be indicated if, in addition to a Vancouver B3 periprosthetic fracture, there are additional larger segmental bone defects extending at least 8 cm into the diaphysis [29]. Since bone regeneration is necessary for integration of the allograft, APC is only recommended for younger patients [27–29]. Wong et al. [28] report 5-year results in 15 type B3 fractures treated with an allograft. The rate of bony incorporation of the allografts was 93.3%, and loosening of the implanted prostheses was 6.6%. The most common problems associated with this procedure are dislocations and infection (see Chap. 9).

A further prosthesis variant that has been described is the use of tumor prostheses (megaprostheses). They are an option for Vancouver type B3 fractures with significant bone loss in elderly patients because, compared to the use of allografts; for example, they allow for earlier weight bearing of the limb [30, 31]. The remaining bone fragments are secured to the megaprosthesis together with the associated soft tissue structures [30, 31]. This solution has been suggested by some authors for older patients. Again, dislocation and infection are the most common complications of this procedure (see Chap. 9). Klein et al. [32] achieved a Harris hip score of 71 points (56 to 90 points) for 21 proximal femoral replacements in B3 fractures with an average age of 78.3 years (52 to 90 years) and observed 2 dislocations and 2 infections each after an average observation period of 3.2 years. Eight patients (38%) were able to walk without walking aids at the last follow-up.

18.2 Treatment of Vancouver Type B2 Fractures (UCS Type IV.3-B2)

Type B2 fractures require revision of the stem. The fracture should be bridged with the fixation zone of the new stem, i.e., distal to the fracture. In my opinion, cemented stems are only advisable in exceptional cases of osteoporotic bones of older patients where cementless fixation is not possible (Vancouver B3). In general, a cementless revision stem is therefore preferable for Vancouver B2 fractures. The use of distally fixed prosthetic stems is technically easier and provides more reproducible outcomes than proximally fixed stems with concomitant use of strut grafts. As a general rule, the use of distally fixed cementless revision stems is to be recommended, whereby modular revision stems will simplify the surgical procedure (Figs. 18.1a–c and 18.3a–c). The distal component can be used to achieve distal fixation of the stem distal to the fracture in the isthmus of the femur, and then, the proximal trial component can be used to adjust leg length, offset, and anteversion independently of each other before being finalized with the original component.

18.3 Treatment of Vancouver Type B3 Fractures (USC Type IV.3-B3)

The options for type B3 fractures comprise the distal fixation stems with cemented or cementless distal fixation, an allograft prosthesis composite (APC), and the use of a tumor prosthesis (megaprosthesis) as a so-called proximal femoral replacement. Regardless of the procedure used, the fractured proximal bone of the femur should always be preserved and "wrapped" around the implanted prosthesis (Fig. 18.4a–c).

Cemented prosthesis revision is not recommended for type B3 fractures because of the thin, sclerotic bone bed and associated poor cementing qualities. These fractures can be treated with cementless revision stems and additional augmentation. This augmentation is achieved either by a combination of impaction grafting and strut grafting or by means of a proximal allograft with or without additional strut grafting [5, 6, 28, 33–36]. These techniques are more suitable for younger patients [28]. In older patients (> 80 years), such fractures can be treated with tumor prostheses (proximal femoral replacement) with the bone fragments attached to the prosthesis [30, 31]. The use of these megaprostheses allows earlier loading of the leg, which is advantageous in older patients [31]. However, the prerequisite for the use of tumor prostheses is that the bone distal to the fracture is still sufficiently stable for the implantation of a proximal femoral replacement. If this is not the case, or if the distal femoral region is also fractured, the only remaining solution is the implantation of a intramedullary femoral replacement (push-through prosthesis) with simultaneous replacement of the knee joint. Here too, the bone with the muscles attached should be retained rather than using a extramedullary femoral replacement (total femoral replacement). In general, B3 fractures show a slightly higher risk of revision than B2 fractures [37]. However, Munro et al. [35, 36] did not see any difference in complication rates, survival rates, and clinical scores between B2 and B3 fractures.

18.4 Surgical Techniques of Revision Prostheses in Periprosthetic Fractures

An analysis of the literature on the treatment of periprosthetic fractures Vancouver types B2 and B3 reveals differences in the surgical techniques and in the cementless implants used (Table 18.2):

When using proximal fixation stems without cement, the fixation point is in the region of the fracture. This will result in a poorer quality of primary stem fixation. For example, Invaco et al. [18] reported stem loosening in a quarter of their cases using this technique and Sledge et al. [20] found a subsidence of the stem in over a quarter of their cases.

Cementless stems with distal fixation in the isthmus have the advantage that they bridge the fracture area with their anchorage zone. Therefore, the stability of the stem is not affected by the quality of the osteosynthesis and the fracture can heal without undesirable load effects (Figs. 18.1a–c, 18.3a–c, and 18.4a–c). Modular revision stems also have the advantage, even in periprosthetic fractures, of allowing the two surgical objectives to be achieved in a separately controlled manner during revision, namely firm distal fixation of the prosthesis in the isthmus of the femur with bridging of the fracture using the distal stem component and correct adjustment of the leg length, offset, and antetorsion in the second step with the proximal component of the prosthesis.

The distally fixed prosthetic stem can be implanted in two different ways.

Technique 1: In the first technique, the fracture is first reducted and the position of the fragments

Table 18.2 Overview of the various surgical techniques and stems used for stem revision in Vancouver B2 and B3 fractures

Author	N (B2/B3)	ETO	OP-Tech.	Stem	Follow-up [month]	Union	HHS	Subsidence	Dislocation	Fracture	Infection	Loosening
Incavo [18]	8/0	–	1	1	49	87.5%	67.6	–	0%	37.5%	0%	25%
Sledge [20]	7/0	+	1	1,2	33	100%	83	28.6%	0%	0%	0%	0%
O'Shea [38]	10/12	+	2	2	33.7	91%	≈ 75	9.1%	0%	0%	4.5%	0%
Invaco [18]	4/0	–	1	2	49	100%	78.3	–	0%	0%	0%	25%
Moran [39]	4/0	–	1	2	24	100%	87	–	0%	0%	0%	0%
Ko [40]	12/0	+	2	3	58.5	100%	≈80	16.6%	0%	8.3%	8.3%	0%
Levine [41]	12/5	+	2	2,4 (in B3)	44.5	100%	–	17.6%	5.8%	5.8%	5.8%	0%
Park [42]	16/11	In 2	1	4	57.6	92.6%	84.7	7.4%	0%	7.4%	3.7%	7.4%
Mulay [43]	10/12	+	2	4	24	91%	69	77.3%	22.7%	4.5%	4.5%	0%
Neumann [44]	35/20	In 4	1	4	67	100%	72	3.8%	3.8%	0%	1.9%	4%
Munro [35, 36]	30 /17	+	2*	4	54	98%	76	8.5%	4%	4%	2%	2%
Fink [45]	22/10	+	2	4	32.2	100%	81.6	0%	3.4%	0%	0%	0%
Amenabar [46]	66/10	+	2	4	74.4				5.3%	2.6%	1.3%	6.6%
Van Laarhoven [47]	70/12	?	?	4	34.8	94.3%		8.1%	18%		4.6%	0%

ETO extended trochanteric osteotomy
Surgical technique 1 = reduction and retention of the fragments before implantation of the stem
Surgical technique 2 = transfemoral, implantation of the stem and then cerclage of the fragment around the stem; * = additional strut grafts for Vancouver B3
Stem 1 = with proximal fixation; Stem 2 = nonmodular, distal fixation, fully porous-coated; Stem 3 = nonmodular, distal fixation, tapered; Stem 4 = modular, distal fixation, tapered

is held with cerclages or reduction forceps. The prosthetic stem is then implanted endofemorally.

Technique 2: In the second technique, the proximal fragment (usually spiral-shaped) is first exposed up to its tip via a transfemoral approach (extended trochanteric osteotomy). Then, the fixation bed of the revision prosthesis is prepared in the distal fragment under visual control and the revision stem is implanted in the distal fragment, bridging the fracture site. Finally, the proximal fragments are repositioned on the prosthetic stem using cerclages. In the case of modular stems, in situ assembly and osteosynthesis of the proximal fracture fragments around the implanted stem are completed only after a successful trial fitting has been carried out.

The disadvantage of the first technique is that it is not possible to reliably verify the location of the fixation zone of the prosthetic stem. This means that the bridging of the fracture with the fixation zone is not verifiable either. Thus, even after the implementation of the principles of distal stem fixation in endofemoral implantation (see Chap. 7), the fixation zone of the endofemorally implanted stem is likely to be at least partially in the region of the fracture, making it much more difficult to achieve reproducible outcomes with this technique. Although Moran et al. [39] did not see any complications in a small number of cases when using distally fixed stems with this implantation technique, Invaco et al. [18] reported loosening in one of four cases and Park et al. [42] reported loosening, subsidence, and intraoperative fracture in approximately 7% of cases.

The main advantage of the abovementioned implantation technique 2 using the transfemoral approach is that the fixation bed of the new prosthesis can be prepared directly under visual control and any remaining cement residues can be removed relatively easily. This also reduces the risk of further fractures or perforations [48]. The disadvantage of this technique is that the osteotomy of the transfemoral approach enlarges the access and three fragments are created from the two fracture-related fragments. However, in our own study, as well as in the relevant literature, this enlargement of the access was not seen as a disadvantage and the healing rate of the fracture was not affected by it [45] (Table 18.2).

Our own study involved 22 Vancouver B2 and 10 B3 fractures and 19 cemented and 13 cementless stems. Two additional cup revisions were performed due to cup loosening, otherwise the existing cup was left in place or an inlay exchange (23 times) was performed. According to the classification of Paprosky et al. [49], 10 cases had a type II defect, 15 cases had a type IIIA defect, and 7 cases had a type IIIB defect. The interval between primary implantation and periprosthetic fracture was 4.9 ± 5.1 (1–20) years.

Radiographic studies 6 months after surgery showed fracture healing and bony consolidation of the bone in all cases. The average fracture healing time was 14.5 ± 5.2 weeks (8–24 weeks). According to the Engh classification [50] for biological fixation of the stem, bony ingrowth fixation was observed in 28 cases and stable fibrous fixation in 4 cases. The distal fixation zone in the isthmus of the femur in cases with Paprosky II and IIIA defects, where no additional distal locking was required, was 4.5 ± 1.1 cm (3.1–6.2 cm). No subsidence of the revision stem or breakage of the locking screws was seen during the study period.

Intraoperative blood loss averaged 990 ± 570 mL and ranged from 460 to 2000 mL. The Harris hip score increased continuously after surgery: 3 months postoperatively, it was 59.2 ± 14.6 points, 6 months postoperatively 66.9 ± 14.8 points, 9 months postoperatively 72.1 ± 15.4 points, 12 months postoperatively 75.2 ± 14.9 points, 18 months postoperatively 77.6 ± 15.9 points, and 24 months postoperatively 81.6 ± 16.5 points. One dislocation occurred 6 weeks postoperatively, which was treated conservatively and one deep vein thrombosis. According to the classification of Beals and Tower [3], all outcomes of this study were considered to be excellent.

As already mentioned, another surgical option is the distal locking technique. Here, the fracture is bridged with a prosthetic stem, which is then locked distally like an intramedullary nail. Once the fracture has healed, the distal locking screws can be removed (6–9 months postoperatively) and the stem left to subside in order to achieve proximal stem fixation. The problem with this technique is that distal fixation with secondary osteointegration does not occur due to the very low 0.6° taper of the stem used and fixation with locking screws alone is not effective. Therefore, it is not possible to control how well and for how long the locking screws will fix the prosthesis and not break. After breakage or removal of the screws, the proximal fixation quality of the stem through secondary subsidence cannot be controlled either. Although Eingärtner et al. [25] report a 100% healing rate and no stem loosening in 12 Vancouver B1 and B2 fractures with a 2-year follow-up, we believe that the technique we describe above has the advantage over that described by Eingärtner in that the individual surgical steps and the fixation of the stem can be controlled with respect to location and quality. For example, in a later study of 41 periprosthetic fractures of the Vancouver A to C types, Eingärtner et al. [26] reported a revision rate of 12% when this technique was used.

18.5 Failed Osteosynthesis of Vancouver B1 Fractures (UCS Type IV.3-B1)

Based on the very good results with the surgical approach we have used in the treatment of Vancouver B2 and B3 periprosthetic fractures in terms of fracture healing rate, stem stability, dislocation rate, intraoperative fracture rate, and clinical outcomes, we also believe that this technique is indicated for prosthesis revision in the event of failure of a technically correct osteosynthesis in a Vancouver B1 fracture (at the level of the fixed prosthesis stem). Despite the correct execution of these osteosyntheses, failures with plate fractures have been observed as the result of the position of the fracture (transverse fracture) and/or the bone quality. Depending on the study, these failures range from 0 to 25% [51]. Lindahl et al. [52] found a rate of 6.6% in an analysis of the Swedish Prosthesis Registry, and Dehghan et al. [53] found a frequency of 5% in a meta-analysis.

For failed osteosynthesis of Vancouver B1 fractures, it is helpful to select a procedure from the various treatment options that can predictably and reproducibly deliver favorable outcomes. If there are obvious surgical–technical errors, such as osteosynthesis plates that are too short or screws in the fracture area, it appears advantageous to perform a reosteosynthesis (e.g., with double plating or additional strut graft) [54–56]. However, if the reasons for failure are more to do with poor bone quality or fracture pattern, the alternative surgical procedures such as reosteosynthesis with double plates or plate and strut graft do not in my opinion present reproducible chances of success [57]. In these cases of failed osteosynthesis, we choose to switch to a modular revision stem, as this generally has a lower complication rate compared to plate osteosynthesis for Vancouver B1 fractures, and therefore, the chances for success in these reoperations appear to be higher [58]. In addition, plate osteosyntheses cannot normally be subjected to 100% weight bearing. However, partial weight bearing is rarely possible in the mostly elderly patients, and this may have contributed to the failure of their previous osteosyntheses in the first place [59]. In contrast, a prosthesis with cone-in-cone fixation in an isthmus with good bone quality is stable under full weight bearing (Fig. 18.5a–c).

In our own study, 14 patients with failed osteosyntheses of Vancouver B1 fractures were prospectively examined with a minimum follow-up period of 2 years (2–10 years, mean 4 ± 1.7 years) [60] (Fig. 18.5a–c). The patients comprised 11 women and 3 men with an average age of 72.4 ± 13.5 (65–90) years. The interval between primary implant surgery and periprosthetic B1 fracture was 5.9 ± 4.1 (1–10) years. The body mass index at the time of surgery was 27.7 ± 5.0 (20.9–35.4). In accordance with the fracture pattern, there were 10 Paprosky type IIIA defects and 4 type IIIB defects, where the fracture passed through the isthmus of the femur with less than 3 cm of intact isthmus. In these latter cases, additional distal locking was carried out (Fig. 18.6a–c).

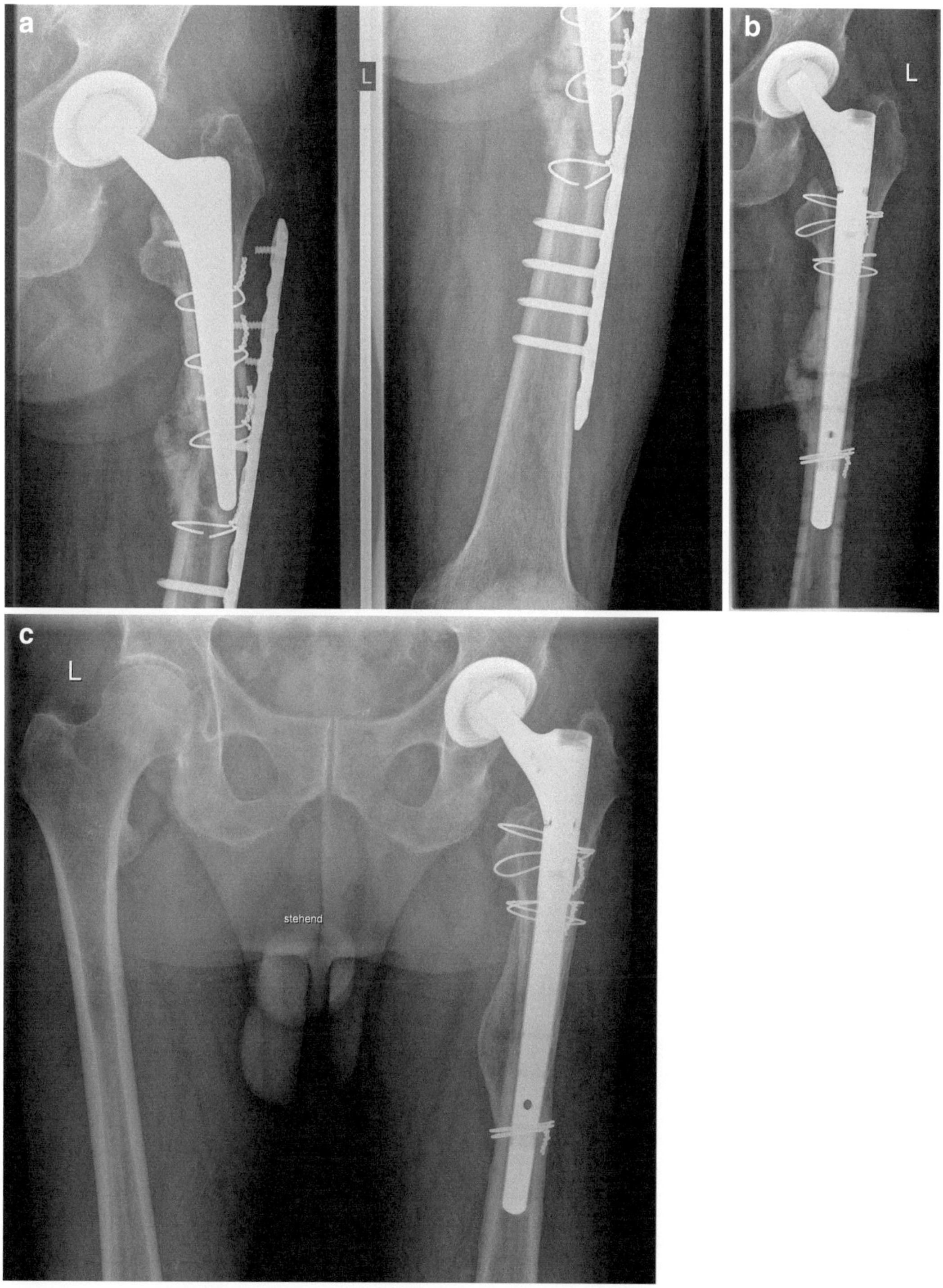

Fig. 18.5 (**a**) Failed plate osteosynthesis of a Vancouver type B1 fracture with plate fracture. (**b**) Radiograph 10 days after transfemoral stem revision using a Revitan Curved (Zimmer Biomet, Winterthur, Switzerland). (**c**) Radiograph 6 months after surgery showing bony consolidation of the fracture

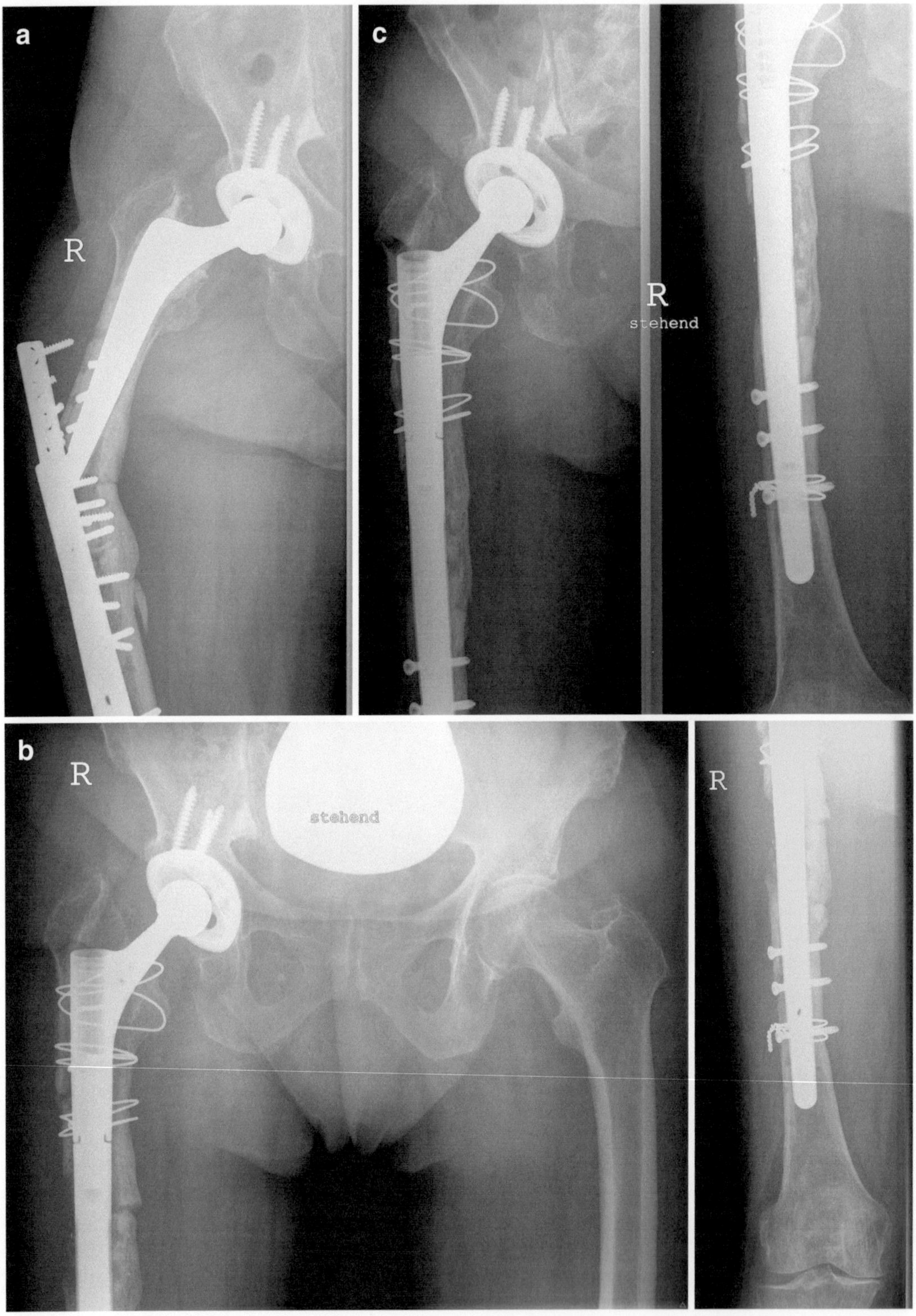

Fig. 18.6 (**a**) Failed double-plate osteosynthesis of a Vancouver type B1 fracture with plate fracture. (**b**) (**b1** and **b2**): Radiograph 10 days after transfemoral stem revision using a Revitan Curved (Zimmer Biomet, Winterthur, Switzerland). (**c**) Radiograph 12 months after surgery showing bony consolidation of the fracture

The evaluation of radiographs showed that in all cases, within 6 months of the procedure, there was osseous consolidation of the fracture and of the bony flap created during the transfemoral approach. The average fracture healing time was 15.5 ± 5.7 weeks (10–24 weeks). In accordance with the Engh classification [50] for biological fixation of the stem, bony ingrowth fixation was observed in all cases. The distal fixation zone in the isthmus of the femur in cases with Paprosky IIIA defects where no additional distal locking was required was 4.6 ± 1.4 cm (3.1–6.1 cm). No subsidence of the revision stem or fracture of the locking screws (in the 4 cases with Paprosky IIIB defects) was observed during the study period.

The average intraoperative blood loss was 980 ± 430 mL, ranging from 470 to 2000 mL. The Harris hip score increased continuously after surgery: 3 months postoperatively, it was 61.2 ± 15.7 points, 6 months postoperatively 67.3 ± 14.4 points, 12 months postoperatively 75.9 ± 15.3 points, and 24 months postoperatively 81.5 ± 16.8 points. According to the classification of Beals and Tower [3], all outcomes of this study could be considered to be excellent.

Thus, even in failed plate osteosyntheses of Vancouver B1 fractures changing the procedure to a transfemorally implanted, distal fixation, modular, tapered revision stem resulted in reproducibly good results in terms of stable fixation of the stem, subsidence of the stem, fracture healing, and clinical outcome. Extending the access with a proximal longitudinal osteotomy of the femur during transfemoral access promotes fracture healing and osteointegration of the stem by stimulating additional callus formation.

References

1. Duncan DP, Masri BA. Fractures of the femur after hip replacement. Instr Course Lect. 1995;44:293–304.
2. Duncan CP, Haddad FS. The unified classification system (UCS): improving our understanding of periprosthetic fractures. Bone Joint J. 2014;96-B:713–6.
3. Beals RK, Tower SS. Periprosthetic fractures of the femur. An analysis of 93 fractures. Clin Orthop. 1996;327:238–46.
4. Fink B, Fuerst M, Singer J. Periprosthetic fractures of the femur associated with hip arthroplasty. Arch Orthop Trauma Surg. 2005;125:433–42.
5. Haddad FS, Duncan CP, Berry DJ, Lewallen DG, Gross AE, Chandler HP. Periprosthetic femoral fractures around well-fixed implants: use of cortical onlay allografts with or without a plate. J Bone Joint Surg. 2002;84-A:945–50.
6. Tsiridis E, Haddad FS, Gie GA. Dal-Miles plates for periprosthetic femoral fractures. A critical review of 16 cases. Injury. 2003;34:107–10.
7. Adolphson P, Jonsson U, Kalen R. Fractures of the ipsilateral femur after total hip arthroplasty. Arch Orthop Trauma Surg. 1987;106:353–7.
8. Cooke PH, Newman JH. Fractures of the femur in relation to cemented hip prostheses. J Bone Joint Surg. 1988;70-B:386–9.
9. Namba RS, Rose NE, Amstutz HC. Unstable femoral fractures in hip arthroplasty. Orthop Trans. 1991;15:753.
10. Bethea JS, DeAndrade JR, Fleming LL, Lindenbaum SD, Welch RB. Proximal femoral fractures following total hip arthroplasty. Clin Orthop. 1982;170:95–106.
11. Lindahl H, Malchau H, Herberts P, Garellick G. Periprosthetic femoral fractures classification and demographics of 1049 periprosthetic femoral fractures form the Swedish National Hip Arthroplasty Register. J Arthroplasty. 2005;20:857–65.
12. Lindahl H, Garellick G, Regner H, et al. Three hundred an twenty-one periprosthetic femoral fractures. J Bone Joint Surg Am. 2006;88-A:1215–22.
13. Abdel MP, Cotino U, Mabry TM. Management of periprosthetic femoral fractures following total hip arthroplasty. Int Orthop. 2015;39:2005–10.
14. Springer BD, Berry DJ, Lewallen DG. Treatment of periprosthetic femoral fractures following total hip arthroplasty with femoral component revision. J Bone Joint Surg Am. 2003;85-A:2156–62.
15. Kyle RF, Crickard GE III. Periprosthetic fractures associated with total hip arthroplasty. Orthopedics. 1998;21:982–4.
16. Jukkala-Partio K, Parito EK, Solovieva S, Paavilainen T, Hirvensalo E, Alho A. Treatment of periprosthetic fractures in association with total hip arthroplasty—a retrospective comparison between revision stem and plate fixation. Ann Chir Gyn. 1998;87:229–35.
17. Schmidt AH, Kyle RF. Periprosthetic fractures of the femur. Orthop Clin North Am. 2002;33:143–52.
18. Incavo SJ, Beard DM, Pupparo F, Ries M, Wiedel J. One-stage revision of periprosthetic fractures around loose cemented total hip arthroplasty. Am J Orthop. 1998;27:35–41.
19. Lewallen DG, Berry DJ. Periprosthetic fracture of the femur after total hip arthroplasty: treatment and results to date. Instr Course Lect. 1998;47:243–9.
20. Sledge JB 3rd, Abiri A. An algorithm for the treatment of Vancouver type B2 periprosthetic proximal femoral fractures. J Arthroplasty. 2002;17:887–92.
21. Wang J-W, Wang C-J. Periprosthetic fracture of the femur after hip arthroplasty: the clinical out-

come using cortical strut allografts. J Orthop Surg. 2000;8:27–31.
22. Weeden SH, Paprosky WG. Minimal 11-year follow-up of extensively porous-coated stems in femoral revision total hip arthroplasty. J Arthroplasty. 2002;17 Suppl:134–7.
23. Fink B, Grossman A, Schubring S, Schulz MS, Fuerst M. Short-term results of hip revisions with a curved cementless modular stem in association with the surgical approach. Arch Orthop Trauma Surg. 2009;129:65–73.
24. Tangsataporn S, Safir OA, Vincent AD, Abdelbary H, Gross AE, Kuzyk PRT. Risk factors for subsidence of a modular tapered femoral stem used for revision total hip arthroplasty. J Arthroplasty. 2015;30:1030–134.
25. Eingartner C, Volkmann R, Pütz M, Weller S. Uncemented revision stem for biological osteosynthesis in periprosthetic femoral fractures. Int Orthop. 1997;21:25–9.
26. Eingartner C, Ochs U, Egetemeyer D, Volkmann R. Treatment of periprosthetic femoral fractures with the Bicontact revision stem. Z Orthop Unfall. 2007;145:29–33.
27. Rasouli MR, Porat MD, Hozack WJ, Parvizi J. Proximal femoral replacement and allograft prosthesis composite in treatment of periprosthetic fractures with significant proximal bone loss. Orthop Surg. 2012;4:203–10.
28. Wong P, Gross AE. The use of structural allografts for treating periprosthetic fractures about the hip and knee. Orthop Clin North Am. 1999;30:259–64.
29. Kellett CF, Boscainos PJ, Maury AC, et al. Proximal femoral allograft treatment of Vancouver type-B3 periprosthetic femoral fractures after total hip arthroplasty. Surgical technique. J Bone Joint Surg Am. 2007;89-A(Suppl 2):S68–79.
30. Dorotka R, Windhager R, Kotz R. Periprosthetic femoral fractures in total hip prosthesis implantation. Functional and radiological comparison between plate osteosynthesis and proximal femur replacement. Z Orthop. 2000;138:440–6.
31. Wilson D, Masri BA, Duncan CP. Periprosthetic fractures: an operative algorithm. Orthopedics. 2001;24:869–70.
32. Klein GR, Parvizi J, Rapuri V, Wolf CF, Hozack WJ, Sharkey PF, Purtill JJ. Proximal femoral replacement for the treatment of periprosthetic fractures. J Bone Joint Surg Am. 2005;87-A:1777–81.
33. Aigner C, Marschall C, Reischl N, Windhager R. Cortical strut grafts, an alternative to conventional plating in periprosthetic fractures of the femur. Z Orthop. 2002;140:328–33.
34. Brady OH, Garbuz DS, Masri BA, Duncan CP. The treatment of periprosthetic fractures of the femur using cortical onlay allograft struts. Orthop Clin North Am. 1999;30:249–57.
35. Munro JT, Masri BA, Garbuz DS, Duncan CP. Tapered fluted modular titanium stems in the management of Vancouver B2 and B3 periprosthetic fractures. Bone Joint J. 2013;95-B(Suppl A):17–20.
36. Munro JT, Garbuz DS, Masri BA, Duncan CP. Tapered fluted titanium stems in the management of Vancouver B2 and B3 periprosthetic femoral fractures. Clin Orthop Relat Res. 2014;472:590–8.
37. Kahn T, Grindlay D, Olliviere BJ, Scammell BE, Manktelow ARJ, Pearson RG. A systematic review of Vancouver B2 and B3 periprosthetic femoral fractures. Bone Joint J. 2017;4(Suppl B):17–25.
38. O'Shea K, Quinlan JF, Kutty S, Mulcahy D, Brady OH. The use of uncemented extensively porous-coated femoral components in the management of Vancouver B2 and B3 periprosthetic femoral fractures. J Bone Joint Surg Br. 2005;87-B: 1617–21.
39. Moran MC. Treatment of periprosthetic fractures around total hip arthroplasty with an extensively coated femoral component. J Arthroplasty. 1996;11:981–8.
40. Ko PS, Lam JJ, Tio MK, Lee OB, Ip FK. Distal fixation with Wagner revision stem in treating Vancouver type B2 periprosthetic femur fractures in geriatric patients. J Arthroplasty. 2003;13:446–52.
41. Levine BR, Della Valle CJ, Lewis P, Berger RA, Sporer SM, Paprosky W. Extended trochanteric osteotomy for the treatment of Vancouver B2/B3 periprosthetic fractures of the femur. J Arthroplasty. 2008;23:527–33.
42. Park M-S, Lim Y-J, Chung W-C, Ham D-H, Lee S-H. Management of periprosthetic femur fractures treated with distal fixation using a modular femoral stem using an anterolateral approach. J Arthroplasty. 2009;24:1270–6.
43. Mulay S, Hassan T, Birtwistle S, Power R. Management of types B2 and B3 femoral periprosthetic fractures by a tapered, fluted, and distally fixed stem. J Arthroplasty. 2005;20:751–6.
44. Neumann D, Thaler C, Dorn U. Management of Vancouver B2 and B3 femoral periprosthetic fractures using a modular cementless stem without allografting. Int Orthop. 2012;36:1045–50.
45. Fink B, Grossmann A, Singer J. Hip revision arthroplasty in periprosthetic fractures of Vancouver type B2 and B3. J Orthop Trauma. 2012;26:206–11.
46. Amenabar T, Rahman WA, Avhad VV, Vera R, Gross AE, Kuzyk PR. Vancouver type B2 and B3 periprosthetic fractures treated with revision total hip arthroplasty. Int Orthop. 2015;39:1927–32.
47. Van Laarhoven SN, Vles GF, van Haaren EH, Schotanus MGM, van Hemert WLW. Tapered, fluted, modular, titanium stems in Vancouver B periprosthetic femoral fractures: an analysis of 87 consecutive revisions. Hip Int. 2021;31(4):555–61. https://doi.org/10.1177/1120700020904933.
48. Fink B. Revision arthroplasty in periprosthetic fractures of the proximal femur. Oper Orthop Traumatol. 2014;26:455–68.
49. Paprosky WG, Greidanus NV, Antoniou J. Minimum 10-year results of extensively porous-coated stems in revision hip arthroplasty. Clin Orthop Relat Res. 1999;369:230–42.

50. Engh CA, Glassman AH, Suthers KE. The case of porous-coated hip implants: the femoral side. Clin Orthop Relat Res. 1990;261:63–81.
51. Boesmmueller S, Baumbach S, Hofbauer M, Wozasek GE. Plate failure following plate osteosynthesis in periprosthetic femoral fractures. Wien Klin Wochenschr. 2015;127:770–8.
52. Lindahl H, Malchau H, Oden A, Garellick G. Risk factors for failure after treatment of a periprosthetic of the femur. J Bone Joint Surg Br. 2006;88:26–30.
53. Dehghan N, McKee MD, Nuth A, Ristevski B, Schemitsch EH. Surgical fixation of Vancouver type B1 periprosthetic femur fractures: a systematic review. J Orthop Trauma. 2014;28:721–7.
54. Frohberg L, Troelsen A, Brix M. Periprosthetic Vancouver type B1 and C fractures treated by locking-plate osteosynthesis. Fracture union and reoperations in 60 consecutive fractures. Acta Orthop. 2012;83:648–52.
55. Graham SM, Moazen M, Leonidou A, Tsiridis E. Locking plate fixation for Vancouver B1 periprosthetic femoral fractures: a critical analysis in 135 cases. J Orthop Sci. 2013;18:426–36.
56. Moloney GB, Westrick ER, Siska PA, Tarkin IS. Treatment of periprosthetic femur fractures around a well-fixed hip arthroplasty implant: span the whole bone. Arch Orthop Trauma Surg. 2014;134:9–14.
57. Leonidou A, Moazen M, Lepetsos P, Graham SM, Macheras GA, Tsiridis E. The biomechanical effect of bone quality and fracture topography on locking plate fixation in periprosthetic femoral fractures. Injury. 2015;46:213–7.
58. Laurer HL, Wutzler S, Possner S, Geiger EV, Saman AE, Marzi I, Frank J. Outcome after operative treatment of Vancouver type B and C periprosthetic fractures: open reduction and internal fixation versus revision arthroplasty. Arch Orthop Trauma Surg. 2011;131:983–9.
59. Moazen M, Mak JH, Etchels LW, Jin Z, Wilcox RK, Jones AC, Tsiridis E. Periprosthetic femoral fractures—a biomechanical comparison between Vancouver type B1 and B2 fixation methods. J Arthroplasty. 2014;29:495–500.
60. Fink B, Oremek D. Hip revision arthroplasty for failed osteosynthesis in periprosthetic Vancouver B1 fractures using a cementless, tapered, modular revision stem. Bone Joint J. 2017;99-B(4 Suppl B):11–6.

19 Femoral Spacers in Septic Two-Stage Revision

Contents

19.1 **Type of the Spacer** ... 262

19.2 **Fixation of the Spacer** ... 263

19.3 **Local Antibiotics in the Spacer** ... 266

19.4 **Duration of the Spacer Period and Systemic Antibiotic Therapy** ... 269

19.5 **Aspiration Before Reimplantation** ... 269

19.6 **Type of Prosthesis Used for Reimplantation** ... 273

References ... 273

Periprosthetic infections are serious complications of total hip arthroplasty with an incidence of 1–2% [1–3]. In the case of early infections that occur within 4 weeks after implantation, the implant can usually be left in place and only the articulating changeable pieces (head, inlay) have to be replaced in an immediate operation that includes radical debridement of the joint. In the case of a late infection (later than 4 weeks after surgery), all foreign material has to be removed. In such cases, a distinction can be made between one- and two-stage septic revisions. The two-stage septic revision includes an initial operation with removal of all foreign material and radical debridement and mostly implantation of a spacer containing antibiotics. This is followed by an intermediate phase of usually 6–12 weeks either with a spacer or with a Girdlestone situation. Thereafter, an implantation of a prosthesis, either cemented or cementless, will be performed, followed by 6–12 weeks of antibiotic therapy [1]. In one-stage septic revision, after removal of all foreign material and radical debridement, a new, usually cemented, prosthesis is implanted in the same operation using antibiotic-containing cement. However, knowledge of the microorganism causing the infection and its antibiogram is essential for this procedure [1, 4–6]. This concept leads to success rates that are as high as those achieved in two-stage septic revisions [7, 8].

The two-stage septic revision is still the most commonly used method for the treatment of periprosthetic late infections. The disadvantage of the two-stage concept is that two surgeries are necessary. The advantage is that surgical debridement is performed twice, with the second operation allowing the eradication of any residual organisms remaining after the first debridement. Antibiotics tailored to the sensitivity of the pathogen are added to the cement of the spacer although

B. Fink, *Femoral Revision Arthroplasty*, https://doi.org/10.1007/978-3-030-84821-7_19

an admixture of more than 10% of the cement leads to a weakening of the mechanical properties of the spacer. However, since the cement of the spacer is not intended for permanent fixation of an endoprosthesis, its mechanical properties are not of primary importance at this stage so large quantities of antibiotics can indeed be added to the cement. Two-stage revision concepts for infected hip endoprostheses have achieved success rates of 90–100% [9–12].

In two-stage septic revisions, a spacer containing antibiotics is usually fitted for 6–12 weeks before the final prosthesis is implanted. The function of the spacer is to release the antibiotic into the infected bed of the prosthesis on the one hand, while on the other hand it is designed to minimize soft tissue contractions and maintain soft tissue tension so ensuring appropriate functionality [9]. This makes the reimplantation of the new prosthesis in the second step technically easier compared to the Girdlestone situation in which the leg is shortened and there is marked formation of scar tissue in the former joint [1].

There are many questions regarding the one- and two-stage procedures that still need to be answered, and existing procedures are based more on empirical results than on data from prospective or randomized studies with high levels of evidence. For this reason, the following aspects of two-stage revision are treated very differently by different groups: the type of spacer, the type of antibiotic used in the spacer, the duration of the spacer period, the duration of systemic antibiotic treatment, aspiration before reimplantation, and the type of reimplantation (cemented or cementless).

19.1 Type of the Spacer

There are several different types of spacers: static and mobile spacers, monoblock and two-piece mobile spacers, preformed spacers (e.g., Spacer G, TECRES, Verona, Italy), and spacers that are individually manufactured in the operating room (e.g., StageOne Select, Zimmer Biomet, Warsaw, IN, USA, or Prostalac, DePuy Synthes, Warsaw, IN, USA) (Fig. 19.1a–c).

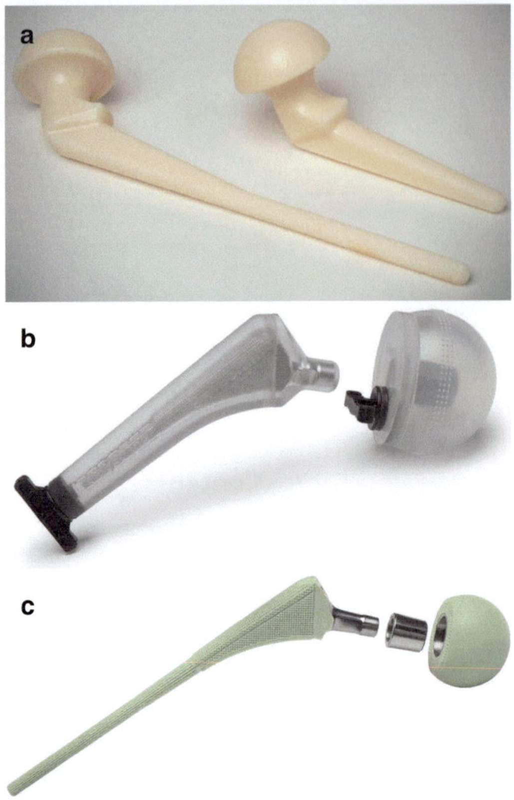

Fig. 19.1 (**a**) Spacer G (TECRES, Verona, Italy), non-modular hemispacer. (**b**) Mold of the StageOne Select Spacer (Zimmer Biomet, Warsaw, IN, USA), which is created as a modular hemispacer on the operating table. (**c**) Operator-created StageOne Select spacer (Zimmer Biomet, Warsaw, IN, USA)

Antibiotic-loaded beads form a kind of spacer that does not have a specific articulating surface and thus represent a more or less static spacer that merely fills the gap created by the removal of the affected prosthesis. The disadvantage of this procedure is that the beads used are typically preformed beads that contain only gentamycin or vancomycin [13, 14]. Leg shortening and instability occur in the same way as in a Girdlestone situation and cause problems with mobilization. The reimplantation of a prosthesis is also often complicated by scarring, tissue contraction, and an osteoporosis that results from inactivity [15–18]. In addition, during mobilization, the beads have a tendency to break and zirconium dioxide particles may become abraded, a process which can lead to third body wear after reimplantation of the final prosthesis. For these reasons, Disch et al. [19] chose not to use local antibiotic carriers after removal of the infected prosthesis during two-stage revision and to leave a Girdlestone situation for an average of 13 months. They observed a significant reduction in quality of life in 32 hips during the Girdlestone phase and a re-infection rate of 6.3% during the 41.3 months of follow-up.

Mobile spacers can be divided into hemi- and articulating spacers. The hemispacers (only on the femoral side) can be designed as monoblock (e.g., Spacer G, TECRES, Verona, Italy) or modular devices (e.g., StageOne Select, Zimmer Biomet, Warsaw, IN, USA). The disadvantages of these spacers include fracture of the spacer, dislocations, and bone resorption at the acetabulum [17, 20]. The hemispacer induces bone resorption at the acetabulum because the hard cement has to articulate against the infection-related osteoporotic bone. This is avoided with two-piece articulating spacers by giving the spacer a joint surface of its own. However, this cement-based articular surface in the two-piece spacer can lead to the release of abrasion-induced cement particles, which must be removed during the reimplantation by debridement and synovectomy [19, 21].

19.2 Fixation of the Spacer

The femoral component of the spacer is associated with the risk of spacer breakage. This risk is particularly high when the femoral component is made of cement alone. Jung et al. [22] found a fracture rate of 10.2% in 88 hip spacers. We recommend that the spacer should consist of a metal core encased in cement, as is the case with commercially available spacers. Another risk is related to the possibility of dislocation of the spacer from the femoral bone (either with or without fracture). Jung et al. [22] reported a dislocation rate of 17%. In order to avoid this complication, we recommend that the prepared spacer is not simply inserted into the femur, but rather that it is fixed in the metaphysis of the femur with cement [1].

We use an articulating spacer in which the acetabular component consists of cement containing a special mixture of antibiotics tailored to the pathogen. The spacer stem component is made from a low-cost cemented prosthesis stem model. Prior to implantation, the stem is smeared with the patient's own blood and then coated with antibiotic-supplemented cement (with a special mixture of antibiotics tailored to the pathogen), applied about 6 min after mixing. These measures are taken to weaken the cementation in order to ease the removal of the spacer during the second stage of the revision. The two components of the spacer are linked via a metal headpiece [1, 10] (Fig. 19.2). An analysis of the synovial membranes obtained during the second operation to remove the spacer has revealed abraded particles of the cement, which include zirconium dioxide particles [21]. However, it can

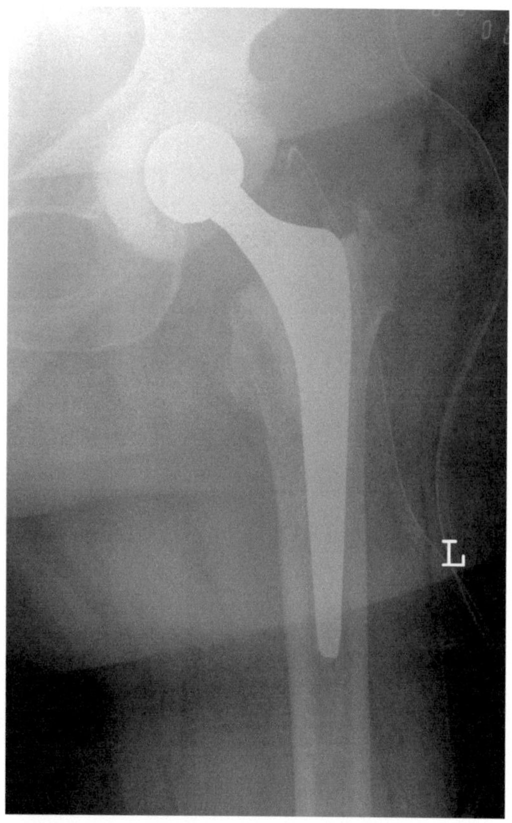

Fig. 19.2 Interim prosthesis as a mobile spacer consisting of a cemented stem (with deliberately poor cementation), which articulates with a metal head in a cement cup

be assumed that all types of spacers produce abrasion-induced cement particles. This only underlines the necessity of radical debridement of the joint area at the time of prosthesis implantation during the second stage of the revision [21]. The use of zirconium-free spacer cement (Heraeus Medical GmbH, Wertheim, Germany) aims to circumvent this problem of abraded particles containing zirconium dioxide.

Another important factor in deciding which type of spacer to use is the extent of the bone defect, which in some cases may also be caused by explantation of the infected prosthesis. The removal of well-fixed cemented or cementless infected femoral implants is a challenge for the surgeon. The infected prosthesis bed must be radically debrided, whereby the functionally important bone areas such as the greater trochanter, where the gluteal muscles are attached, must be spared as much as possible. For this reason, we prefer the transfemoral approach for the removal of firmly fixed infected femoral components. This approach allows effective debridement of the infected prosthetic bed and the frequently present osteolytic areas, while minimizing damage to the greater trochanter, the vasto-gluteal sling, the gluteal muscles, and the femoral isthmus, which is a fixation site for the new prosthesis during the second stage of surgery. The endofemoral approach for removal of the femoral component does not always allow reproducible debridement of the osteolytic regions and carries a higher risk of femoral fracture. The transfemoral approach avoids this risk. Consequently, we carry out the operation endofemorally only if the removal of the stem and, if necessary, the cement, as well as the necessary debridement, can be performed without complications of this kind. However, if problems are anticipated during preoperative planning or during intraoperative procedures, we choose the transfemoral approach or switch to it during surgery. In transfemoral revision, however, it is important that the spacer is long enough and extends beyond the limits of the resulting bony flap (2 diaphyseal widths) so that the entire construction is sufficiently stable. Some commercially available spacers are longer (Spacer G up to 211 mm, StageOne up to 200 mm, and Prostalac up to 240 mm). If even greater lengths are required (e.g., after removal of an infected cementless long revision stem with a correspondingly long bony flap), long cemented prosthetic stems may have to be converted to spacers and cemented in with an appropriately "poorer" cementation (Figs. 15.5a–c and 19.3a–d).

When using the transfemoral approach, we prefer to close the bony flap with cerclage wires to avoid migration of the flap or its dislocation, as recommended by Morshed et al. [23] (Fig. 19.4a). Two double cerclages are introduced with the flap open, the spacer is smeared with blood, coated with cement that contains antibiotics tailored to the pathogen and has been left to stand for 6–7 min, inserted into the distal femur, and then the bony flap of the transfemoral access is closed by tightening the cerclages. Any excess cement is then removed. During the second stage of the procedure, we reopen the flap by removing the cerclage wires so that we can perform a second radical debridement of the prosthetic bed and ensure that the distally fixed, cementless, modular revision stem is correctly fixed in the isthmus of the femur distal to the osteotomy (Fig. 19.4b,c).

To analyze the outcome of this procedure for revision of infected hip prostheses, 76 two-stage septic revisions were prospectively followed with a mean follow-up period of 51.2 ± 23.2 (24–118) months, in which the transfemoral approach was used and the bony flap was fixed with cerclage wires in the first stage and reopened in the second stage [24]. The rate of bony consolidation of the flap after reimplantation was 98.7%, and a successful outcome without re-infection was reported in 93.4% of cases. Subsidence of the stem was 6.6% and dislocation 6.6%. Aseptic loosening of the implants was not observed. The Harris hip score was 62.2 ± 12.6 points with the spacer and 86.6 ± 15.5 points 2 years after implantation of the new implant. Nine fractures (11.8%) of the flap occurred during surgery due to osteolytic or osteoporotic weakness of the flap and were osteosynthesized with double-looped cerclages. All healed without further intervention [24]. Our data show that the transfemoral approach is a safe method for the septic revision

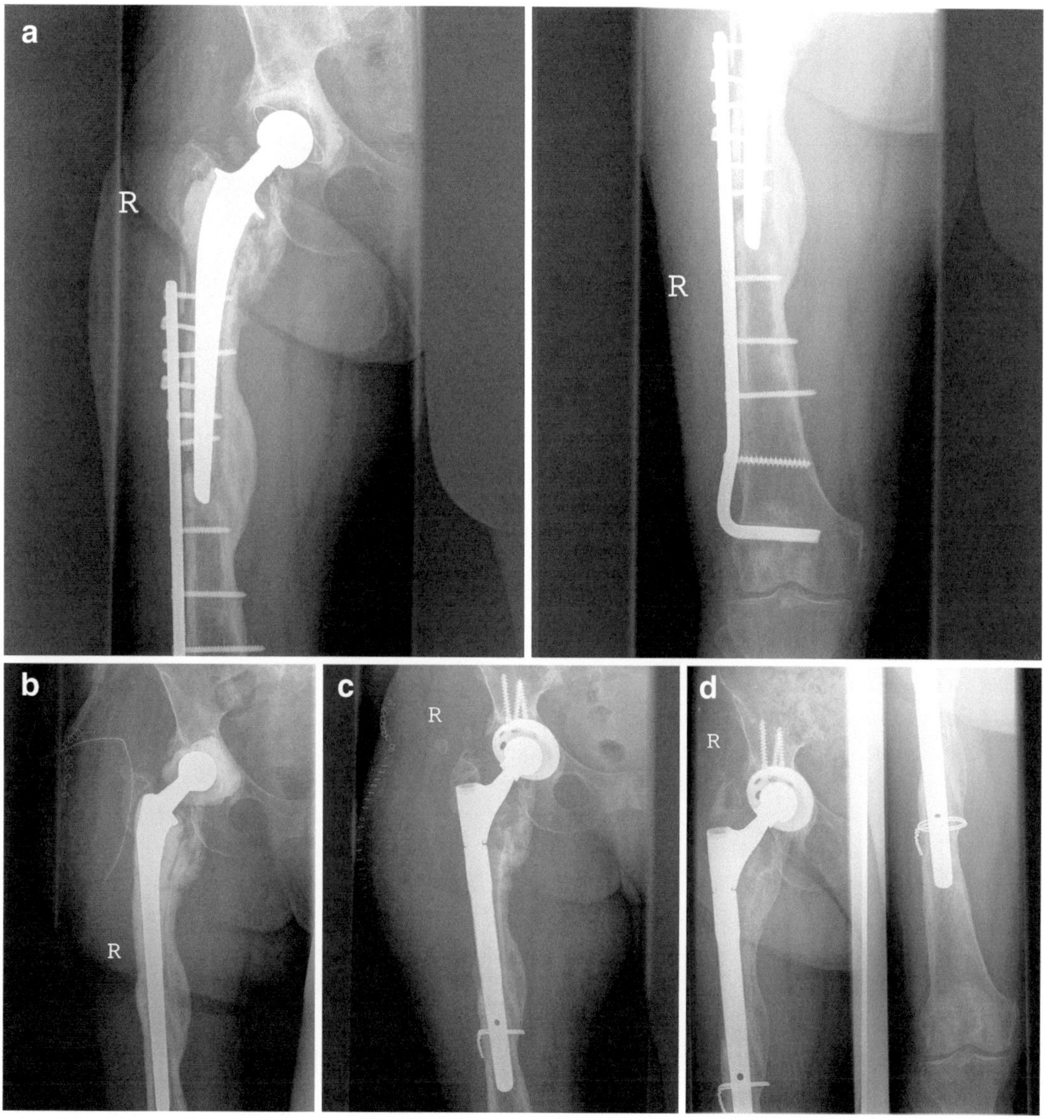

Fig. 19.3 (**a1** and **a2**) Extramurally implanted cemented prosthesis with plate osteosynthesis for the treatment of a periprosthetic fracture, which is infected with Enterococcus faecalis, and a sequestrum. (**b**) Postoperative radiograph after transfemoral removal of the implants, debridement and sequestrectomy and implantation of a cement-coated long cemented stem and a cement cup as spacer. (**c**) Postoperative radiograph after transfemoral implantation of a modular revision stem Revitan Curved and an Allofit-S cup (Zimmer Biomet, Winterthur, Switzerland). (**d**) Radiograph 1 year after surgery shows an unchanged position of the prosthesis and only slight proximalization of the greater trochanter

of fixed cemented or cementless hip prostheses and that the use of cerclage wires to close the osteotomy flap in the first stage does not result in higher re-infection rates. Similarly, reopening the transfemoral access in the second stage does not result in reduced healing of the flap. However, it must be remembered that the integrity of the muscles on the bony flap is important for the vascularization of the flap.

A further problem associated with spacer implantation is caused by bone defects in the acetabulum. This can lead to situations in which sta-

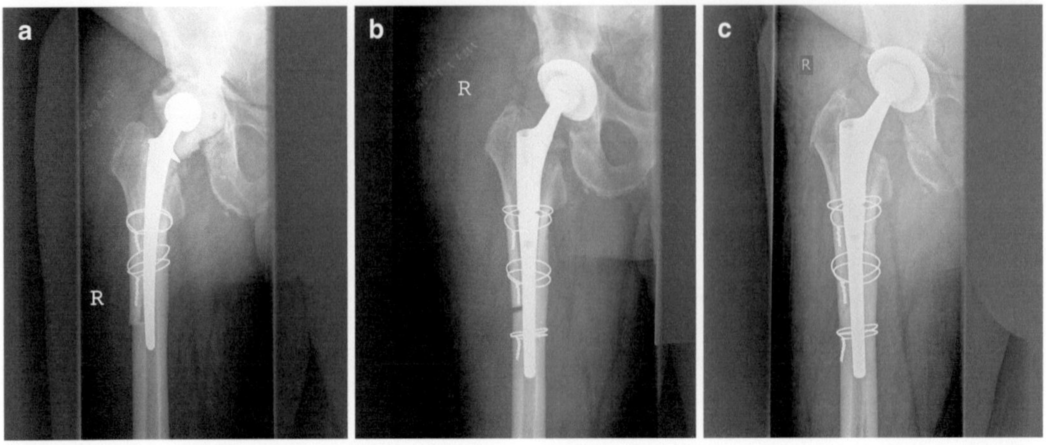

Fig. 19.4 (**a**) Interim prosthesis as spacer implanted via a transfemoral approach. (**b**) Postoperative radiograph after transfemoral reimplantation of a modular revision stem and Allofit cup (ZimmerBiomet, Winterthur, Switzerland). (**c**) Radiograph 6 months after surgery showing complete consolidation of the osteotomy and osteointegration of the implants

ble fixation of the cup spacer or a monoblock spacer is not possible. In such cases, and if the infecting organism can be identified, we perform a one-stage revision in which the acetabular cup defect is stabilized by using a complete cup, a Burch–Schneider cage, or a cup cage construct and cementing a polyethylene cup into it (Fig. 19.5a, b). However, sometimes it is also necessary to perform a two-stage revision of the femoral component using the transfemoral approach to explant a septic prosthesis. When a large acetabular cup defect is present, we perform a combination of a one-stage revision of the acetabular component and a two-stage revision of the femoral component (Fig. 19.6a–d). We analyzed 35 such cases with a follow-up period of 42.2 ± 17.2 (24–84) months and identified successful outcomes without recurrence of the infection in 97.1% of all cases. The Harris hip score was 61.2 ± 12.8 points after the first operation and 82.4 ± 15.7 points 2 years after the second stage [25].

19.3 Local Antibiotics in the Spacer

In order for the antibiotic activity of the spacer to be effective, it is important that the local antibiotic concentration is higher than the minimum inhibitory concentration for the pathogens causing the periprosthetic infection and that this level is maintained throughout the spacer period. Otherwise, there is a risk of recurrence of the infection and the appearance of resistant microorganisms. There are very few publications dealing with the elution of antibiotics from the spacer cement in vivo over a period of several weeks. Masri et al. [26] followed 49 patients for a mean period of 118 days between spacer implantation and explantation and found sufficiently high concentrations of the antibiotics vancomycin and tobramycin. Similarly, Hsieh et al. [27] examined 46 patients after a mean period of 107 days and found adequate levels of vancomycin and aztreonam. Bertazzoni Minelli et al. [28] examined 20 patients and showed sufficient elution of the antibiotics gentamycin and vancomycin immediately after spacer implantation, followed by a constant release over a period of 3–6 months. In our own in vivo study, the antibiotic concentration in the membranes surrounding 14 spacers containing gentamycin and clindamycin as well as vancomycin was measured at the site of subsequent implantation of a new prosthesis. Six weeks after spacer implantation, antibiotic levels in spacer membranes were regularly found to be higher than the minimum inhibitory concentration for the bacteria that had caused the periprosthetic infection [29].

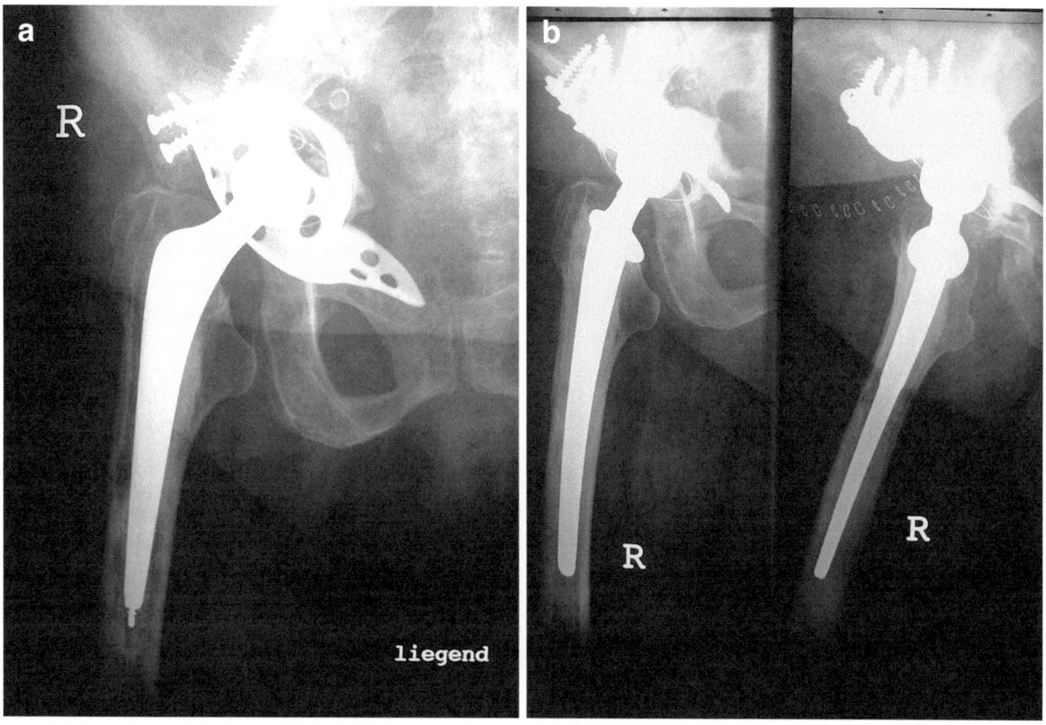

Fig. 19.5 (**a**) Periprosthetic infection with osteolysis in the femur and a major cup defect that does not allow the use of a spacer. (**b**) Radiographs 7 days after surgery after one-stage septic replacement with a cemented SPII stem (Waldemar Link, Hamburg, Germany) and Burch-Schneider cage and cemented Müller flat profile cup (ZimmerBiomet, Winterthur, Switzerland)

Not all antibiotics can be used for admixture in the cement, as they must be available in powder form, water-soluble, and thermostable. The most commonly used are gentamycin, clindamycin, vancomycin, tobramycin, aztreonam, ampicillin, and ofloxacin [30–32]. Most published studies always involve the same antibiotics in the cement. Some authors regularly use vancomycin and tobramycin as local antibiotics because they have a broad spectrum of activity [13, 33]. However, not all bacteria can be successfully treated with those antibiotics (e.g., some Gram-negative organisms). This is also the disadvantage of commercially produced ready-to-use spacers that only contain gentamycin, vancomycin, or sometimes both. This is also an argument for the preoperative determination of the antibiotic resistance pattern of the respective bacteria and the selection of specific antibiotics for treatment. Masri et al. [34] reported a success rate of 89.7% in their retrospective study with bacteria-specific antibiotics mixed into the cement of a PROSTALAC® spacer (DePuy Synthes, Warsaw, IN). We used this concept for custom-made spacers and did not see any re-infection of 36 cases during a minimum follow-up of 2 years [10].

Different antibiotics are released by the spacers at different rates and also affect each other when in combination [4]. The use of two antibiotics leads to a synergistic effect, and the elution of the individual components is better than that of the individual antibiotic alone [30, 35–38]. Many surgeons today use cement with gentamycin and clindamycin in combination (e.g., Copal, Heraeus Medical GmbH, Wertheim, Germany) instead of gentamycin alone, because the combination exhibits better kinetics of antibiotic elution. A third antibiotic (usually vancomycin) is often added according to the organism specificity as defined by an antibiogram [1, 36]. This concept

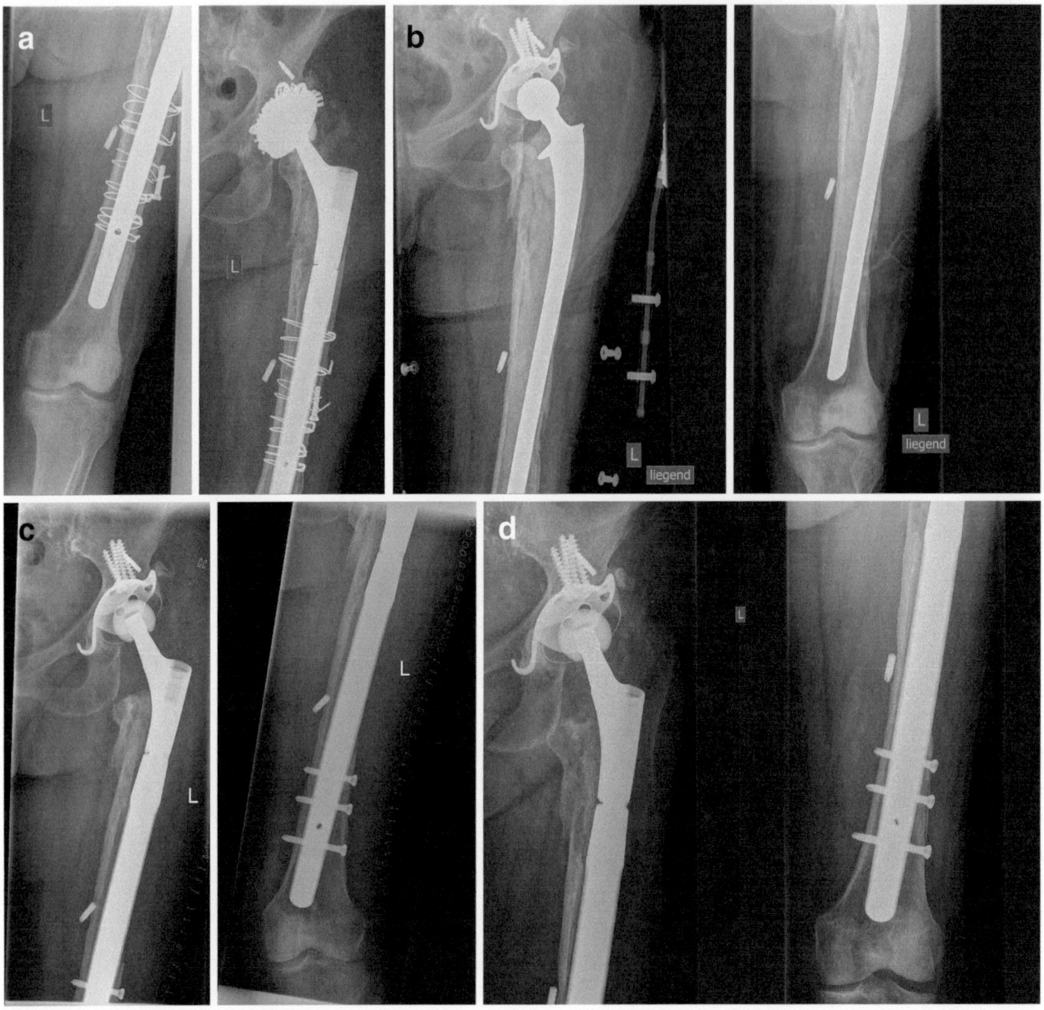

Fig. 19.6 (**a**) Infected modular revision prosthesis and coarsely structured cup after extramural stem revision with loss of the greater trochanter. (**b1** and **b2**) Removal of infected implants and a septic one-stage cup revision with implantation of an interim stem and a permanent cup system consisting of a complete shell and cemented Müller flat profile cup (ZimmerBiomet, Winterthur, Switzerland). (**c1** and **c2**) Radiograph 7 days after a septic two-stage stem revision changing the stem to the modular revision stem Revitan Curved with distal locking (ZimmerBiomet, Winterthur, Switzerland). (**d**) Radiograph 1 year after surgery with distal bony osteointegration of the stem

allowed us and others to achieve an eradication rate between 93.5 and 100%, implying that sufficient antibiotic concentration was in fact available in the tissues surrounding the spacer [1, 20, 29]. However, in our in vivo study, the addition of vancomycin did not result in an increase in the release of the antibiotics gentamycin and clindamycin present in Copal bone cement [29]. Furthermore, hand-mixed cement leads to a better elution of antibiotics than cement mixed under vacuum. This is due to the fact that hand-mixed cement contains air bubbles that increase the total surface area from which the antibiotics elute. However, the mechanical properties (e.g., fracture resistance) of the hand-mixed cement are poorer than those of the vacuum-mixed cement although the mechanical properties of the spacer cement do not necessarily have to be similar to those of the cement used to fix the implants [39]. I therefore recommend the addition of several organism-specific antibiotics to the spacer cement. This concept enabled us to show that the local antibiotic concentrations were still above the relevant minimum inhibitory concentrations 6 weeks after implantation. Furthermore, we observed a very low recurrence rate of infection in the clinical setting, at or around 0% [10, 24, 25, 29]. Thus, the antibiotic-containing spacer not only fulfills a mechanical function, but also plays an important role in the treatment of periprosthetic infections.

19.4 Duration of the Spacer Period and Systemic Antibiotic Therapy

The period between the two stages of a two-stage revision and that of the systemic antibiotic therapy varies greatly between studies. They range from a few days to several years for the duration of the spacer period and from 2 weeks to several months for the duration of systemic antibiotic therapy after reimplantation (Tables 19.1 and 19.2). Many authors determine the time of reimplantation of a prosthesis based on clinical parameters and clinical chemistry data or perform joint aspiration prior to surgery [12, 20, 34, 40]. Other authors have a more or less rigid procedural plan [11, 14, 43]. Due to these differences in the procedure, not only between studies but also within studies, it is not possible to decide how long the time between the two operations should be, and thus for how long the spacers should remain in place and how long the antibiotics should be administered. This also seems to underline the importance of surgical debridement for the therapeutic success of the two-stage revision. However, most surgeons choose a spacer period of 6–12 weeks and systemic antibiotic therapy of 6–12 weeks after reimplantation (Tables 19.1 and 19.2).

19.5 Aspiration Before Reimplantation

There are no comparative studies in the literature that consider this aspect of the therapeutic concept. In order to be able to make a reproducible assessment of the microbiological results of a joint aspiration as a basis for deciding whether or not reimplantation can be performed, antibiotic treatment must be discontinued for a period of at least 2 weeks, preferably for 4 weeks [52]. Since the recommended bacterial cultivation period is 2 weeks, aspiration of the joint before reimplantation results in a delay of this operation of between 4 and 6 weeks [53]. In our study of local antibiotic concentrations in the spacer membranes, we could show that, 6 weeks after spacer implantation, antibiotic levels were higher than the minimum inhibitory concentrations. However, it is unclear whether this would also be true after another 4–6 weeks. Nevertheless, the fact that an effective antibiotic level could be present in the tissue at the time of aspiration suggests that the prognostic value of the whole procedure of joint aspiration before reimplantation is overestimated. This hypothesis is supported by the study of Preininger et al. [54] for two-stage revisions of infected knee endoprostheses, in which a sensitivity of only 21% was found for aspiration of the spacer synovial fluid prior to reimplantation. Moreover, Hoell et al. [55] found a sensitivity of only 5% for aspiration before reimplantation of hip and knee two-stage revisions. Furthermore, Parvizi et al. [56] state as a consensus opinion of experts that diagnostic aspiration should not be performed prior to reimplantation for the purpose of demonstrating freedom from infection. For this reason, we refrain from this procedure and rely solely on clinical observation and monitoring of CRP levels. Previous experience has shown

Table 19.1 Outcomes of two-stage cemented revision of infected total hip arthroplasties

Author	N	Follow-up	Spacer/beads	Local antibiotics	Duration of intravenous antibiotic	Interval until reimplantation	Antibiotics after reimplantation	Freedom from infection	Aseptic loosening
McDonald [40]	82	5.5 years	None (Girdlestone)	None	26.1 (4–59 days)	1.5 years (6 days–6.2 years)	No antibiotic in cement	87%	
Colyer [41]	37	2.7 years	None (Girdlestone)	None	6 weeks parenteral	6 weeks (4–214 weeks)	2 weeks parenteral, 3 months oral	84%	
Garvin [11]	32	≥2 years, 4.1 years	Beads	Gentamycin	6 weeks parenteral	6 weeks		91%	0%
Lieberman [12]	32	40 (24–80) months	Beads Spacer	Gentamycin Tobramycin Vancomycin	6 weeks (20–49 days)	8,8 weeks (3 weeks–32 months)		91%	
Younger [42]	48	43 (24–63) months	Spacer	Gentamycin	3 weeks parenteral, 3 weeks oral	13 weeks (5–42 weeks)	3 weeks parenteral, 3 weeks oral	94%	0%
Leunig [17]	12	2.2 years	Spacer	Gentamycin		4 (2–7) months		100%	
Evans [43]	23		Spacer	Gentamycin	6 weeks	12 months	None	95.7%	
Hsieh [16]	24	4.2 years	Spacer	Specific: Vancomycin Piperacillin Aztreonam Teicoplanin	2 weeks parenteral, 4 weeks oral	11–17 weeks, until CRP normal	1 week parenteral	100%	0%
Matar [44]	29	5 (2–9) years	Spacer	Vancomycin Gentamycin	1 week parenteral 5 weeks oral	12 weeks	None	96.5%	

Table 19.2 Outcomes of two-stage cementless revision of infected total hip arthroplasties, * = combination of another local antibiotic with tobramycin, Mo = months, ** = 13 of 22 reimplantations cementless; stem subsid = stem subsidence; nm = nonmodular; pf = proximal fixation

Author	N	Follow-up	Spacer/beads	Local antibiotics	Duration of intravenous antibiotic	Interval until reimplantation	Antibiotics after reimplantation	Freedom from infection	Aseptic loosening
Wilson [45]	22/ 13**	≥3 years, 48 months	Resection arthroplasty	None	3 weeks parenteral	6–12 weeks	3 days parenteral	91%/100% cementless	7.6% stem loosening
Nestor [46]	34	47 (24–72) months	Resection arthroplasty	None	≥4 weeks parenteral	8 (3–19) months	Various	82%	18% stem
Fehring [13]	25	41 (24–98) months	Beads	Tobramycin in 16 cases	6 weeks parenteral	4.8 months		92%	0%
Haddad [14]	50	5.8 (2–8.7) years	Beads + cement ball	Gentamycin	5 days parenteral and then oral	3 weeks	≥ 3 months	92%	8% stem subsidence
Koo [47]	22	41 (24–78) months	Spacer Beads	Vancomycin Gentamycin Cefotaxime	6 weeks	6–12 weeks		95%	5% cup loosening 30% stem subs.
Hofmann [32]	27	76 (28–148) months	Old stem and new polyethylene cup	Tobramycin	6 weeks parenteral, in 17 cases additional 6 weeks oral			94%	0%
Kraay [33]	33	≥ 2 years	Spacer in 16 cases	Tobramycin in 16 cases	≥6 weeks parenteral	7.4 (3–37) months		92%	9% cup 0% stem
Masri [34]	29	≥ 2 years	Prostalac spacer	Tobramycin Tobramicin Vancomycin Cefuroxime Penicillin*	6 weeks parenteral or in combination with oral	12 weeks	5 days intravenous	90%	0%
Yamamoto [48]	17	38 months	Spacer	Gentamycin Vancomycin	>3 weeks		1 week parenteral, oral until CRP normal	100%	
Fink [10]	36	≥ 2 years	Spacer	Specific: Gentamycin Clindamycin Vancomycin Ampicillin Ofloxacin	2 weeks parenteral, 4 weeks oral	6 weeks	2 weeks parenteral, 4 weeks oral	100%	6% stem subsidence 0% loosening

(continued)

Table 19.2 (continued)

Author	N	Follow-up	Spacer/beads	Local antibiotics	Duration of intravenous antibiotic	Interval until reimplantation	Antibiotics after reimplantation	Freedom from infection	Aseptic loosening
Berend [49]	189	53 (24–180) months	Spacer (70% articulating, 30% nonarticulating)	Vancomycin + Gentamycin or Vancomycin + Tobramycin)	6 weeks parenteral	≥6 weeks	2 days	83%	
Camurcu [50]	41	54 (24–96) months	Spacer	Teicoplanin	≤2 weeks parenteral, 8 (4–20) weeks in total	6 (1–13) months	≤4 weeks	95.1%	5% cup 0% stem
Akgün [51]	84	33,1 (24–48) months	Mostly Girdlestone	None	61 ± 29.8 days	61 ± 29.8 days	2 weeks parenteral 10 weeks oral	90.5%	

that the CRP drops to a level between 10 and 30 mg/L within 2 or 3 weeks of surgery. A normal level of less than 5 mg/L is not expected when a spacer is implanted. However, if the CRP level does not drop to the abovementioned range of values within 3 weeks, or if there is persistent wound exudation, or if other signs and symptoms indicate a deep-seated infection, we do not carry out a reimplantation, but instead change the spacer with concomitant debridement of the prosthesis bed.

19.6 Type of Prosthesis Used for Reimplantation

Although the use of a cemented prosthesis for reimplantation has the advantage that antibiotics can be added to the cement, there are no obvious differences in the re-infection rate observed between cemented and cementless prostheses at reimplantation (Tables 19.1 and 19.2). Therefore, the measures used in the first stage of surgery, which include radical debridement and local and systemic antibiotic treatment to maintain infection-free status, appear to be more decisive for the treatment of periprosthetic infections than the type of implant used in reimplantation. Since optimal interdigitation of the cement requires cancellous bone and this is not found after debridement of the femur, it is likely that the quality of long-term fixation of the cemented prosthesis to smooth bone surfaces will be compromised. Although there are no reports of aseptic loosening of cemented implants after two-stage septic revision surgery, we know that the rate of loosening of cemented revision stems under such conditions is much higher than that of cementless stems [10, 57]. We therefore use cementless revision stems for reimplantation, and it is the disadvantages of cemented reimplantation that have led us to choose a two-stage procedure instead of the one-stage procedure for revision of the hip joint.

With the concept described here, study results of 100% and 93.5% freedom from infection were achieved [10, 24, 25]. These results suggest that our concept for septic revision will continue to provide reproducibly good clinical outcomes.

References

1. Fink B. Revision of late periprosthetic infections of total hip endoprostheses: pros and cons of different concepts. Int J Med Sci. 2009;6:287–95.
2. Li C, Renz N, Trampuz A. Management of periprosthetic joint infection. Hip Pelvis. 2018;30:138–46.
3. Pulido L, Ghanem E, Joshi A, Purtill JJ, Parvizi J. Periprosthetic joint infection: the incidence, timing, and predisposing factors. Clin Orthop Relat Res. 2008;466:1710–5.
4. Cui Q, Mihalko WM, Shields JS, Ries M, Saleh KJ. Antibiotic-impregnated cement spacers for the treatment of infection associated with total hip or knee arthroplasty. J Bone Joint Surg Am. 2007;89:871–82.
5. Garvin KL, Hanssen AD. Infection after total hip arthroplasty. Past, present, and future. J Bone Joint Surg Am. 1995;77-A:1576–88.
6. Hanssen AD, Osmon DR. Evaluation of a staging system for infected hip arthroplasty. Clin Orthop Relat Res. 2002;403:16–22.
7. George DA, Logoluso N, Castellini G, Gianola S, Scarponi S, Haddad FS, Drago L, Romano CL. Does cemented or cementless single-stage exchange arthroplasty of chronic periprosthetic hip infections provide similar infection rates to a two-stage? A systematic review. BMC Infect Dis. 2016;16:553.
8. Svensson K, Rolfson O, Kärrholm J, Mohaddes M. Similar risk of re-revision in patients after one- or two-stage surgical revision of infected total hip arthroplasty: an analysis of revisions in the Swedish hip arthroplasty register 1979–2015. J Clin Med. 2019;10:485.
9. Burnett RS, Kelly MA, Hanssen AD, Barrack RL. Technique and timing of two-stage exchange for infection in TKA. Clin Orthop Relat Res. 2007;464:164–78.
10. Fink B, Grossmann A, Fuerst M, Schafer P, Frommelt L. Two-stage cementless revision of infected hip endoprostheses. Clin Orthop Relat Res. 2009;467:1848–58.
11. Garvin KL, Evans BG, Salvati EA, Brause BD. Palacos gentamycin for the treatment of deep periprosthetic hip infections. Clin Orthop Relat Res. 1994;298:97–105.
12. Lieberman JR, Callaway GH, Salvati EA, Pellicci PM, Brause BD. Treatment of the infected total hip arthroplasty with a two-stage reimplantation protocol. Clin Orthop Relat Res. 1994;301:205–12.
13. Fehring TK, Calton TF, Griffin WL. Cementless fixation in 2-stage reimplantation for periprosthetic sepsis. J Arthroplasty. 1999;14:175–81.
14. Haddad FS, Muirhead-Allwood SK, Manktelow AR, Bacarese-Hamilton I. Two-stage uncemented revision

hip arthroplasty for infection. J Bone Joint Surg Br. 2000;82-B:689–94.
15. Hsieh PH, Chen LH, Chen CH, Lee MS, Yang WE, Shih CH. Two-stage revision hip arthroplasty for infection with a custom-made, antibiotic-loaded, cement prosthesis as an interim spacer. J Trauma. 2004;56:1247–52.
16. Hsieh PH, Shih CH, Chang YH, Lee MS, Shih HN, Yang WE. Two-stage revision hip arthroplasty for infection: comparison between the interim use of antibiotic-loaded cement Ketten and a spacer prosthesis. J Bone Joint Surg Am. 2004;86-A:1989–97.
17. Leunig M, Chosa E, Speck M, Ganz R. A cement spacer for two-stage revision of infected implants of the hip joint. Int Orthop. 1998;22:209–14.
18. Mitchell PA, Masri BA, Garbuz DS, Greidanus NV, Duncan CP. Cementless revision for infection following total hip arthroplasty. Instr Course Lect. 2003;52:323–30.
19. Disch AC, Matziolis G, Perka C. Two-stage operative strategy without local antibiotic treatment for infected hip arthroplasty: clinical and radiological outcome. Arch Orthop Trauma Surg. 2007;127:691–7.
20. Hsieh PH, Shih CH, Chang YH, Lee MS, Yang WE, Shih HN. Treatment of deep infection of the hip associated with massive bone loss: two-stage revision with an antibiotic-loaded interim cement prosthesis followed by reconstruction with allograft. J Bone Joint Surg Br. 2005;87:770–5.
21. Fink B, Rechtenbach A, Buchner H, Vogt S, Hahn M. Articulating spacers used in two-stage revision of infected hip and knee prostheses abrade with time. Clin Orthop Relat Res. 2011;469:1095–102.
22. Jung J, Schmid NV, Kelm J, Schmitt E, Anganostakos K. Complications after spacer implantation in the treatment of hip joint infections. Int J Med Sci. 2009;6:265–73.
23. Morshed S, Huffman GR, Ries MD. Extended trochanteric osteotomy for 2-stage revision of infected total hip arthroplasty. J Arthroplasty. 2005;20:294–301.
24. Fink B, Oremek D. The Transfemoral approach for removal of well-fixed femoral stems in 2-stage septic hip revision. J Arthroplasty. 2016;31:1065–71.
25. Fink B, Schlumberger M, Oremek D. Single-stage acetabular revision during two-stage THA revision for infection is effective in selected patients. Clin Orthop Relat Res. 2017;475:2063–70.
26. Masri BA, Duncan CP, Beauchamp CP. Long-term elution of antibiotics from bone-cement: an in vivo study using the prosthesis of antibiotic-loaded acrylic cement (PROSTALAC) system. J Arthroplasty. 1998;13:331–8.
27. Hsieh PH, Chang YH, Chen SH, Ueng SW, Shih CH. High concentration and bioactivity of vancomycin and aztreonam eluted from simplex cement spacers in two-stage revision of infected hip implants: a study of 46 patients at an average follow-up of 107 days. J Orthop Res. 2006;24:1615–21.
28. Bertazzoni Minelli E, Benini A, Magnan B, Bartolozzi P. Release of gentamycin and vancomycin from temporary human hip spacers in two-stage revision of infected arthroplasty. J Antimicrob Chemother. 2004;53:329–34.
29. Fink B, Vogt S, Reinsch M, Buchner H. Sufficient release of antibiotic by a spacer 6 weeks after implantation in two-stage revision of infected hip prostheses. Clin Orthop Relat Res. 2011;469:3141–7.
30. Anagnostakos K, Kelm J, Regitz T, Schmitt E, Jung W. In vitro evaluation of antibiotic release from and bacteria growth inhibition by antibiotic-loaded acrylic bone cement spacers. J Biomed Mater Res B Appl Biomater. 2005;72:373–8.
31. Hoff SF, Fitzgerald RH Jr, Kelly PJ. The depot administration of penicillin G and gentamycin in acrylic bone cement. J Bone Joint Surg Am. 1981;63-A:798–804.
32. Hofmann AA, Goldberg TA, Tanner AM, Cook TM. Ten-year experience using an articulating antibiotic cement hip spacer for the treatment of chronically infected total hip. J Arthroplasty. 2005;20:874–9.
33. Kraay MJ, Goldberg VM, Fitzgerald SJ, Salata MJ. Cementless two-staged total hip arthroplasty for deep periprosthetic infection. Clin Orthop Relat Res. 2005;441:243–9.
34. Masri BA, Panagiotopoulos KP, Greidanus NV, Garbuz DS, Duncan CP. Cementless two-stage exchange arthroplasty for infection after total hip arthroplasty. J Arthroplasty. 2007;22:72–8.
35. Baleani M, Persson C, Zolezzi C, Andollina A, Borrelli AM, Tigani D. Biological and biomechanical effects of vancomycin and meropenem in acrylic bone cement. J Arthroplasty. 2008;23:1232–8.
36. Ensing GT, van Horn JR, van der Mei HC, Busscher HJ, Neut D. Copal bone cement is more effective in preventing biofilm formation than Palacos R-G. Clin Orthop Relat Res. 2008;466:1492–8.
37. Penner MJ, Masri BA, Duncan CP. Elution characteristics of vancomycin and tobramycin combined in acrylic bone-cement. J Arthroplasty. 1996;11:939–44.
38. Simpson PM, Dall GF, Breusch SJ, Heisel C. In vitro elution and mechanical properties of antibiotic-loaded SmartSet HV and Palacos R acrylic bone cements. Orthopäde. 2005;34:1255–62.
39. Hanssen AD, Spangehl MJ. Practical applications of antibiotic-loaded bone cement for treatment of infected joint replacements. Clin Orthop Relat Res. 2004;427:79–85.
40. McDonald DJ, Fitzgerald RH Jr, Ilstrup DM. Two-stage reconstruction of a total hip arthroplasty because of infection. J Bone Joint Surg Am. 1989;71:828–34.
41. Colyer RA, Capello WN. Surgical treatment of the infected hip implant. Two-stage reimplantation with a one-month interval. Clin Orthop Relat Res. 1994;298:75–9.
42. Younger AS, Duncan CP, Masri BA, McGraw RW. The outcome of two-stage arthroplasty using a custom-made interval spacer to treat the infected hip. J Arthroplasty. 1997;12:615–23.
43. Evans RP. Successful treatment of total hip and knee infection with articulating antibiotic components: a

modified treatment method. Clin Orthop Relat Res. 2004;427:37–46.
44. Matar HE, Stritch P, Emms N. Two-stage revisions of infected hip replacements: subspecialisation and patient-reported outcome measures. J Orthop. 2019;16:179–81.
45. Wilson MG, Dorr LD. Reimplantation of infected total hip arthroplasties in the absence of antibiotic cement. J Arthroplasty. 1989;4:263–9.
46. Nestor BJ, Hanssen AD, Ferrer-Gonzalez R, Fitzgerald RH Jr. The use of porous prostheses in delayed reconstruction of total hip replacements that have failed because of infection. J Bone Joint Surg Am. 1994;76-A:349–59.
47. Koo KH, Yang JW, Cho SH, Song HR, Park HB, Ha YC, Chang JD, Kim SY, Kim YH. Impregnation of vancomycin, gentamycin, and cefotaxime in a cement spacer for two-stage cementless reconstruction in infected total hip arthroplasty. J Arthroplasty. 2001;16:882–92.
48. Yamamoto K, Miyagawa N, Masaoka T, Katori Y, Shishido T, Imakiire A. Cement spacer loaded with antibiotics for infected implants of the hip joint. J Arthroplasty. 2009;24:83–9.
49. Berend KR, Lombardi AV Jr, Morris MJ, Bergeson AG, Adams JB, Sneller MA. Two-stage treatment of hip periprosthetic joint infection is associated with a high rate of infection control but high mortality. Clin Orthop Relat Res. 2013;2013(471):510–8.
50. Camurcu Y, Sofu H, Buyuk AF, Gursu S, Kaygusuz MA, Sahin V. Two-stage cementless revision total hip arthroplasty for infected primary hip arthroplasties. J Arthroplasty. 2015;30:1597–601.
51. Akgün D, Müller M, Perka C, Winkler T. High cure rate of periprosthetic hip joint infection with multidisciplinary team approach using standardized two-stage exchange. J Orthop Surg Res. 2019;14:78.
52. Mont MA, Waldman BJ, Hungerford DS. Evaluation of preoperative cultures before second-stage reimplantation of a total knee prosthesis complicated by infection. A comparison-group study. J Bone Joint Surg Am. 2000;82-A:1552–7.
53. Schäfer P, Fink B, Sandow D, Margull A, Berger I, Frommelt L. Prolonged bacterial culture to identify late periprosthetic joint infection: a promising strategy. Clin Infect Dis. 2008;47:1403–9.
54. Preininger B, Janz V, von Roth P, Trampuz A, Perka CF, Pfitzner T. Inadequacy of joint aspiration for detection of persistent periprosthetic infection during two-stage septic revision knee surgery. Orthopedics. 2017;40(4):231–4.
55. Hoell S, Moeller A, Gosheger G, Hardes J, Dieckmann R, Schulz D. Two-stage revision arthroplasty for periprosthetic joint infections: what is the value of cultures and white cell count in synovial fluid and CRP in serum before second stage reimplantation? Arch Orthop Trauma Surg. 2016;136:447–52.
56. Parvizi J, Gehrke T, Chen AF. Proceedings of the international consensus on periprosthetic joint infection. Bone Joint J. 2013;95-B:1450–2.
57. Wirtz DC, Niethard FU. Etiology, diagnosis and therapy of aseptic hip prosthesis loosening—a status assessment. Z Orthop Ihre Grenzgeb 1997;135:270–280.

Postoperative Rehabilitation 20

Contents

20.1 **Cemented Revision and Cement-in-Cement Revision** 277
20.2 **Impaction Grafting** 277
20.3 **Cementless Revision** 277
20.4 **Allograft Prosthesis Composite (APC)** 278
20.5 **Proximal Femoral Replacement** 278
20.6 **Total Femoral Replacement** 278
References 278

20.1 Cemented Revision and Cement-in-Cement Revision

In this case, as with cemented primary implantation, full weight bearing is possible immediately after surgery and postoperative treatment is carried out in the usual manner as described for primary arthroplasty.

20.2 Impaction Grafting

Since the incorporation of the bone graft into the host bone surrounding it appears to be critical for the durability of the entire construct, most investigators carry out a very long period of incremental weight bearing up to full weight bearing after 4 to 6 months [1]. During the early years of their study, te Stroet et al. [1] even prescribed bed rest for 6 weeks after surgery. In the second six weeks, a mobilization with 10 to 15 kg partial weight bearing was allowed and in the next six weeks with 50 % of the body weight.

20.3 Cementless Revision

On the one hand, the postoperative follow-up depends on whether a femoral osteotomy and/or a transfemoral approach was carried out. On the other hand, the bone quality, the age of the patient, and the quality of the press-fit fixation achieved intraoperatively all play a role. Thus, this surgical guide cannot reach any generally applicable conclusions. As a rule, however, partial weight bearing is recommended for approximately 6 weeks after surgery. If a transfemoral approach was chosen, the load should not exceed 20 kg for about 6 weeks and further weight bearing should be done stepwise until

B. Fink, *Femoral Revision Arthroplasty*, https://doi.org/10.1007/978-3-030-84821-7_20

full weight bearing is achieved within 3 months. During this time, follow-up radiographs are recommended 6 and 12 weeks after surgery. Furthermore, during the first 6 weeks of transfemoral access, flexion should not exceed 70 to 80 degrees in order not to endanger the healing of the bony flap.

20.4 Allograft Prosthesis Composite (APC)

Postoperative follow-up treatment depends on the type of fixation of the prosthesis in the host bone:

- In the case of cementless implantation, a partial weight bearing of approximately 20 kg should be applied until the first signs of incorporation of the allograft are radiologically visible. Some authors recommend a low partial weight bearing for 3 months [2].
- Full weight bearing can be permitted with cemented implantation.
- Active abduction and aggressive physiotherapy with muscle training should be avoided for the first 3 months.

20.5 Proximal Femoral Replacement

Even with a proximal femoral replacement, the follow-up treatment depends on the way it is fixed in the rest of the femur:

- Immediate full weight bearing is permitted when the usual cemented fixation is carried out in the distal femur.
- In the case of cementless fixation, a stepwise increase in weight bearing is necessary, analogous to the procedure for cementless revision prostheses with distal fixation.
- The increased tendency for dislocation should be taken into account in the first three months after surgery with regard to the permitted range of motion, and any movements that might promote dislocation should be avoided.

20.6 Total Femoral Replacement

The total femoral replacement can be subjected to full weight bearing immediately. Due to the increased tendency to dislocate, dislocation-promoting movement should be avoided for 3 months and the extent of movement should be limited as necessary.

References

1. Te Stroet MAJ, Rijen WHC, Gardeniers JWM, van Kampen A, Schreurs BW. The outcome of femoral component revision arthroplasty with impaction allograft bone grafting and a cemented polished Exeter stem. A prospective cohort study of 208 revision arthroplasties with a mean follow-up of ten years. Bone Joint J. 2015;5:771–9.
2. Maury AC, Pressman A, Cayen B, et al. Proximal femoral allograft treatment of Vancouver type-B3 periprosthetic femoral fractures after total hip arthroplasty. J Bone Joint Surg Am. 2006;88:953–8.

Management of Complications 21

Contents

21.1 Complications Associated with the Transfemoral Approach (Extended Trochanteric Osteotomy) 279
21.2 Proximalization of the Bony Flap 280
21.3 Subsidence of a Cementless Revision Stem 281
21.4 Intraoperative Fracture of the Greater Trochanter 285
21.5 Postoperative Fracture of the Greater Trochanter 286
21.6 Intraoperative Perforation of the Femur 286
21.7 Intraoperative Fissures and Periprosthetic Fractures of the Femoral Shaft 287
21.8 Postoperative Periprosthetic Fracture of the Femoral Shaft 289
21.9 Hematoma 289
21.10 Periprosthetic Infection 289
21.11 Dislocations 290
21.12 Prosthesis Stem Fracture and/or Fracture of the Junction between Modular Components 290
References 295

21.1 Complications Associated with the Transfemoral Approach (Extended Trochanteric Osteotomy)

When the bony flap is opened, osteolysis of the flap area may cause fractures of the flap. Since the fragments are located in the soft tissue composite of the vastus lateralis muscle, only an additional double cerclage is required to hold the fragments individually when closing the flap (Fig. 21.1a, b). An intraoperative trochanteric rupture or fracture can also be stabilized with a transosseous fiber wire cerclage, which is guided through the most cranially located double cerclage. Since the vasto-gluteal sling is retained in the transfemoral approach (extended trochanteric osteotomy) and the traction forces of the gluteus musculature are neutralized by those of the vastus lateralis muscle, there is a low risk of

B. Fink, *Femoral Revision Arthroplasty*, https://doi.org/10.1007/978-3-030-84821-7_21

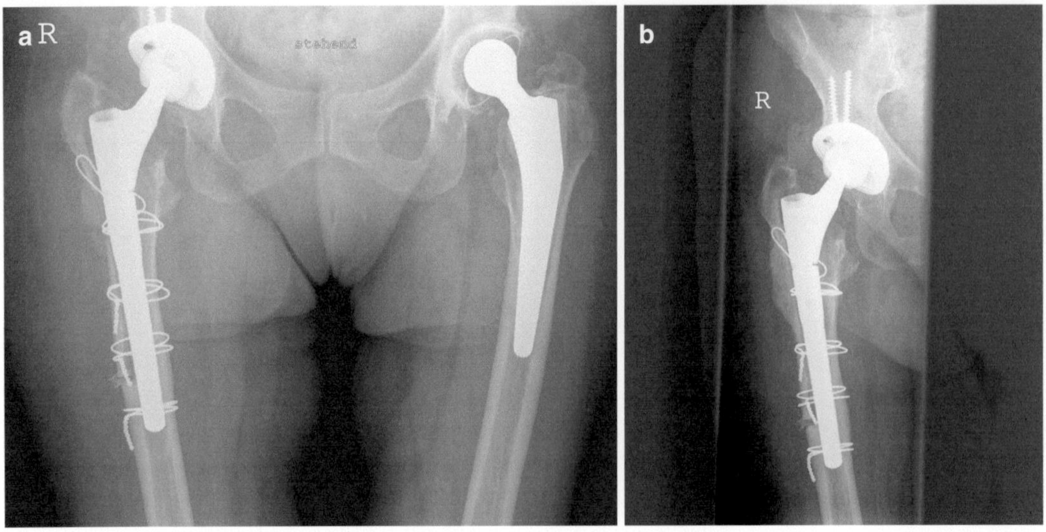

Fig. 21.1 (**a**) Radiograph 3 months after transfemoral prosthesis revision on the right side. An intraoperative fracture of the flap because of osteolysis was osteosynthesized with cerclages. (**b**) Radiograph 6 months after surgery showing complete bony consolidation of the fracture

dislocation of the greater trochanter. After surgery, trochanteric ruptures occur rarely and if they occur than below the tuberculum innominatum. As a rule, they do not lead to a significant dislocation, are usually stable (because of the intact vasto-gluteal sling), and will heal back to the bone (Fig. 21.2a, b). A prolonged partial weight bearing of approximately 10 kg for 8 weeks is recommended. Weekly radiological checks should be performed to verify the location of the trochanter. However, if a secondary dislocation occurs, osteosynthesis of the trochanter with cerclages, tension band, or, if necessary, a claw plate is necessary.

Closure of the flap can be difficult, especially with straight revision stems. For this reason, we prefer a curved revision stem for transfemoral access as well, since the curved stem follows the anatomical shape of the femur and does not produce a quasi-offset elevation as straight stems do. This higher offset causes the more frequent occurrence with straight stems of difficulties in the closure of the flap. We generally prefer to close the flap with cerclages or cables. In our opinion, simply suturing the flap together with the intermuscular septum, as originally described by Heinz Wagner, leads to less stable closure, which in turn leads to dislocation of the flap [1]. In our experience, a certain gap to the flap of up to 1 cm can be accepted. This gap will be closed by the subsequent callus formation. If bone shavings were retained during the operation (when the cup or femur was reamed), these can be introduced into the gap. However, it is important to check that no cement residues remain in the trochanteric region that might impede closure of the flap. Interfering bone protrusions in the trochanteric region should also be removed. We advise against excessive thinning of the greater trochanteric region with the intention of improving closure of the flap. It carries the high risk of bone weakening with subsequent unintentional trochanteric fracture.

21.2 Proximalization of the Bony Flap

The loosening of a prosthetic stem often causes the stem to subside, thereby causing a shortening of the leg, which in turn causes a shortening of the gluteal muscles if left untreated for a lengthy period of time. This in turn leads to a proximalization of the bony flap when the correct leg length is restored during revision surgery. This can result in a gap between the reaffixed flap and

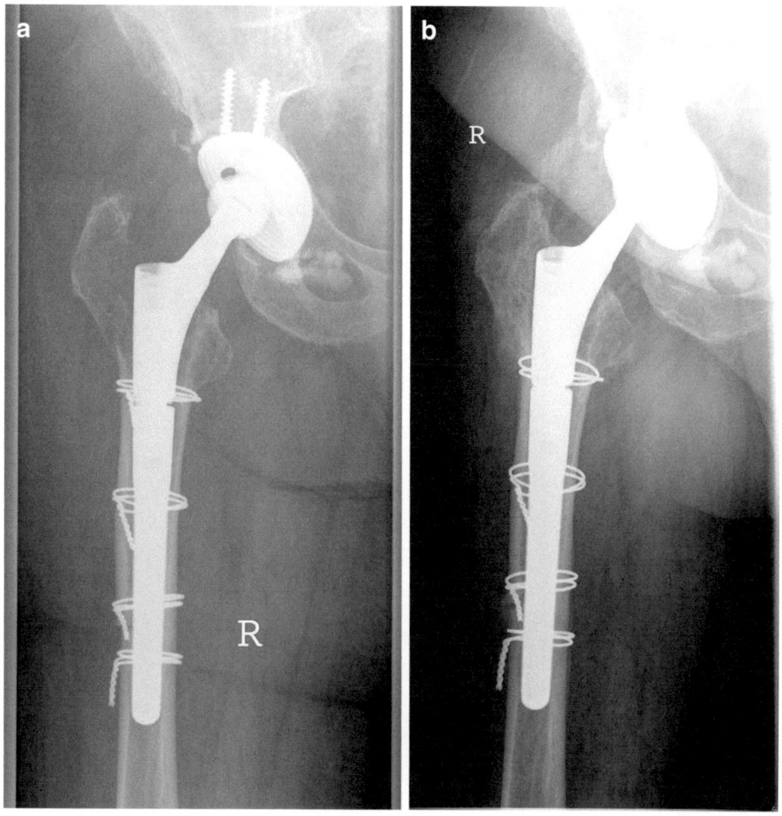

Fig. 21.2 (**a**) Nondisplaced fracture of the greater trochanter after surgery caused by an osteolytic weakening of this area. (**b**) Radiograph 3 months later. The greater trochanteric fracture has healed with callus formation after conservative therapy

the femur at the distal end of the flap (Fig. 21.3a–c). This gap can also be filled with bone chips or bone shavings obtained from the intraoperative reaming procedure. However, even without this filling, the gap is usually closed by callus formation within the first few months of surgery. The tendency to proximalize is particularly pronounced in the case of short flaps, since only a small portion of the vastus lateralis muscle remains on the flap as a counterpart to the gluteal musculature that pulls the flap cranially and ventrally.

If, on the other hand, the flap is proximalized after surgery has been completed, this is mostly the result of an insufficient closure or rare breakage of the cerclage wires, which leaves the flap unstable. This is mentioned in 7.4% of >1 cm, including 1.4% with more than 2 cm in 612 revisions by Abdel et al. [2]. In this rare complication, too much activity-related stress was exerted on the flap and its fastenings. In most cases, not only a proximalization occurs, but also a ventralization of the flap due to the pulling of the gluteal muscles occurs, which can lead to impingement. In this case, a revision with a new closure of the flap is required.

21.3 Subsidence of a Cementless Revision Stem

Subsidence of the stem occurs if the prosthesis has not been firmly fixed. This is caused by the choice of a stem design that is not suitable for the bone defect (e.g., a proximally fixing revision stem for a proximally deficient femur of the Paprosky III type) or a stem diameter that is too thin, which only has a three-point fixation in the femur instead of a circular cylinder-in-cylinder, cone-in-cylinder, or cone-in-cone fixation. Such a three-point fixation does not result in sufficient bone contact, and thus, subsidence occurs (Fig. 21.4a, b). Hancock et al. [3] investigated the relationship between subsidence and the choice

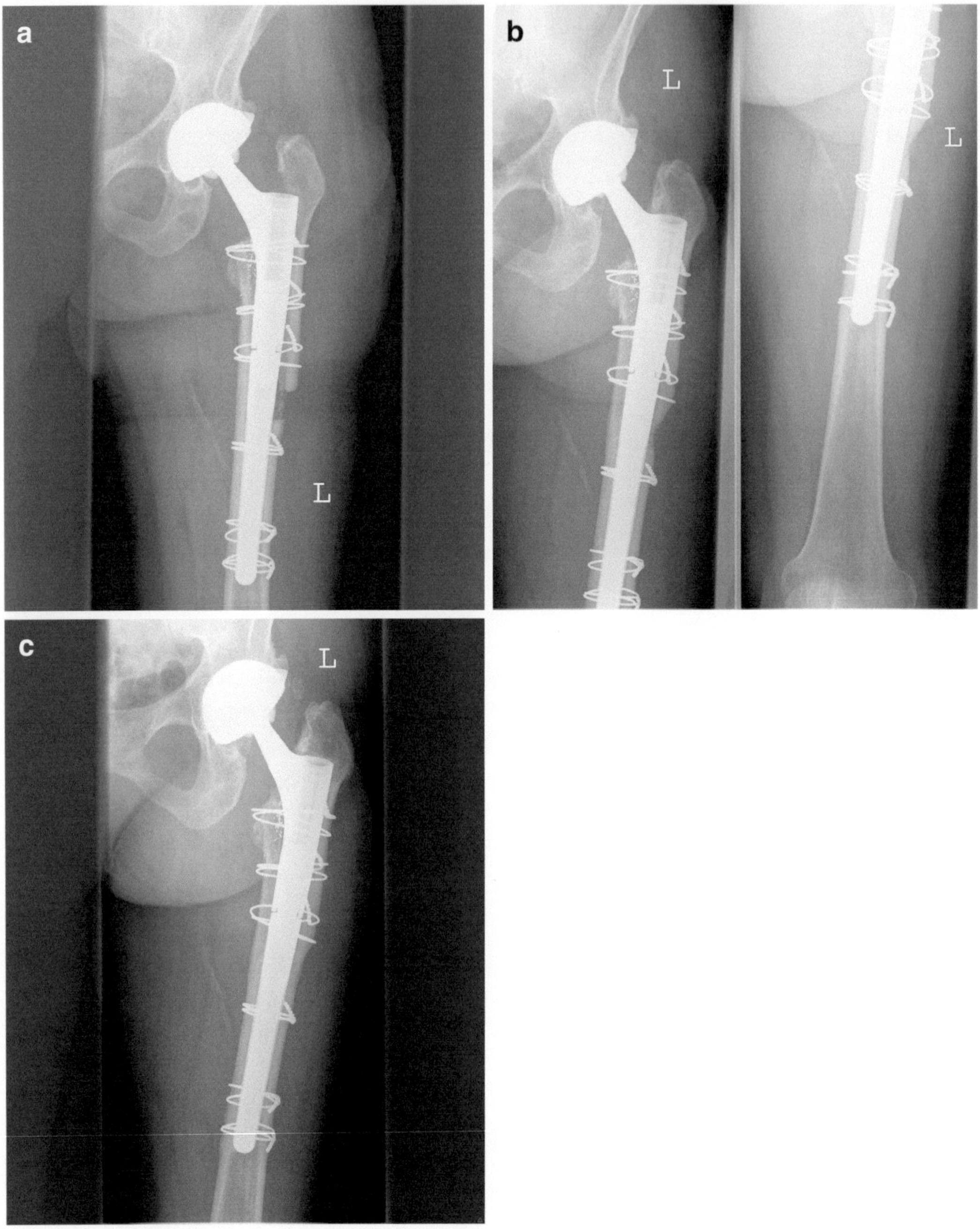

Fig. 21.3 (**a**) Radiograph 2 weeks after surgery after transfemoral stem revision. A gap has developed between the flap and distal femur due to gluteal muscle traction. This gap was filled with milling debris intraoperatively. Two additional double cerclages were applied distally because of a fissure that developed during surgery. (**b**) Radiograph 3 months after surgery: After partial weight bearing of 10 kg for 6 weeks and subsequent stepwise loading, bony consolidation of the flap, and osteointegration of the stem without subsidence has occurred. The former gap under the flap is already closed up with bone. (**c**) Radiograph 1 year after surgery. Complete closure of the old gap and unchanged position of the stem without subsidence

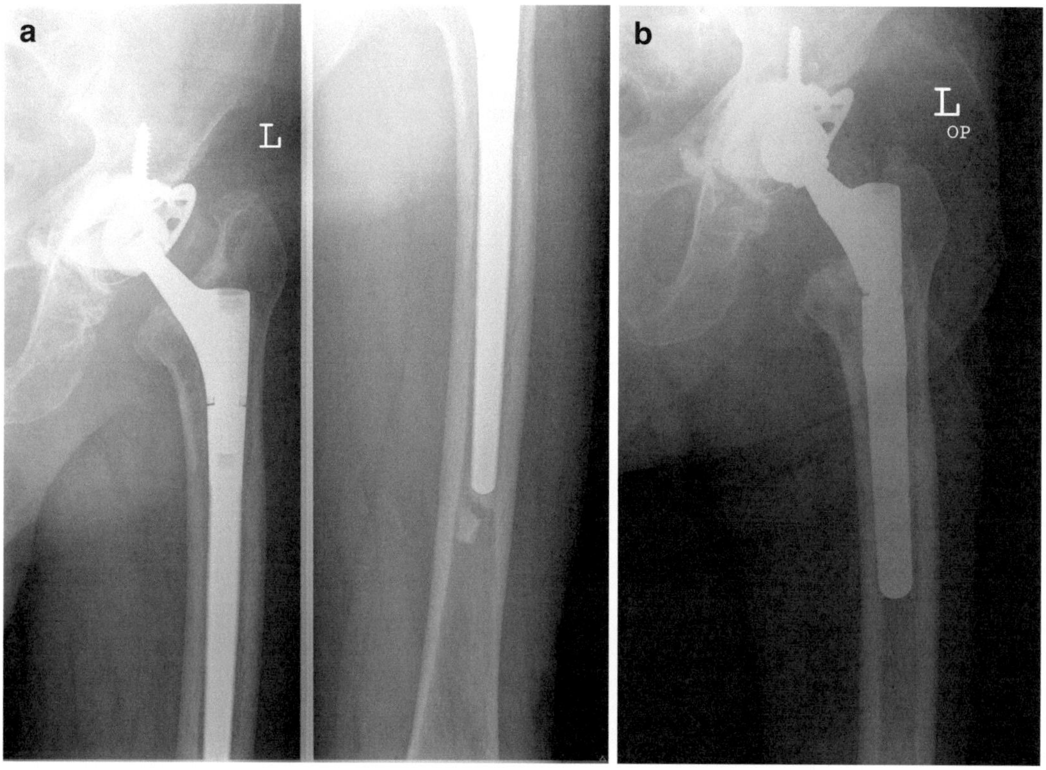

Fig. 21.4 (**a**) Modular revision stem implanted extramurally using the endofemoral approach and tabletop assembly of the modular components (Revitan Curved, Zimmer Biomet, Winterthur, Switzerland). The stem is too thin and too long, has failed to become fixed, and is showing subsidence. (**b**) Radiograph 6 months after revision surgery to a 6 mm thicker and 6 cm shorter revision stem Revitan Curved

of a stem that was too thin and found a significant negative relationship between stem thickness and the degree of subsidence of the stem. Therefore, it can be generally stated that a significant subsidence of the stem of 5 or more millimeters is caused by the choice of too thin stems. The subsidence occurs in the first months following surgery [4, 5]. To avoid this, a revision system adapted to the bone defect must be selected, whereby in my opinion Paprosky III and IV defects should only be treated with distally fixed stem systems. On the other hand, it is important to avoid technical miscalculations that could lead to the selection of an implant that is too thin and/or to subsidence. These include the following:

1. A deviation of the femur axis is not corrected by a transfemoral approach (extended trochanteric osteotomy): Especially when implanting a straight revision stem that is too thin, a three-point fixation with little bone contact occurs instead of a circular fixation (Fig. 21.5). Subsidence of the stem then occurs with increasing postoperative weight bearing. Park et al. [6] found a significantly higher incidence of subsidence of the modular straight tapered revision stem after endofemoral implantation (13%) compared with transfemoral implantation (0%).
2. Assembly on the table of modular revision stems during endofemoral implantation: Premature bone contact of the proximal component prevents firm seating of the distal component in the prepared fixation bed. If the proximal bone flexes after surgery because of its elasticity, the stem will subside and usually slide into the prepared fixation bed, where it may become firmly fixed (Fig. 21.4a, b). The same phenomenon can also occur with straight, nonmodular revision stems [7]. This

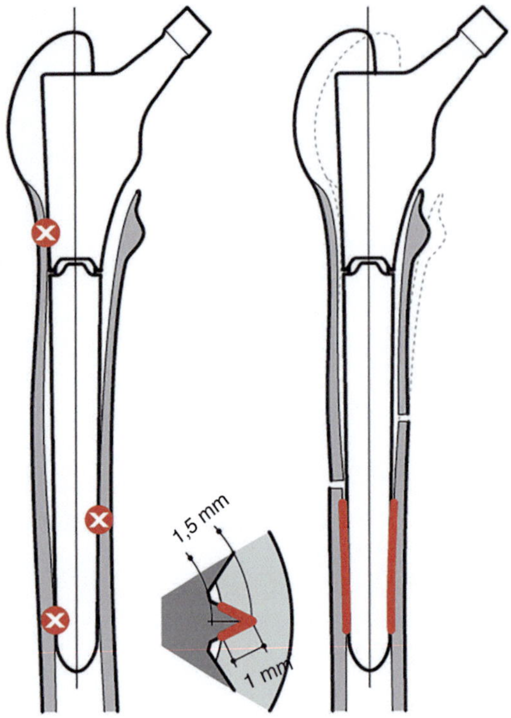

Fig. 21.5 Left: Exposure of a three-point fixation that led to subsidence. Right: Exposure of the distal cone-in-cone anchorage that was achieved by using a transfemoral approach in the same situation as on the left (with permission of Zimmer Biomet, Winterthur, Switzerland)

phenomenon can be avoided with modular, distal fixation stems by first positioning the final distal component in the prepared distal fixation bed and then creating space for the firm implantation of the proximal component (usually with a hollow reamer). This also reduces the risk of unintentional trochanteric fractures.

3. The choice of too long straight revision stems: The longer a straight revision stem implanted in the curved femur is, the smaller the contact surface of the stem with the bone, and the more likely a three-point fixation with subsidence is to occur (Fig. 21.6).
4. The fixation zone is too short: Depending on the distal revision stem used and the fixation principle, the length of the fixation zone in the isthmus of the femur may vary. For cylinder-in-cylinder, scratch-fit fixation of extensively porous-coated stems, the minimum is 4 cm, and for cone-in-cone fixation of titanium stems with a taper of 2 degrees, the minimum is 3 cm [4]. If there is only an intact fixation zone less than the respective minimum fixation distance due to defects or fractures, subsidence of the stem will result. In these cases, in addition to the conventional fixation, other fixation principles such as distal locking devices are required to avoid stem subsidence [8].

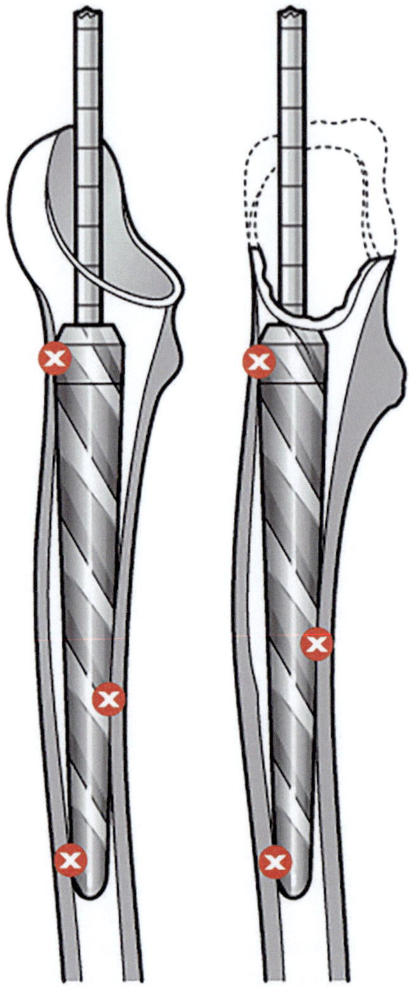

Fig. 21.6 Exposure of the three-point fixation when using a long straight revision stem in the curved femur (with permission of Zimmer Biomet, Winterthur, Switzerland)

Depending on the study and definition of subsidence itself (some authors argue for 5 mm and above, some only from at least 10 mm), subsidence occurs between 0% and 28% of the time (see Tables 6.1, 6.2, 6.3, 6.4, 6.5, 6.6, 6.7, 6.8, 6.9, and 6.10 in Chap. 6). If the stem becomes tightly wedged further distally, it usually becomes firmly fixed. If this does not lead to any problems, such as dislocation or impingement, no further measures are required. Differences in leg length should, however, be compensated by insoles or shoe adjustments. However, a revision is necessary if the patient experiences problems. If the distal component becomes firmly attached, only a revision of the proximal component may be necessary. An analysis of 812 Link MP stems in the Swedish Prosthesis Register by Weiss et al. [9] with an average follow-up of 3.4 years revealed a revision rate of 5%, with more than half of these cases receiving a revision of the proximal component because of stem subsidence. However, when progressive subsidence occurs (Fig. 21.4a), the stem will become loose and cause pain. Therefore, it must be exchanged for a thicker stem (usually also shorter) (Fig. 21.4b).

21.4 Intraoperative Fracture of the Greater Trochanter

Intraoperative fractures of the greater trochanter occur when increased pressure and/or force is applied to the trochanter during endofemoral removal of the old prosthesis, or preparation of the new prosthesis bed or implantation of the new prosthesis. Meek et al. [10] reported 5.7% of 211 prosthesis revisions resulted in a trochanteric fracture when using an extensively porous-coated cobalt chromium stem. The following factors affect the risk of unintentional trochanteric fracture:

1. Anatomy of the proximal femur: Bone or scar tissue may have formed over the shoulder of the prosthetic stem being replaced. This must be removed before the old stem is driven out proximally. Otherwise, there is a risk of an unintentional trochanteric fracture. An overhang of the greater trochanter may also block the way for the old stem to be removed. Here, space must be carefully created in the trochanter in order to remove the stem. If the overhang is significant, an extended trochanteric osteotomy (transfemoral approach) is recommended to avoid the risk of unintentional fracture of the greater trochanter.
2. The chosen surgical approach: The anterior approaches do not allow straight entry into the femoral canal. Access into the femoral shaft must be made in an arc from the ventral. This leads to increased pressure on the greater trochanter during preparation of the fixation bed and implantation of the new stem, which increases the risk of fracture. Regis et al. [11] found a fracture of the greater trochanter in 77.7% (7 of 9) of the Wagner SL revision stems implanted via the anterolateral approach.
3. The shape of the proximal portion of the prosthesis: Prostheses with a laterally protruding shoulder sometimes go deep into the greater trochanteric region during implantation, thus increasing the pressure on the greater trochanter and, as a result, the risk of fracture. Such stems should be avoided if the trochanter is thinned and at risk of fracture.

Intraoperative fractures of the greater trochanter require osteosynthesis. Depending on the size and location of the fracture, once the stem has been implanted endofemorally, the osteosynthesis can be performed using tension band wiring or a trochanteric claw plate in the same way as for a preoperative trochanteric fracture. In the latter case, it is important that the plate is not only attached to the proximal femur by cerclages; at least one screw placed distally to the fracture is required to achieve rotational stability of the osteosynthesis (Fig. 21.7a, b). In some cases, these plate systems allow screws to be angled past the prosthetic stem. Where this is not possible, either monocortical screws or cerclages are required, attached to the plate with eyelets or clips. If a transfemoral revision has been performed, an intraoperative trochanteric fracture of

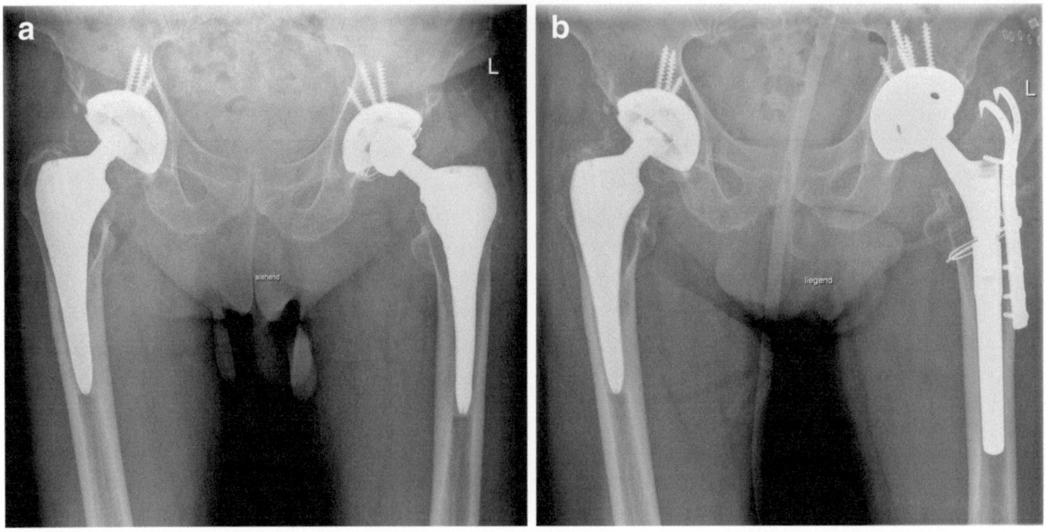

Fig. 21.7 (**a**) Prosthesis loosening with an older dislocated fracture of the left greater trochanter after recurrent dislocations. A PE liner had been cemented into the press-fit shell. (**b**) Postoperative radiograph after endofemoral prosthesis revision to a modular revision stem Revitan Curved and a Trabecular Metal Multihole Shell (Zimmer Biomet, Warsaw, IN, USA) and osteosynthesis of the greater trochanteric fracture with a periplate claw plate (Merete Medical GmbH, Berlin, Germany)

the flap may occur because of osteolysis-related weakening of the bone. After closing the flap, the trochanter is held in place with either a double cerclage or a transosseous fiber wire, which is then guided under the most proximal double cerclage (Fig. 21.1a, b).

21.5 Postoperative Fracture of the Greater Trochanter

Postoperative fractures of the greater trochanter arise as a result of incomplete fractures that were induced intraoperatively and then became evident through the muscle traction during postoperative mobilization of the patient. Abdel et al. [2] observed a postoperative fracture of the greater trochanter in 41 out of 612 hips (7%). The intervention depends on the extent of dislocation of the greater trochanter. If the vasto-gluteal sling is intact and thus the counterpart to the gluteal muscles, i.e., the vastus lateralis muscle, is functionally intact, the greater trochanter will typically not dislocate. Thus, a conservative therapy can be initiated. A partial weight bearing of approximately 10–20 kg should be initiated, and active abduction should be avoided for at least 6 weeks. Weekly radiological checks should be performed to verify that the trochanter does not dislocate secondarily and that fracture healing has begun (Fig. 21.2a, b). Secondary trochanteric dislocation requires surgical treatment (as with intraoperative trochanteric fractures). It is important that this trochanteric dislocation is detected and treated early to prevent shortening of the gluteal muscles. Cranially positioned trochanteric structures that have been dislocated for months are very difficult or impossible to reposition caudally, resulting in permanent gluteal muscle weakness.

21.6 Intraoperative Perforation of the Femur

An intraoperative perforation of the femur may result from the attempt to drill through a distal cement plug, via the endofemoral approach from cranial, or through a bony occlusion in the isthmus of the femur, or during preparation of the fixation bed with a straight reamer. Paprosky et al. [12] reported an incidence of intraoperative perforations of 5.9%. The perforation is usually ventral, or with a varus curved stem, lateral or anterolateral. The perforation can be detected with a guidewire from a flexible intramedullary reamer and confirmed by fluoroscopy. Correct preoperative planning and a decision to use a transfemoral approach (extended trochanteric osteotomy) can usually avoid such perforations. If such a perforation has been caused and detected intraoperatively, a switch from endofemoral to transfemoral or other extended access should be made. Since there is usually still sufficiently intact fixation potential in the isthmus of the femur below the perforation, it is primarily important to keep the situation under control after the perforation is discovered and to avoid unintentional enlargement of the perforation or even fracture. This is achieved by opening the proximal femur to the perforation via the transfemoral approach. The rest of the distal cement can then be drilled straight through and removed under visual control, and the fixation bed for the distally fixed revision stem can be created. It is not advisable to create a window and attempt to remove the distal cement through the perforation and the window, since the success of this procedure cannot be predicted with certainty and the isthmus of the femur (i.e., the fixation zone for the stem) is further weakened. The type of fixation or stem to be selected depends on the size of the remaining isthmus fixation zone. For a scratch-fit fixation of an extensively porous-coated stem, an intact isthmus of 4 cm is required and at least 3 cm for a 2° tapered stem with cone-in-cone anchorage. For a 3.5° tapered stem, even 2 cm of the intact isthmus may be sufficient if this remaining bone has a thick and stable cortex. If these conditions are not met, stabilization of the stem can be achieved by a combination of cone-in-cone fixation in the remaining isthmus and distal locking (see Chap. 7, principles of distal fixation).

21.7 Intraoperative Fissures and Periprosthetic Fractures of the Femoral Shaft

Intraoperative fractures of the femur during revision of endoprostheses have been reported with an incidence of 6.3% for cemented stems and between 3 and 26% for cementless stems [10, 13–17]. Abdel et al. [13] found intraoperative fractures during 12% of 5417 hip prosthesis revisions.

Intraoperative fractures are most commonly caused during dislocation of the joint, removal of the implanted stem or cement remnants, preparation of the femoral prosthesis fixation zone, and impaction of the prosthesis (especially the cementless stems) [18–22]. Risk factors are partly responsible for the fractures and should be taken into account by the surgeon. These risk factors can be divided into patient-related and technical risk factors. The first group can be divided into general patient-related and specific patient-related risk factors.

The general patient-related risk factors include primarily metabolic bone diseases that reduce the mechanical properties of bone. These include for example osteoporosis, osteomalcia, renal or hepatic osteodystrophy and Paget's disease [21, 23, 24]. The first two metabolic bone abnormalities are present in rheumatoid arthritis, for example, and therefore, the risk of periprosthetic fractures is significantly increased in these patients [18, 19, 25–28].

Specific patient-related risk factors include, above all, deformities of the femur, such as those found in hip dysplasia or Perthes disease, in old healed femoral neck fractures, after reconversion osteotomies, or associated with metabolic bone diseases such as Paget's disease [23, 29]. However, local osteolyses are also stress risers that increase the risk of fracture [10]. The cortical thickness plays a decisive role, whereby thin cortical bone increases the risk of fractures. Thicker revision stems are also supposed to increase the risk of fractures [10]. However, in my opinion, this is only an indirect result of having contact with the thinner cortical bone. A widened femur or isthmus of the femur automatically requires a thicker stem.

Technical risk factors for intraoperative periprosthetic fractures include the use of cementless stem endoprostheses and the perforation of the femur during, for example, cement removal [16, 23, 29–31].

The risk of intraoperative fissures and fractures varies according to the stem and implantation technique used. They occur more frequently with oversized scratch-fit implanted cylindrical stems (diameter of the stem greater than the last reamer) than with line-to-line (not oversized) implanted conical stems [10, 32]. For example, Meek et al. [10] described a stem fissure or fracture in 26% of 211 prosthesis revisions with scratch-fit implantation of cylindrical nonmodular cobalt–chromium stems. This was significantly more common for oversized stems (thicker than the reamer) than for stems with line-to-line implantation (same size as the last reamer). Richards et al. [32] found scratch-fit implanted, cylindrical, nonmodular cobalt–chromium stems significantly more likely (29 of 114) to be associated with periprosthetic fractures than tapered modular titanium stems (9 of 103) (see tables in Chap. 6). Miner et al. [33] observed isthmus fissures with an incidence of 10.8% in their study of transfemoral implantation of cementless revision stems. The risk of a fissure in the isthmus region depends on the quality of the bone (thickness of the cortical bone in the isthmus) and the taper of the stem used. Huddleston et al. [34] carried out a multicenter study that compared modular revision stems (mostly ZMR stems with 3.5 degrees of taper) to nonmodular revision stems (with 2 degrees of taper) in patients with bone defects ranging from Paprosky I to IIIA; they reported a higher risk (11% versus 7%) of intraoperative fractures for the modular revision stems with the greater taper.

Intraoperative fissures and/or fractures occur when the old stem is extracted or, in most cases, the new nonmodular stem or the distal component of the modular stem system is driven in. If the final implant sits significantly deeper than the trial prosthesis or rasp, a fissure should be suspected. To be on the safe side, the fixation site should be checked with a fluoroscope although fissures are not always visible using this technique. If a transfemoral approach was chosen, the fissure can be seen on the isthmus and its full extent can be exposed. As long as it is only a fissure, it does not pose a real problem. The formation of the fissure indicates sufficient distal press-fit fixation of the revision stem so that it does not need to be removed. On the contrary, removal of the stem would very likely enlarge the fissure or even cause it to fracture. As a precaution, another double cerclage should be applied in the area of the fissure (below the prophylactic cerclage) and only partial weight bearing of 10–20 kg should be allowed for 6–8 weeks (Fig. 21.3a–c). If a fracture has already occurred, a change in procedure is required. The fracture zone must be bridged with the fixation zone of the revision stem that is now to be selected, which is why this new stem will be considerably longer. Usually, it is the fixation zone in the isthmus of the femur that is fractured and the remaining unaffected fixation zone in the isthmus is less than the minimum length for the newly selected stem. Distal interlocking of a longer revision stem, which is then implanted transfemorally, can help as an additive fixation concept in these cases [8]. However, fixation with the locking screws alone is not sufficient. Following transfemoral exposure, the fixation bed is prepared, the distal component is implanted with subsequent distal locking, trial positioning with a proximal trial component is performed, and the two modular components are assembled in situ. Finally, the flap or fracture fragments are closed or repositioned with cerclages around the newly implanted prosthesis (Figs. 16.35, 16.36, and 16.37).

Park et al. [6] found an intraoperative fracture rate of 20% when modular distally fixed straight revision stems were implanted endofemorally and 6% during a transfemoral approach. In addition, anterior cortical perforation occurred in 13% of cases with the endofemoral approach, but not once (0%) with the transfemoral approach.

21.8 Postoperative Periprosthetic Fracture of the Femoral Shaft

Postsurgical periprosthetic fractures of the femur after revision surgery are reported to occur with an incidence of between 1.5 and 4.2% [19, 35–38]. The incidence for cemented stem endoprostheses is between 2.8 and 4 and 1.5% for cementless stem endoprostheses [35–38].

The main cause of postoperative periprosthetic fractures is minor trauma in loosened stem endoprostheses, where the loosening process has led to weakening of the bone. For this reason, a periprosthetic fracture caused by a minor trauma should always make one suspect a prosthesis loosening, even if this is not clearly visible on the radiograph.

The risk factors for postoperative fractures can be divided into general and local risk factors.

Patient-related general risk factors for postsurgery fractures also include metabolic bone diseases with weakening of the mechanical properties of the bone [39, 40].

Local risk factors include loosened implants, heterotopic ossification, and stress risers [23, 41]. Heterotopic ossification leads to an abrupt blockade of movement and usually causes long spiral fractures due to a kind of hypomochlion. Stress risers include old screw holes, osteolyses, perforations, bone windows (for cement removal), leaked cement, the ends of osteosynthesis plates, varus positioning of the stem with peaks of stress at the tip of the prosthesis, and impingement of loose stem implants against the lateral cortex of the femur [23, 41].

Depending on the localization and fixation strength of the prosthesis, osteosynthesis or revision arthroplasty may be required. Periprosthetic fractures at the level of the stem with a firmly seated prosthesis (Vancouver B1 fracture) are rather rare in revision procedures. The stem is usually loosened (Vancouver B2 and B3 fractures), and a prosthesis revision is required. Please refer to Chap. 18 of this book for more information.

21.9 Hematoma

Postsurgery hematomas are rare, occur more often during transfemoral access, and are caused by bleeding from the perforating vessels or bone. Preoperative and intraoperative use of tranexamic acid as well as connecting the drainage tubes to a cell saver after surgery may help to reduce the development of a hematoma. Redon tubes can be removed in exceptional cases on the third day after surgery. After surgery, compression bandaging can help to reduce the extent of the hematoma and passive lymph drainage can speed up the resorption of the hematoma. However, if significant acute bleeding is suspected, the source of the bleeding should be identified with an angio-CT and the appropriate revision performed.

21.10 Periprosthetic Infection

Periprosthetic joint infections (PJI) occur significantly more frequently after revision surgery, averaging around 4% (see tables in Chap. 6), than after primary implantation. The principles of treating early, or acute, and late, or chronic, periprosthetic infections are, of course, also valid after revision surgery. While the implant can be left in place with a high chance of success in the case of early PJI that occurs within 4 weeks of implantation, late PJI requires an implant revision [42]. Early infections require immediate revision with debridement of the wound and irrigation with an antiseptic solution (e.g., Octenisept, Schülke & Mayr, Norderstedt, Germany or LavaSurge, B. Braun, Melsungen, Germany) and exchange of the articulating components. If a transfemoral approach had been used for the initial implantation, it should be reopened with a muscle-sparing procedure, and the flap should be cleaned and rinsed on the inside as well and closed again with new cerclages. The various therapeutic concepts for the treatment of chronic PJI are described in the extensive literature currently available. This is addressed in part in Chap. 19.

21.11 Dislocations

Postoperative dislocations are not uncommon after revision surgery (between 3 and 30%; see tables in Chap. 6) [43, 44]. According to Guo and colleagues [45], 75% of all dislocations occur after revision surgery. The causes of this are complex, and an analysis should be carried out before revision surgery. It is not uncommon for the stabilizing gluteal muscles or vasto-gluteal sling to be damaged, even with the loss of the greater trochanter. The number of previous revision surgeries and the selected surgical approaches is important for this analysis [45]. In a meta-analysis, Guo et al. [45] found a 1.95-fold higher risk of dislocation if 2 or more operations had been performed before and a 2.23-fold higher risk if 3 or more operations had been performed before. With the original Wagner SL revision stem (Zimmer Biomet, Winterthur, Switzerland), dislocations were seen with an incidence of up to 30% (Table 6.5). This was partly due to subsidence but mainly due to the low offset of the original stem of 36 mm and a high centrum collum diaphyseal angle of 145°. Thus, when comparing two conical monoblock prostheses with different offset and CCD angles (145° and 135°), Procenca and Cabral [46] found significantly lower dislocation rates for the stem with a higher offset (3% versus 12%). Modular prostheses tend to reduce the incidence of dislocation because they allow the leg length and anteversion to be adjusted separately and independently of the fixation of the distal component and because many stems have different offset variations of the proximal component [47]. The fact that the dislocation rate is not significantly lower for modular stems than for nonmodular stems, however, is an indication that soft tissue alteration due to previous surgical procedures is the main reason for the dislocations [47] (Tables 6.7, 6.8, 6.9, and 6.10).

If the stem and cup are in the correct position, a conservative treatment can be attempted for the first dislocation, similar to that for primary arthroplasty. If necessary, corrective orthoses can be worn after the first dislocation following revision surgery. Multiple dislocations (at the latest after the third) require further revision surgery. The position of the implants and an impingement-free range of motion must be checked again during the operation. Revision of the head, the proximal prosthetic component, and/or the cup are treatment options. Otherwise, the joint can be stabilized by changing the cup to a dual-mobility cup.

If during trial component positioning, a tendency for dislocation becomes apparent—especially in the case of unchanged acetabular cups with low anteversion and revision via a posterolateral approach—a higher level of antetorsion must be set for the proximal component of a modular stem. The use of elevated-edge inlays is also helpful in these cases, whereby care must be taken to avoid impingement of the stem with the raised edge of the inlay. With longer head systems, stability can be improved to a certain extent by increasing soft tissue tension. If these corrections are not sufficient, a cup exchange with orientation adjustment is required. If the abductors have also been altered as a result of previous operations, revision to a dual-mobility system is recommended [44].

21.12 Prosthesis Stem Fracture and/or Fracture of the Junction between Modular Components

Modular revision stems have the advantage that they allow the individual goals of femoral stem revision to be achieved step by step, in sequence and separately from each other, thus making the results of stem revision controlled and reproducible [7]. The distal component provides a controlled distal fixation in the femoral diaphysis, and then, the proximal trial component is used to select the correct stem length, antetorsion, and offset, which are then reproduced with the implantation of the final proximal component [7]. The disadvantage of modular revision stems lies in the junction of two components that are both subjected to mechanical forces. Failure of this junction of the modular components has been described as disconnection, corrosion, and breakage [5, 48, 49]. The weakest point of the modular junction is the male taper. Breakage of this male taper is mechanically induced by so-called "fretting", which is the term used to describe the repetitive mechanical erosion of the protective oxidized surface of metal components in close contact with each other that results from oscillating micromovements of the two adjacent surfaces [50]. The resulting damage can be caused by wear, fatigue, or corrosion. The process of removing the passive oxide coating by fretting followed by corrosion is called "fretting corrosion"[50]. Modular joints in revision stems are subject to high bending moments because of their offset from the joint force vector (lever effect), especially in situations with poor proximal osseous support. The patient's anatomy and body weight as well as his physical activity influence the bending load on the male taper of the joint [50, 51]. Several years after implantation, fatigue fractures of the male taper of the modular junction may occur in unfavorable situations (long lever arm, high load) [52, 53] (Fig. 21.8b). Lombardi and colleagues found out that a hardening process on the male taper of modular stems with the result of improving the taper strength, the initially relatively high fracture incidence was reduced by a factor of 3.5 [54]. Marshall et al. [55] reported a comparison of 40 modular revision stems without the hardening process and 162 stems that had been hardened with an average follow-up of 17 years for the first group and 7 years for the second group. Nonhardened modular taper joints broke in 15% of cases and hardened ones in 2%.

Krueger et al. [56] analyzed all 113 fractured stems identified in a study of 37,600 implanted modular MRP prostheses (Peter Brehm, Weisendorf, Germany). This corresponds to an incidence of 0.3%. However, it was not possible to analyze radiographs to assess the medial osseous support at the junction. They used the data to identify risk factors for junction fractures, namely a high offset due to a lateralized proximal component and the use of extra-long offset head com-

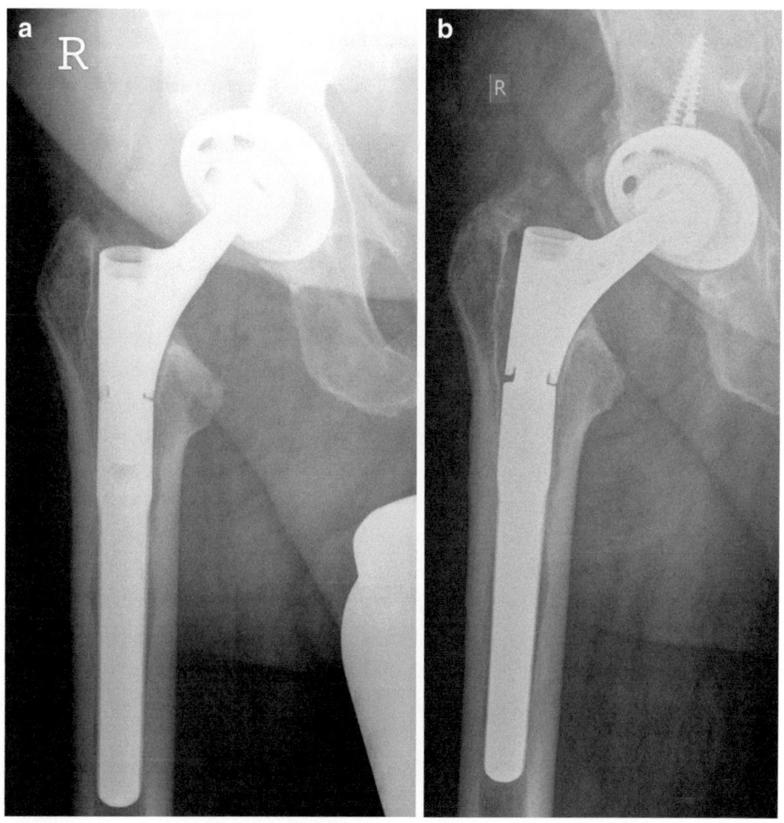

Fig. 21.8 (**a**) Radiograph 4 years after endofemoral revision surgery in a patient with a BMI of 39 using a modular revision stem Revitan Curved (Zimmer Biomet, Winterthur, Switzerland). An oscillation of the proximal component has caused radiolucency seen medial and lateral to the proximal component. The distal component is osseointegrated up to the junction. (**b**) Fracture of the junction 5 years after surgery

ponents. 79% of the fractured junctions had a lateralized proximal component, an extra-long offset head component, or a combination of both. The use of a lateralized proximal component resulted in a 33% increase in bending moment at the junction compared to the standard version of the proximal component [57]. Furthermore, these data analysis revealed that breakages were significantly more frequent in straight versus curved stems (60% vs. 38%), short proximal components versus longer proximal components, males, and patients with high body mass index (BMI) (32 kg/m^2 vs. 27 kg/m^2). It was also found that physical contamination and damage to the junction were evident in one-third of the fractures and that the junction had often not been tightened intraoperatively with the required torque. This should be avoided during surgery, as impurities can promote and facilitate corrosion at the junction [58, 59].

All modular revision stems are biomechanically tested according to DIN-ISO [60]. The test procedure specifies the fixation of the implant at the distal tip and the application of force to the head. This leads to an oscillation of the stem with a peak amplitude at some distance from the junction, which is therefore not exposed to the risk of fracture during this test procedure [52, 60] (Fig. 21.9).

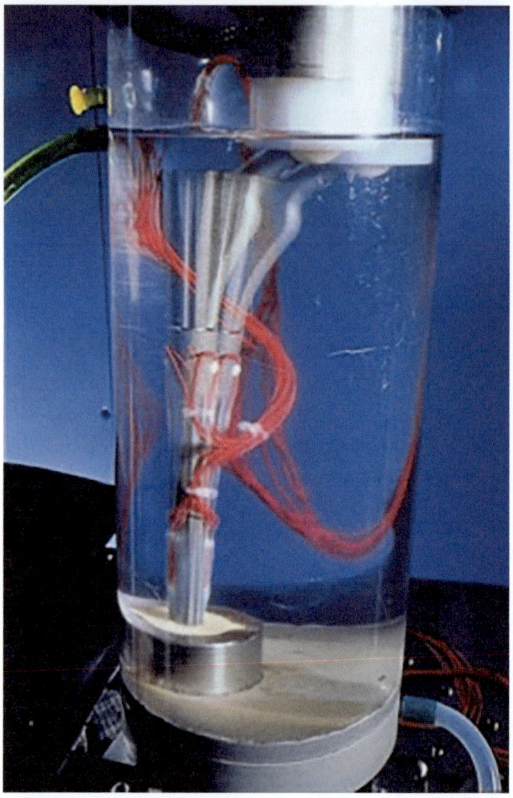

Fig. 21.9 Visualization of the oscillations during a biomechanical durability test of a modular revision stem according to DIN-ISO. The stem combination is clamped distally, and the peak oscillation amplitude is located away from the junction (distally) so that the junction is not subjected to critical stress (with permission of Zimmer Biomet, Winterthur, Switzerland)

An analysis of the rarely occurring fractures of the junction reveals that they also occur in vivo in other situations. A review of the literature (using the keywords "breakage" or "fracture" and "junction" and "modular revision stem") revealed 29 cases of junction fractures associated with a variety of modern modular revision stems, in which an analysis of the combination of the selected modular stem components and the osseous support of the junction could be performed [52, 61–64]. All 29 cases presented the same clinical features: an osseointegrated distal component that is firmly anchored in the bone up to the level of the junction and a lack of medial osseous support for the proximal component (Fig. 21.8b). The significantly more frequent use of short proximal components in the fractured stems in the study by Krüger et al. [56] also supports these findings. Although the cause of a junction fatigue fracture is certainly multifactorial, the scenario just described appears to be the main cause of such a fracture [65]. In this scenario, the peak oscillation amplitude of the entire stem construction is at the level of the junction. Over time, this can lead to a fatigue fracture at this weakest point of the entire construction [52, 63]. Patients with an excessive body weight or body mass index, who undertake intense physical activity and are implanted with high offset stems, have the greatest risk of fatigue fracture [52, 63].

So the goal should be to avoid this situation of oscillation at the level of the junction. The surgeon can play a significant role in this with the appropriate surgical technique:

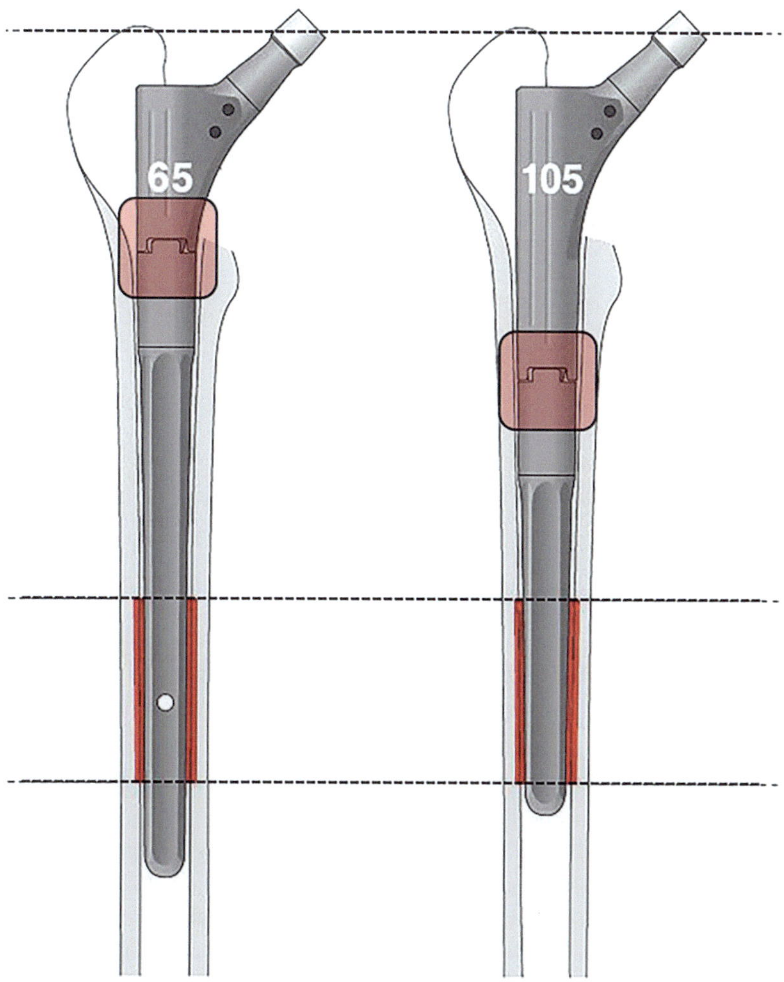

Fig. 21.10 Comparison of two different stem combinations with different positioning of the junction. The combination of a distally short distal and a longer proximal component places the junction further distally into the femur, and there is medial osseous support (with permission of Zimmer Biomet, Winterthur, Switzerland)

1. Using short distal components and fixing them at the tip of the stem in the isthmus of the femur means that the longer proximal component moves the junction more distally into the femur (usually below the trochanter minor) (Fig. 21.10). This provides the junction with medial osseous support and prevents oscillations with a peak amplitude at the level of the junction. This can be achieved, for example, using a transfemoral approach to implant a distally fixed modular revision stem with a taper angle of 2 degrees and press-fit fixation at the distal end of the shortest distal component in the isthmus (Fig. 21.2a, b). In the case of an endofemoral approach, this can be realized, for example, with curved conical stems with a 2-degree taper by means of a three-surface fixation of the stem. Stems with a greater taper have their fixation zone in the isthmus above the tip of the stem [66]. However, even with these stems, the distal component should be as short as possible in order to have the junction in the distal part of the femur and osseous support. Huber and Morlock [67] were able to calculate that the amount of leverage at the junction decreases as the junction is lowered. (Fig. 21.11). Using a realistic three-dimensional model, they calculated the leverage and force effects on the junction and concluded that the optimal length of the proximal component lay between 70 and 90 mm.
2. If there is a gap between the proximal component and the medial bone in the calcar region

Fig. 21.11 Simplified two-dimensional illustration of the lever effect at the junction for different component combinations (according to Michael Morlock, Technical University Hamburg, Harburg, Germany [67])

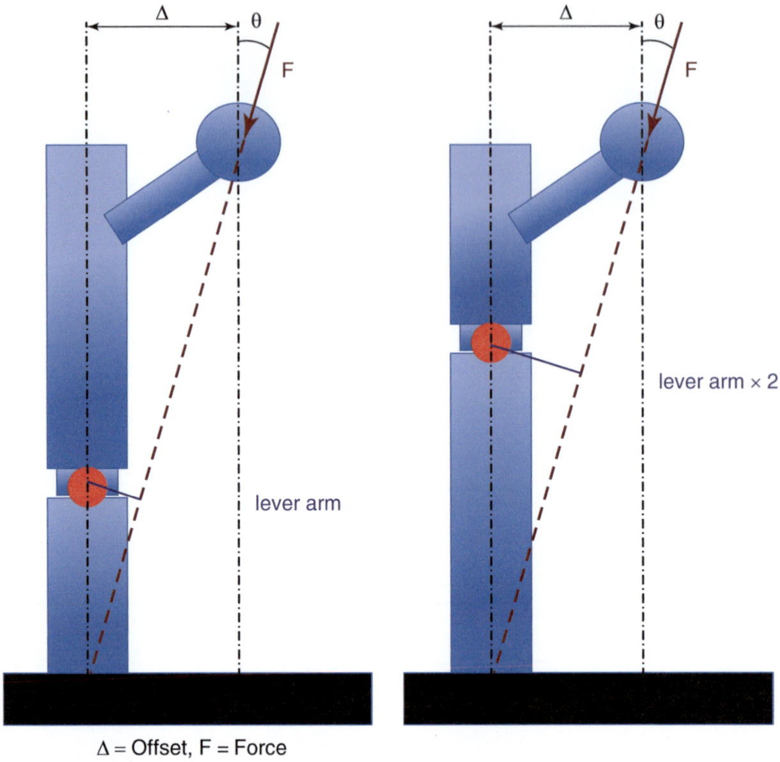

after endofemoral implantation of the modular components, the calcar region should be filled with autologous or homologous bone (Fig. 21.4b). Milling debris can be used here that was obtained during the reaming of the medullary canal and, if appropriate, the cup.
3. In a transfemoral procedure with an extended trochanteric osteotomy, if the axis of the medial femur bone is a significant distance from the proximal bone, the medial femur should also be corrected with a double osteotomy and cerclages used to bring the proximal bone into contact with the proximal component (Fig. 21.12a–c).

In our opinion, these measures move the peak amplitude of the oscillating micromovements of the femoral stem assembly away from the junction and thus significantly reduce the risk of junction fracture.

Furthermore, my hypothesis is supported by the findings of Ladurner et al. [63] who analyzed 54 transfemoral stem revisions and found 3 junction fractures all of which involved a combination of a longer distal and a short proximal component. They were also able to show that bone regeneration after a transfemoral approach proceeds from distal to proximal and that the use of short proximal components results in a longer period of integration and less bone regeneration than combinations with longer proximal components.

In cases of proximal femoral defects, some authors recommend the adjunctive placement of a cortical strut graft on the medial side of the proximal femur in order to protect the junction [68]. We do not perform this procedure because we believe that a large medial bone defect that would be suitable for cortical strut graft deposition does not have the problematic scenario discussed with regard to localization of the oscillation peak amplitude at the level of the junction, but actually has an oscillation peak distal to the junction. In our opinion, the latter does not constitute an elevated risk of fracture for the junction. In an analysis of our case histories, out of 992 implantations of the modular distal fixation revision stem Revitan Curved (Zimmer Biomet, Winterthur, Switzerland), we found 34

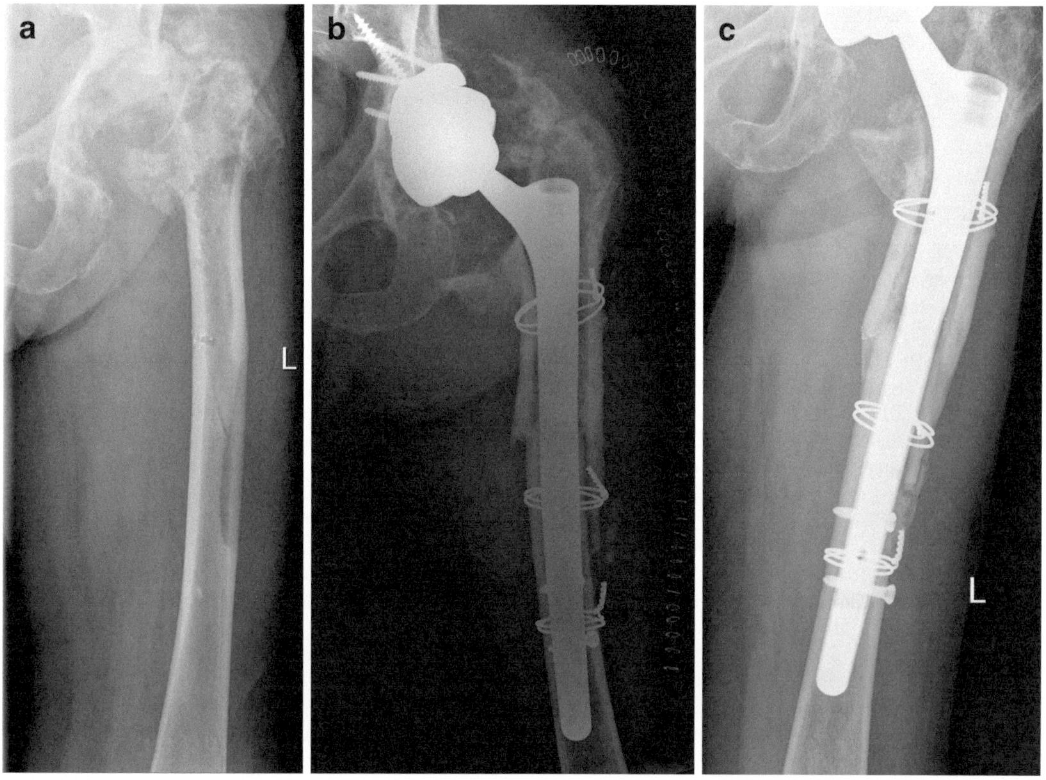

Fig. 21.12 (**a**) Girdlestone situation after extramural prosthesis explantation because of a periprosthetic infection with a lateral bone defect in the isthmus region and varus of the femur. (**b**) Postoperative radiograph after prosthesis revision via a transfemoral approach with the modular revision stem Revitan Curved with distal locking and a trabecular metal cup with graft (Zimmer Biomet, Warsaw, IN, USA). A double osteotomy was performed for axial correction of the femur and medial support of the proximal femoral component. (**c**) Radiograph 6 months after surgery with consolidation of the osteotomies and osteointegration of the stem

cases with a total lack of proximal bone (partly because of revisions of broken megaprostheses). None of these cases resulted in a fracture of the prosthesis stem or junction (Fig. 9.3a–c). Therefore, I suggest that the recommendation made by the manufacturer, that modular revision stems should not be used in the absence of medial support of the proximal component, is not specific enough. The presence of the femoral calcar region can cause a junction fracture if there is a gap separating it from the proximal component in physically active, overweight patients (Fig. 21.8a, b), but the absence of the proximal femoral bone, as just explained, does not (Fig. 9.3a–c).

However, nonmodular monoblock revision stems may also fracture [69, 70]. As with modular revision prostheses, the body weight and physical activity of the patient as well as the diameter of the prosthesis play a decisive role [69, 70]. Therefore, the implantation of a thicker, shorter tapered stem should be preferred to a longer, thinner revision stem for monoblock prostheses as well.

References

1. Wagner H, Wagner M. Femur-Revisionsprothese. Z Orthop. 1993;131:574–7.
2. Abdel MP, Wyles CC, Viste A, Perry KI, Trousdale RT, Berry DJ. Extended trochanteric osteotomy in revision total hip arthroplasty. Contemporary outcomes of 612 hips. J Bone Joint Surg Am. 2021;103:162–73.
3. Hancock DS, Sharplin PK, Larsen PD, Philips FT. Early radiological and functional outcomes for a cementless press-fit design modular femoral stem revision system. Hip Int. 2019;29:35–40.

4. Fink B, Grossmann A, Schubring S, Schulz MS, Fuerst M. Short-term results of hip revisions with a curved cementless modular stem in association with the surgical approach. Arch Orthop Trauma Surg. 2009;129(1):65–73.
5. Fink B, Urbansky K, Schuster P. Mid term results with the curved modular tapered, fluted titanium Revitan stem in revision hip replacement. Bone Joint J. 2014;96-B(7):889–95.
6. Park YS, Moon YM, Lim SJ. Revision total hip arthroplasty using a fluted and tapered modular distal fixation stem with and without extended trochanteric osteotomy. J Arthroplasty. 2007;22:993–9.
7. Fink B. Letter to the editor: is there a benefit to modularity in "simpler" femoral revisions? Clin Orthop Relat Res. 2016;474:2538–9.
8. Fink B, Grossmann A, Fuerst M. Distal interlocking screws with a modular revision stem for revision total hip arthroplasty in severe bone defects. J Arthroplasty. 2010;25:759–65.
9. Weiss R, Stark A, Kärrholm J. A modular cementless stem vs. cemented long-stem prostheses in revision surgery of the hip. A population-based study from the Swedish hip arthroplasty register. Acta Orthop. 2011;82:136–42.
10. Meek D, Garbuz DS, Masri BA, Greidanus NV, Duncan CP. Intraoperative fracture of the femur in revision total hip arthroplasty with a diaphyseal fitting stem. J Bone Joint Surg. 2004;86-A:480–5.
11. Regis D, Sandri A, Bonetti I, Graggion M, Bartolozzi P. Femoral revision with Wagner tapered stem. A ten-to 15 year follow-up study. J Bone Joint Surg Br. 2011;93-B:1320–6.
12. Paprosky WG, Greidanus NV, Antoniou J. Minimum 10-year-results of extensively porous-coated stems in revision hip hip arthroplasty. Clin Orthop Relat Res. 1999;369:230–42.
13. Abdel MP, Houdek MT, Watts CD, et al. Epidemiology of periprosthetic femoral fractures in 5417 revision total hip arthroplasties. Bone Joint J. 2016;98-B:468–74.
14. Christensen CM, Seger BM, Schultz RB. Management of intraoperative femur fractures associated with revision hip arthroplasty. Clin Orthop. 1989;248:177–80.
15. Della Rocca GJ, Leung KS, Pape HC. Periprosthetic fractures: epidemiology and future projections. J Orthop Trauma. 2011;25:S66–70.
16. Fitzgerald RH Jr, Brindley GW, Kavanagh BF. The uncemented total hip arthroplasty: intraoperative femoral fractures. Clin Orthop Relat Res. 1988;235:61–6.
17. Grabuz DS, Masri BA, Duncan CP. Periprosthetic fractures of the femur: principles of prevention and management. Instr Course Lect. 1998;47:237–42.
18. Bogoch ER, Moran EL. Bone abnormalities in the surgical treatment of patients with rheumatoid arthritis. Clin Orthop Relat Res. 1999;366:8–21.
19. Fink B, Fuerst M, Singer J. Periprosthetic fractures of the femur associated with hip arthroplasty. Arch Orthop Trauma Surg. 2005;125:433–42.
20. Fink B. Periprosthetic fractures of the hip. The role of revision arthroplasty. Eur J Orthop Traumatol. 2014;5:37–41.
21. Pellicci PM, Inglis AE, Salvati EA. Perforation of the femoral shaft during total hip replacement. J Bone Joint Surg. 1980;62-A:234–40.
22. Taylor MM, Meyers MH, Harvey JP. Intraoperative femur fractures during total hip replacement. Clin Orthop. 1978;137:96–103.
23. Haddad FS, Masri BA, Garbuz DS, Duncan CP. The prevention of periprosthetic fractures in total hip and knee arthroplasty. Orthop Clin North Am. 1999;30:191–207.
24. Kelley SS. Periprosthetic femoral fractures. J Am Acad Orthop Surg. 1994;2:164–72.
25. Akesson K, Önsten I, Obrant KJ. Periarticular bone in rheumatoid arthritis versus arthrosis. Histomorphometry in 103 hip biopsies. Acta Orthop Scand. 1994;65:135–8.
26. Bogoch E, Hastings D, Gross A, Gschwend N. Supracondylar fractures of the femur adjacent to resurfacing and MacIntosh arthroplasties of the knee in patients with rheumatoid arthritis. Clin Orthop. 1998;229:213–20.
27. Bogoch ER, Moran E. Abnormal bone remodelling in inflammatory arthritis. Can J Surg. 1998;41:264–71.
28. Younger AS, Dunwoody J, Duncan CP. Periprosthetic hip and knee fractures: the scope of the problem. Instr Course Lect. 1998;47:251–6.
29. Tsiridis E, Haddad FS, Gie GA. The management of periprosthetic femoral fractures around hip replacements. Injury. 2003;34:95–105.
30. Schwartz JT, Mayer JG, Engh CA. Femoral fracture during non-cemented total hip arthroplasty. J Bone Joint Surg. 1989;71-A:1135–42.
31. Stuchin SA. Femoral shaft fracture in porous and press-fit total hip arthroplasty. Orthop Rev. 1990;19:153–9.
32. Richards CJ, Duncan CP, Masri BA, Garbuz DS. Femoral revision hip arthroplasty. A comparison of two stem designs. Clin Orthop Relat Res. 2010;468:491–6.
33. Miner TM, Momberger NG, Chong D, Paprosky WL. The extended trochanteric osteotomy in revision hip arthroplasty: a critical review of 166 cases at mean 3-year, 9-month follow-up. J Arthroplasty. 2001;16:188–94.
34. Huddleston JI, Testreault MW, Yu M, Bedair H, Hansen VJ, Choi H-R, Goodman SB, Sporer MD, Della Valle CJ. Is there a benefit to modularity in "simpler" femoral revisions? Clin Orthop Relat Res. 2016;474:415–20.
35. Kavanagh BF. Femoral fractures associated with total hip arthroplasty. Orthop Clin North Am. 1992;23:249–57.
36. Lamb JN, Jain S, King SW, West RM, Pandit HG. Risk factors for revision of polished taper-slip cemented stems for periprosthetic femoral fracture after primary Total hip replacement: a registry-based cohort study from the National Joint Registry for England, Wales,

Northern Ireland and the Isle of Man. J Bone Joint Surg Am. 2020;102:1600–8.
37. Lewallen DG, Berry DJ. Periprosthetic fracture of the femur after total hip arthroplasty: treatment and results to date. Instr Course Lect. 1998;47:243–9.
38. Morrey BF, Kavanagh BF. Complications with revision of the femoral component of total hip arthroplasty: comparison between cemented and uncemented techniques. J Arthroplasty. 1992;7:71–9.
39. Bethea JS, DeAndrade JR, Fleming LL, Lindenbaum SD, Welch RB. Proximal femoral fractures following total hip arthroplasty. Clin Orthop. 1982;170:95–106.
40. Tower SS, Beals RK. Fractures of the femur after hip replacement. The Oregon experience. Orthop Clin North Am. 1999;30:235–47.
41. Larsen E, Menck H, Rosenklint A. Fractures after hemialloplastic hip replacement. J Trauma. 1987;27:72–4.
42. Fink B. Revision of late periprosthetic infections of total hip endoprostheses: pros and cons of different concepts. Int J Med Sci. 2009;6:287–29.
43. Bozic KJ, Kurzt SM, Lau E, Ong K, Vail TP, Berry DJ. The epidemiology of revision total hip arthroplasty in the United States. J Bone Joint Surg Am. 2009;91-A:128–33.
44. Philippot R, Adam P, Reckhaus M, Delangle F, Verdot F, Curvale G, Farizon F. Prevention of dislocation in total hip revision surgery using a dual mobility design. Orthop Traumatol Surg Res. 2009;95:407–13.
45. Guo L, Yang Y, An B, Yang Y, Shi L, Han X, Gao S. Risk factors for dislocation after revision total hip arthroplasty: a systematic review and meta-analysis. Int J Surg. 2017;38:123–9.
46. Procenca A, Cabral R. Revision of the femoral side in total hip replacement. Eur Instr Course Lect. 2005;7:143.
47. Regis D, Sandri A, Bartolozzi P. Stem modularity alone is not effective in reducing dislocation rate in hip revision surgery. J Orthop Traumatol. 2009;10:167–71.
48. Bobyn JD, Tanzer M, Krygier JJ, Dujovne AR, Brookes CE. Concerns with modularity in total hip arthroplasty. Clin Orthop Relat Res. 1994;298:27–36.
49. Atwood SA. Corrosion-induced fracture of a double-modular hip prosthesis. J Bone Joint Surg Am. 2010;92-A:1522–5.
50. Krull A, Morlock MM, Bishop NE. Factors influencing taper failure of modular revision stems. Med Eng Phys. 2018;54:65–73.
51. Lakstein D, Eliaz N, Levi O, Backstein D, Kosashvili Y, Safir O, Gross AE. Fracture of cementless femoral stems at the mid-stem junction in modular revision hip arthroplasty systems. J Bone Joint Surg Am. 2011;93:57–65.
52. Fink B. What can the surgeon do to reduce the risk of junction breakage of modular revision stems. Arthroplasty Today. 2018;31:306–9.
53. Norman P, Iyengar S, Svensson I, Flivik G. Fatigue fracture in dual modular revision total hip arthroplasty stems: failure analysis and computed tomography diagnostics in two cases. J Arthroplasty. 2014;29:850–5.
54. Lombardi AV Jr, Berend KR, Mallory TH, Adams JB. Modular calcar replacement prosthesis with strengthened taper junction in total hip arthroplasty. Surg Technol Int. 2007;16:206–9.
55. Marshall DJ, Berend KR, Morris MJ, Adams JB, Lombardi AV Jr. Results of a modular femoral revision system before and after taper roller hardening in total hip arthroplasty. Surg Technol Int. 2017;30:336–40.
56. Krueger DR, Guenther K-P, Deml MC, Perka C. Mechanical failure of 113 uncemented modular revision femoral components. Risk factors for fracture and failure with a case control comparison analysis. Bone Joint J. 2020;102-B:573–9.
57. Skendzel JG, Baha JD, Urquhart AG. Total hip arthroplasty modular neck failure. J Arthroplasty. 2011;26:338.e1–4.
58. Morlock M, Bünte D, Gührs J, Bishop N. Corrosion of the head-stem taper junction. Are we on the verge of an epidemic? Review article. HHS J. 2017;13:42–9.
59. Lavernia CJ, Baerga L, Barrack RL, et al. The effects of blood and fat on Morse taper disassembly forces. Am J Orthop (Belle Mead NJ). 2009;38:187–90.
60. Schramm M, Wirtz DC, Holzwarth U, Pitto RP. The Morse taper junction in modular revision hip replacement--a biomechanical and retrieval analysis. Biomed Tech (Berl) 2000;45(4):105–109.
61. Duncan ST, Hayes CB, Nunley RM. Fracture at the modular junction of a cementless revision hip system: a case report. JBJS Case Connect. 2016;6:e48.
62. Herold F, Eijer H. Fracture of a femoral revision stem following a technical failure. Case Rep Orthop. 2018;2018:9691627.
63. Ladurner A, Zdravkovic V, Grob K. Femoral bone restoration patterns in revision total hip arthroplasty using distally fixed modular tapered titanium stems and an extended trochanteric osteotomy approach. J Arthroplasty. 2018;33:2210–7.
64. Rieger B, Ilchmann T, Bollinger L, Stoffel KK, Zwicky L, Clauss M. Mid-term results of revision total hip arthroplasty with an uncemented modular femoral component. Hip Int. 2018;28:84–9.
65. Rueckl K, Sculco PK, Berliner J, Cross MB, Koch C, Boettner F. Fracture risk of tapered modular revision stems: a failure analysis. Arthroplasty Today. 2018;4:300–5.
66. Van Houwelingen AP, Duncan CP, Masri BA, Greidanus NV, Garbuz DS. High survival of modular tapered stems for proximal femoral bone defects at 5 to 10 years follow-up. Clin Orthop Relat Res. 2013;471:454–62.
67. Huber G, Morlock MM. Which length should the neck segment of modular revision stems have? Clin Biomech. 2021; in press.
68. Lim CT, Amanatullah DF, Huddleston JI 3rd, Hwang KL, Maloney WJ, Goodman SB. Cortical strut allograft support of modular femoral junctions dur-

ing revision total hip arthroplasty. J Arthroplasty. 2017;32:1586–92.
69. Landa J, Benke M, Dayan A, Pereira G, Di Cesare PE. Fracture of fully coated echelon femoral stems in revision total hip arthroplasty. J Arthroplasty. 2009;24:322.e13–8.
70. Locker PH, Arthur J, Edmiston T, Puri R, Levine BR. Fracture of a titanium non-modular femoral stem after revision total hip arthroplasty. A case report and review of the literature. Bull Hosp Jt Dis. 2018;76:278–84.

22 Explanation of Terms

Content

References 301

- **Barnejtt–Nordin Index**: It is defined as a score for quantifying a reduction in cortical thickness of the femur caused by osteoporosis. Also, it is used to quantify proximal bone regeneration or stress shielding of the femur [1] (Fig. 22.1).
- **Beals and Tower Criteria**: It describes the postoperative outcome after treatment of a periprosthetic femoral fracture [2].

Outcome	Prosthesis		Fracture
Excellent	Firmly fixed, stable	and	Healed with minimal deformity without shortening
Good	Firmly fixed after minimal subsidence	or	Healed with moderate deformity with shortening
Poor	Loose	or	Nonunion, infection, new fracture with severe deformity and shortening

- **Corrosion:** Corrosion describes the reaction of a metallic material with its environment that causes a measurable change in the material (corrosion phenomenon) and can lead to impairment of the function of a component or an entire system (corrosion damage). In most cases, this reaction is electrochemical, but in some cases it can also be chemical or metallurgical in nature.
- **Engh classification:** It describes the degree of osteointegration of a cementless hip prosthesis [3].
  - **Bony ingrowth fixation:** complete bony osteointegration
  - **Stable fibrous fixation:** incomplete bony osteointegration with at least partially connective tissue stable fixation of the implant without migration
  - **Questionable fixation:** questionably stable fixation because of increased radiolucent margins
  - **Unstable fixation:** definite loosening with migration or change in position of the implant.
- **Fretting:** This describes a tribological phenomenon that occurs with components under a high level of stress in which repeated local adhesion or seizing followed by separation of two articulating surfaces occurs because of inadequate lubrication. The resulting friction causes the generation of abraded particles.

B. Fink, *Femoral Revision Arthroplasty*, https://doi.org/10.1007/978-3-030-84821-7_22

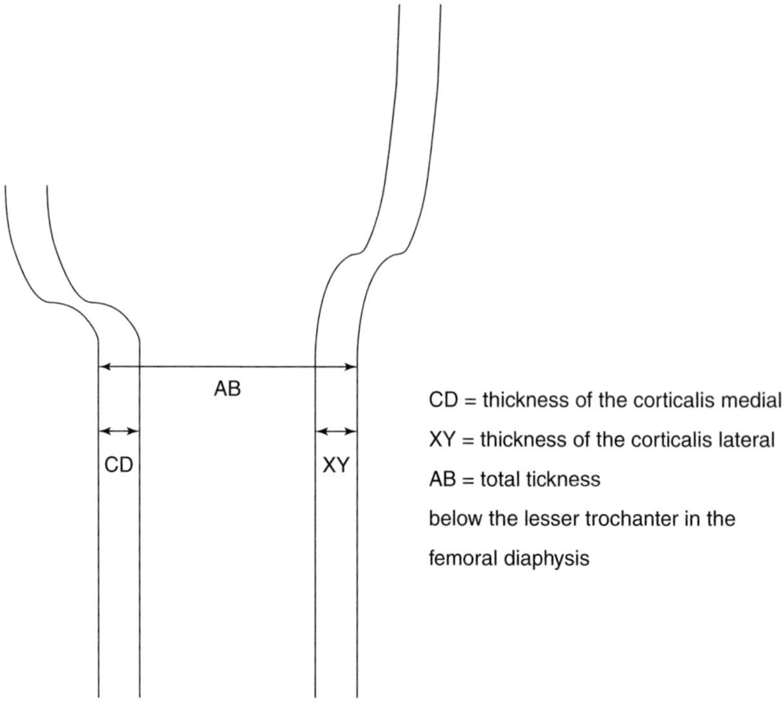

Fig. 22.1 Barnett and Nordin Index calculation [1]: BN = sum of the thickness of the medial (CD) and lateral cortex (XY) just below the greater trochanter, where it becomes parallel, divided by the total thickness of the shaft (AB), multiplied by 100

- **ICM Definition:** ICM is International Consensus Meeting, at which experts met in Philadelphia in 2013 and 2018 to address important issues surrounding periprosthetic infection and each time developed a new definition for periprosthetic late infection [4].
- **In situ assembly:** It is an assembly of modular prosthesis components within the patient's surgical site (as opposed to tabletop assembly).
- **Interface:** This designates the connecting layer of two different material surfaces (e.g. bone–cement, cement–prosthesis, prosthesis–bone).
- **Junction:** It is the connection between two components of a modular stem prosthesis. It usually comprises a male and a female part.
- **Modulus of Elasticity:** The modulus of elasticity is a parameter used in material engineering to describe the relationship between stress and strain in the deformation of a solid body. The modulus of elasticity increases with the resistance that a material presents to its elastic deformation. A stem prosthesis made of a material with a high modulus of elasticity such as cobalt–chromium is thus more rigid than the same component made of a material with a low modulus of elasticity such as titanium.
- **Stress shielding:** It is defined as reduction in bone density in the vicinity of a prosthetic stem due to the transfer of typical stresses from the bone to the implant. The bone around the implant is exposed to less stress because of the stiffness of the implant, and the bone decreases in density by virtue of Wolff's law. The phenomenon is visible on a radiograph some years after surgery and occurs more often with cementless prosthetic stems than with cemented ones. The stiffer the implant, the stronger this process becomes. It is therefore more frequently observed in cementless cobalt–chromium revision stems than in the more elastic titanium stems, which have a lower modulus of elasticity.
- **Strut graft:** It is an allogeneic cortical bone graft several centimeters in length that serves as an external biological scaffold or

plate for the treatment of diaphyseal periprosthetic fractures or for biological bridging and augmentation of bone defects. It is fixed to the corresponding bone with cerclages.

- **Subsidence:** It is postsurgical sinking or downward slippage of a cementless prosthetic stem. In most cases, this is referred to as subsidence when the stem sinks by more than 5 mm. The stem can then become fixed at a deeper point and be firmly osseointegrated. Otherwise, it is referred to as progressive subsidence, which indicates a lack of fixation and osteointegration of the stem and is tantamount to loosening of the stem.
- **Tabletop assembly:** It is an assembly of modular prosthesis components on the operating table (as opposed to in situ assembly).
- **Taper:** It is sometimes known as conicity, and taper describes the angle of a conically shaped object. The dimension is given in degrees or percent.

References

1. Barnett E, Nordin BE. The radiological diagnosis of osteoporosis: a new approach. Clin Radiol. 1960;11:166–74.
2. Beals RK, Tower SS. Periprosthetic fractures of the femur. An analysis of 93 fractures. Clin Orthop Relat Res. 1996;327:238–46.
3. Engh CA, Glassman AH, Griffin W, Mayer JG. Results of cementless revision for failed cemented hip arthroplasty. Clin Orthop Relat Res. 1988;235:91–110.
4. Parvizi J, Tan TL, Goswami K, Higuera C, Della Valle C, Chen AF, Shohat N. The 2018 definition of periprosthetic hip and knee infection: an evidence-based and validated criteria. J Arthroplast. 2018;33:1309–14.

MIX
Papier aus verantwortungsvollen Quellen
Paper from responsible sources
FSC® C105338

If you have any concerns about our products,
you can contact us on
ProductSafety@springernature.com

In case Publisher is established outside the EU,
the EU authorized representative is:
Springer Nature Customer Service Center GmbH
Europaplatz 3, 69115 Heidelberg, Germany

Printed by Libri Plureos GmbH
in Hamburg, Germany